Teaching Guide for EMT PREHOSPITAL CARE

Mark C. Henry, MD
Associate Professor and Chairman
Department of Emergency Medicine
School of Medicine
State University of New York at Stony Brook
Stony Brook, New York

Edward R. Stapleton, EMT-P
Director of Prehospital Care and Education
University Hospital
Instructor
Department of Emergency Medicine
School of Medicine
State University of New York at Stony Brook
Stony Brook, New York

Richard L. Judd, PhD, NREMTA, EMSI
Executive Dean and Professor of Emergency Medical Sciences
Central Connecticut State University
and
Allied Medical Staff
New Britain General Hospital
New Britain, Connecticut

W. B. SAUNDERS COMPANY
Harcourt Brace Jovanovich, Inc.
Philadelphia London Toronto Montreal Sydney Tokyo

W. B. SAUNDERS COMPANY
Harcourt Brace Jovanovich, Inc.
The Curtis Center
Independence Square West
Philadelphia, PA 19106

Editor: Margaret M. Biblis
Developmental Editor: Shirley Kuhn
Production Manager: Carolyn Naylor

TEACHING GUIDE FOR EMT: PREHOSPITAL CARE ISBN 0-7216-4619-2

Printed in the United States of America

Last digit is print number: 9 8 7 6 5 4 3 2 1

Teaching Guide for EMT: Prehospital Care

The education of EMTs can be both rewarding and challenging experience for the EMS instructor. Lecture preparation represents the most difficult and time consuming aspect of an instructor's work. Reviewing objectives, selecting the appropriate learning activities, organizing equipment and planning the organization of content and audiovisuals can be a formidable task.

This instructors guide represents our efforts in researching and organizing material for the EMT student. Our educational philosophy is rooted in the idea that individuals learn better when provided with the rationale and meaningfulness of material. We cannot expect our students to memorize every grouping of signs and symptoms related to their range of prehospital encounters. By understanding the "whys" and "hows" of emergency care the students will have the most solid basis for assessments, decision making and actions needed to save the patient's life.

The Teaching Guide for EMT Prehospital Care is designed to provide maximum support for the instructor in achieving these goals. The lectures closely follow the organization of the book and the related Study and Review manual. This structure provides the consistency and reinforcement needed to assure acquisition and retention of essential information for your students.

The guide follows the same approach chapter by chapter; materials and equipment for the lesson, behavioral objectives, reading preparation for the instructor, suggested learning activities and a detailed content outline for each topic. Although the DOT curriculum provides the basis for training in most states we recognize that some states vary the approach based on their perceived needs. Topics are intentionally separated to allow for varied approaches to EMT training. Each topic has a distinct section so that instructors who follow the "DOT approach", as well as, instructors who vary in sequence or scope can easily adapt with this teaching guide. Additionally, a DOT reading list can be found in the appendix to match student reading assignments to the DOT sequence.

Approach to Lecture Preparation

We recommend the following approach when using this teaching guide:

1. Carefully read the related chapter in EMT Prehospital Care. The pages pertaining to each topic follow the learning activities in the instructors guide. Be sure to review the illustrations, tables, procedures and protocols which summarize much of the key information. If you are not clear on a particular point you may want to review the optional suggested reading material for clarification.

2. Review the behavioral objectives at the beginning of the section in the teaching guide and consider the related learning activities. Are the learning activities best suited to achieve the objectives? You may want to develop your own learning activities to enhance the presentation. A discussion of suggested learning activities can be found in the appendix.

3. Thoughtfully review the content outline. The content outline is a comprehensive guide for the instructor that closely follows the organization of the textbook chapter. During the lecture, the content outline can be used to keep track of the presentation. You may want to make notes in the margin to add information or clarify concepts for yourself. The related slide set is keyed to the content outline at every level with the chapter and slide number i.e. **(Slide 2-5)**. View the slides while reviewing the content outline to become familiar with the correlation of the teaching point and slide. Slides may consist of illustrations, tables or text. Every attempt was made to provide a clear relationship between the content and the related audiovisual.

   The content outline can also be used as a student handout. It was intentionally separated from the learning activities and instructor material section so that it can be xeroxed for this purpose. This is very helpful for students who have poor note taking skills.

4. Finally, review the exam questions at the end of the chapter. They include both multiple choice and matching questions that evaluate and reinforce basic information or the so-called "enabling objectives" of learning and "terminal objectives" or the specific assessment and treatment decisions expected from the EMT. Multiple choice and matching items were used to simulate the most common formats used in program and certifying examinations. These items are designed to provide the essential knowledge needed to understand and remember key building blocks of information that lay the foundation for clinical application. They also reflect a similar distribution of items presented in the study and review manual to again provide maximum consistency and reinforcement.

When appropriate, examinations are followed by performance sheets for the essential skills learned in class. These skill sheets are adapted from state and national agencies and reflect the state-of-the-art performance standards. The performance sheets were designed to be straight forward and to the point and not cluttered with excess information. They reflect the same approaches presented in the textbook with related illustrations.

The protocols in the textbook are a great summary resource for students. You should bring this to the students attention to maximize the effectiveness of the tool. Obviously, they should be reviewed first to assure that they reflect local and state standards in your region.

Summary

We hope that you find this guide helpful in organizing your programs. We have tried to make it as accurate and as practical as possible and we welcome your feedback.

We wish to thank the following contributors for their efforts:

Donna Stapleton, R.N.C.
Obstetrical Nurse
Good Samaritan Hospital
West Islip, New York
Paramedic and EMT Instructor
Booth Memorial Medical Center

Eric Niegelberg, EMT-P
EMS Coordinator
University Hospital
Paramedic Instructor
State University of New York
at Stony Brook

Peter Andryuk, EMT-P
Paramedic Instructor
EMS Academy
New York City Emergency Medical Services

A thank you to the Laerdal Medical Corporation for use of the ECG strips contained within chapter six and a special thanks to Jo Ann Broumay for her assistance in preparing the manuscript.

Mark C. Henry, MD
Edward R. Stapleton, EMT-P
Richard Judd, Ph. D.

Developing Effective Learning Activities

Overview

The National EMT Curriculum, familiar to EMT instructors, provides an organized instructor's guide that furnishes objectives, equipment and audiovisual requirements, preparation tasks, administrative matters, instructor note section and a content outline. Suggestions for learning activities are also provided. However, recommended objectives and learning activities are exclusively lecture, demonstration, practice and testing. This may be related to the limited available time. These type of objectives and learning activities generally promote rote learning. Additionally, the lecture or lecture-demonstration format tends to be non-participatory. This can work to the detrimental of the EMT candidate since exclusive lecture format (particularly in three hour sessions) can discourage class participation and result in poor retention. The use of alternate learning activities can provide a motivational boost to an EMT program and also may achieve a higher level of learning. Following is a review of various teaching strategies and a discussion of their advantages, disadvantages and suggestions for application in an EMT Program.

The Lecture

Lecture format is the traditional teaching strategy that allows for presentation of a lot of information over a relatively short period of time. Lectures are well suited to explain material that is straightforward. Since audience participation is limited, large groups can learn in a lecture format. It is an effective format to disseminate information.

The common mistake is to use the lecture format exclusively. Because the student is usually in a passive role, it makes it more difficult to teach more complex topics which require synthesis and application. More complex topics benefit from learning activities that involve the learner, such as discussion, role playing, and application of knowledge to case histories.

Group Discussion

Group discussion is effective for learning clinical knowledge, problem solving, and the development of new ideas. It has broad application within the EMT program. Group discussion can be integrated within a lecture presentation to allow the students a more active role. For example, students can be presented with a clinical scenario and asked to apply information from readings and lecture to assess the problem and propose treatment. Students might explore feelings and personal reactions to topics such as child abuse, terminal illness, ethics, professionalism; where value formation is part of the instructor's goal. In addition, this method allows students to learn from each other.

Another powerful use of discussion is to apply recently acquired information to "new" problems. For example, after presenting the pathophysiology of disease states, such as tension pneumothorax, the students might be asked to devise a treatment for this condition based on their understanding of anatomy and physiology. This is a powerful way to improve understanding and retention.

Things that will improve the effectiveness of group discussion include:

1. The structure and focus of the discussion must be maintained. Discussions that are random and haphazard can accomplish very little and provide negative feedback to the participants.

2. Adequate time must be allocated to sufficiently explore the scope of the topic.

3. A non-evaluative climate is essential to avoid suppression of opinion. It is helpful to initially accept and record all ideas to permit free exchange. Rejection of ideas or solutions can occur later in the session when the group has become more comfortable and secure. This style of discussion is called brainstorming and can be extremely effective in the achievement of higher order cognitive and affective objectives.

Tutorials

The tutorial is a valuable learning activity for clarifying and reinforcing information presented in class. The tutorial can consist of intensive one to one review by an instructor or fellow student or a group format where students work together to clarify and strengthen concepts. One on one tutorials requires an empathetic and sensitive facilitator to be effective. A threatening atmosphere can hamper the concentration of the student due to stress and poor self esteem.

Tutorial format is also very appropriate for the acquisition of psychomotor skills. Students who have achieved basic competency may even work among themselves to master skills, provided provisions for validity and feedback are developed (i.e., critical performance sheets). Otherwise incorrect learning can occur and provide an obstacle for mastery.

Role Playing

Students can be placed into clinical and patient roles to practice skills and knowledge. This is a very useful tool to synthesize and apply knowledge. It can be very enjoyable and rewarding if the scenarios are constructed with the students ability in mind. Care should be taken to have clear objectives with each scenario.

There should be no confusing or complicated problems that foster failure. Critique should be non-threatening and whenever possible, focus on the correct performance as a medium for reinforcing skills and knowledge.

Role playing provides the closest experience to actual application in the field. If done properly, it can engender confidence in the student for actual clinical experience. However, if the scenarios are difficult, it can provide negative feedback and hinder classroom participation.

Case Study

An oral or written account of an incident is analyzed by the students. This type of learning activity assumes knowledge on the part of the student and is useful as the end of a lesson segment or later in the course. The instructor must carefully decide the key relevant points of the case to guide in the analysis and critique that follows the presentation of facts. This will avoid tangents that confuse the objectives of the discussion.

The case history also allows the instructor to synthesize information and puts the students in the position to work at higher levels of cognitive learning (synthesis and analysis). It also portrays the relevance of information by placing it within a real clinical circumstance. Case history or call review is the foundation of continuing education since it targets the specific performance of field personnel. When the EMT who participated in the call is present, it is essential to be sensitive during critique. Since reviews often focus on the wrong things done in a given circumstance, it can create a "negative" learning environment. It is important to emphasize and reinforce correct performance as well as pointing out areas for improvement.

Summary

The above represents a review of some common and useful learning activities. They are by no means comprehensive. Games, computer assisted learning, workbooks and independent research are other common approaches that should be considered when designing your EMT program. Obviously some of these methods are time consuming and may have limited application in your course. However, every attempt should be made to provide diversified and appropriate learning strategies in your program. Admittedly, it is difficult to predict the success of one method over the other but a carefully selected strategy is likely to be superior to a strict lecture type format.

Suggested Reading

Davies, I.K. Competency Based Learning: Technology, Management and Design. McGraw Hill. New York, NY 1973.

Mager, R.F. Preparing Instructional Objectives. Pitman Management and Training, a Division of Pitman Learning, Inc. Belmont, CA Second Edition.

TEACHING GUIDE FOR EMT PREHOSPITAL CARE

Chapter 1

INTRODUCTION TO PREHOSPITAL EMERGENCY CARE

Materials and Equipment for Lesson

1. Registration material
2. Pretest (optional)
3. Reading list
4. Policy and procedures
5. Sign-in sheet
6. Handouts
   - Content outline
   - Local and state laws, protocols, medical control
   - Standards, hospital destination standards
   - Local radio codes
7. Slide projector, overhead projector, flipchart and/or blackboard
8. Slides or overhead transparencies
9. Film related to EMS systems or EMT work.

Section 1

Course Overview

Suggested Learning Activities
Introduce staff and have students introduce themselves.   **Using lecture format with handouts, provide overview of program EMT by brainstorming and discussion.**

Content

I. Introductions
   A. Introduce and explain the roles of the following persons
      1. Course administrator
      2. Medical director
      3. Instructor coordinator(s)
      4. Lab instructors
      5. Other appropriate staff
   B. Have the students introduce themselves and state their goals for the program

Chapter 1

Content

I. Course overview
   A. Review the following matters pertaining to the program
      1. Course outline
      2. Policy and procedures
      3. Clinical rotations information
      4. Layout of classroom and facility
      5. Starting and completion times
      6. Reading assignment
      7. Examinations and evaluations
         a) Practical
         b) Written
         c) Clinical
      8. State requirements for certification
         a) Written
         b) Practical
         c) Clinical
         d) Fees
      9. State recertification requirements
         a) Continuing education
         b) Refresher training
         c) Challenge testing
         d) Fees
      10. Other requirements
   B. Course purpose (discuss these and other reasons)
      1. Professional advancement
      2. Service to the community
      3. Value of skills in personal life
      4. Ability to deal with human issues in your work
      5. Exiting and interesting field
   C. Suggest methods for organizing learning
      1. Time management
      2. Participation in class
      3. Active listening
      4. Questions
      5. Reading
         a) Skim major heading
         b) Read summary
         c) Detailed reading
         d) Self and peer evaluation
         e) Workbook
         f) Class handouts
      6. Notes
         a) Organizational methods for taking notes
         b) Tape recorders
         c) Rewriting notes at home
      7. Tutoring
         a) Peer tutoring
         b) Program tutoring or review sessions

Section 2

EMS Systems

Objectives
(Slide 1-1)

At the conclusion of the lesson the student will be able to:

1. **Define an EMS system.**
2. **Discuss the history of EMS in relation to the following:**
   - War
   - Technology
   - Physician's role
   - Civilian evolution
   - Trauma
3. **State the statistical significance of heart disease and accidents in relation to the EMS system.**
4. **List 5 components of an EMS system and explain their role.**
5. **Discuss the differences between the following levels of EMT's:**
   - EMT-A
   - EMT-I
   - EMT-P
6. **List 5 functions of a dispatch communication system.**
7. **Define medical control.**
8. **List 5 elements of off-line medical control.**
9. **List 4 primary and 3 other responsibilities of an EMT.**

Instructor Preparation

Reading preparation for the lesson:

EMT Prehospital Care, Chapter 1, pages 3-15
Local regulations and protocols
State regulations and laws
Policy and procedure manual

Optional reading:

Henry M, Stapleton E: EMT's and Medical Control. JEMS, 1985:1(1);32-34

Subcommittee on Medical Control, Committee on Emergency Medical Services, Assembly of Life Sciences: Medical Control in Emergency Medical Service Systems. National Research Council, National Academy Press, 1981

Suggested Learning Activities

Using slides or transparencies discuss the components of an EMS system.

Have the students identify the roles and responsibilities of an EMT by brainstorming and discussion.

Content

III. Overview of EMS **(Slide 1-2)**
- A. EMT is often first medical professional to see patient
- B. You serve several functions:
  - 1. Assure a safe environment
  - 2. Gather and evaluate decision-making facts
  - 3. Provide treatments
  - 4. Mobilize other resources, i.e., rescue
  - 5. Select hospital
  - 6. Communicate with dispatch and hospital
- C. Part of a system to effect survival of ill and injured

IV. EMS systems
- A. Definitions:
  - 1. Emergency = An unforeseen combination of circumstances or the resulting state that calls for immediate action. A pressing need.
  - 2. Medical = Relating to or concerned with physicians or the practice of medicine.
  - 3. Service = The occupation or function of serving; a contribution to the welfare of others.
  - 4. System = A regular interacting or interdependent group of items forming a unified whole.
  - 5. Emergency Medical Services System (EMSS) is the planned **(Slide 1-3)** configuration of community resources and personnel necessary to provide immediate medical care to patients who have suffered sudden or unexpected illness or injury.
- B. Historical perspective **(Slide 1-4)**
  - 1. EMS dates back to "good Samaritan"
  - 2. Battlefields as a laboratory **(Slide 1-5)**
    - a) EMS development occurred over past 20-30 years
    - b) First formal provision of EMS on battlefields
    - c) Napoleonic Wars
      - (1) Dominique Jean (Baron de) Larrey
      - (2) Ambulance volantes (flying field hospital)
    - d) Civil War
      - (1) Dr. Jonathan Letterman
      - (2) Horse-drawn ambulances
    - e) World War I
      - (1) Introduction of traction splint
      - (2) Significant decrease in mortality
    - f) World War II
      - (1) Introduction of air ambulance
      - (2) Further reduction in mortality
    - g) Korean War
      - (1) Helicopters first used
      - (2) Rapid evacuation increased survival
    - h) Vietnam
      - (1) Reinforced value of rapid transport
      - (2) Early surgery for trauma victims

Content

- i) Death rates of battle casualties
  - (1) 8% in World War I
  - (2) 2.5% in Korea
  - (3) Less than 2% in Vietnam

3. Civilian evolution **(Slide 1-6)**
   - a) Varied from area to area
     - (1) Rural
       - (a) Undertaker
       - (b) Volunteer fire service
     - (2) Urban
       - (a) Hospitals
       - (b) Fire service
       - (c) Police
   - b) Early services
     - (1) Cincinnati Hospital in the mid-1860s
     - (2) Michael Reese motorized ambulance 1899
   - c) Pre World War II, physicians provided EMS
   - d) Physicians still used i.e. Soviet Union
4. Trauma as an impetus for EMS **(Slide 1-7)**
   - a) Accidents - leading cause of death 1 to 37 years; automobile caused surge in trauma deaths
     - (1) 1900 seventh leading cause of death
     - (2) Today - third leading cause of death
     - (3) Automobile accidents - more than 45%
   - b) Simple steps were needed prehospital
     - (1) Application of bleeding control
     - (2) Safe patient handling
     - (3) Immobilization
     - (4) CPR
     - (5) Rapid transportation
   - c) As a by-product medical care was improved
5. Technology and knowledge **(Slide 1-8)**
   - a) CPR was taught in 1960
   - b) Portable defibrillators - mid-sixties
   - c) Biotelemetry late 1960s made ALS possible
     - (1) Defibrillation, pharmacology, and advanced airway procedures
     - (2) Paramedics under physician direction
6. The physician and EMS **(Slide 1-9)**
   - a) Physician societies played lead role
     - (1) Academy of Orthopaedic Surgeons
     - (2) American College of Surgeons
   - b) EMT curriculum was initiated through physician groups
   - c) Physicians worked in early systems
   - d) France, Soviet Union, Germany use physicians
7. The Landmark Paper
   - a) 1966, The National Academy of Sciences
     - (1) "Accidental Death and Disability: The Neglected Diseases of Modern Society."
     - (2) 1973, Federal money developed EMS systems

Content

8. The emergence of the EMT **(Slide 1-10)**
    a) Prior to 1960s, training varied
    b) Personnel varied
        (1) Undertakers in some regions
        (2) Volunteer fireman
        (3) First aid training
        (4) Hospitals in urban areas

V. Components of an EMS system
  A. Important facts **(Slide 1-11)**
    1. Heart disease leading cause of death
        a) 540,00 deaths
        b) 350,000 deaths occur outside the hospital
    2. Accidents
        a) 110,000 deaths due to trauma
        b) Leading cause for patient 1-37
    3. Other major EMS cases
        a) Airway obstruction
        b) Pediatric emergencies
        c) Poisoning
        d) Environmental emergencies
        e) Shortness of breath
        f) Medical emergencies
            (1) Diabetic emergencies
            (2) Stroke
            (3) Anaphylaxis
        g) Childbirth
  B. Component #1 - Self help **(Slide 1-12)**
    1. Self recognition of signs and symptoms
    2. Access the EMS system
    3. Some basic measures of self help
  C. Component #2 - Lay rescuers and first responders
    1. First person to recognize an emergency
    2. Provide CPR and first aid skills
    3. Heart Association and Red Cross are leaders
    4. Lay rescuer
        a) Taught in public and private schools
        b) Worksite training
        c) Community programs
        d) High risk family members
    5. First responders
        a) Police, fire personnel
        b) Formal response to EMS
        c) Rescue skills with minimal equipment

Content

D. Component #3 - emergency medical technicians **(Slide 1-13)**
    1. More than 400,000 EMT's U.S.
    2. EMT is the foundation for prehospital care
    3. Definition - successfully completed DOT minimum
    4. Original EMT - safe handling and transportation
    5. Modern day - more dynamic role
        a) Evolves with knowledge and technology
        b) Original EMT courses - 24 hours
        c) Current - 110 hour minimum
        d) Future - ?
    6. Advanced levels **(Slide 1-14)**
        a) EMT-D
            (1) Adds defibrillation skill
            (2) Impacts main problem - cardiac arrest
        b) EMT-I provide additional skills
            (1) Intravenous therapy
            (2) Advanced airway
            (3) Minimal pharmacology
            (4) Commonly used in volunteer systems
        c) EMT-paramedic
            (1) Completed DOT curriculum
            (2) Performs advanced techniques
                (a) EKG interpretation
                (b) Drug therapy
                (c) Invasive airway techniques
                (d) Pharmacology
                (e) Defibrillation

E. Component #4 - emergency departments **(Slide 1-15)**
    1. Serve as the "intersection" of the EMS system; provide stabilizing care
    2. Emergency physicians provide leadership role
        a) Team leader in E.D.
        b) Medical control for prehospital personnel
    3. Standards for E.D.'s have advanced over 20 years
        a) Provide structured advanced care
            (1) Trauma
            (2) Cardiac
            (3) Pediatric

F. Component #5 - critical care units/OR **(Slide 1-16)**
    1. Provide additional lifesaving treatments
    2. Closely monitor to avoid subsequent problems
    3. Specialty critical care facilities
        a) Cardiac
        b) Respiratory
        c) Neonatal
        d) Surgical
        e) Burns
        f) Hyperbaric

Content

G. Component #6 - Rehabilitation **(Slide 1-17)**
   1. Ultimate EMS goal - return patient to community
   2. Specialized long-term care is often needed
   3. Physical and rehabilitation is essential
   4. In-patient and out-patient models

H. Component #7 - Communications **(Slide 1-18)**
   1. Coordination and communication is essential
   2. 911 system plays central role
   3. Elements
      a) The dispatch system
         (1) "Central nervous system"
            (a) Single access number
            (b) Categorizes and prioritizes calls
            (c) Dispatches ambulances
            (d) Coordinates with other agencies
            (e) Communicates with hospital
            (f) Coordinates disaster operations
         (2) Dispatchers national training program
      b) Ambulance-to-hospital communications
         (1) Physician directs care
         (2) Biotelemetry
         (3) Notification of patient conditions
      c) Discuss the structure of the local communications system
         (1) Dispatch
         (2) Ambulance to hospital
         (3) Communication with other agencies

I. Component #8 - Categorization **(Slide 1-19)**
   1. Hospitals are categorized according to resources
   2. Trauma centers, burn centers, replant
   3. Provides highly specialized care
   4. EMT's must know local system of categorization

J. Discuss local categorization structure

K. Component #9 - Medical Control **(Slide 1-20)**
   1. Accountability of EMT by physician
   2. Essential to assure quality of care
   3. Most systems have ALS but not BLS
   4. On-line
      a) Direct supervision of EMT
      b) Biotelemetry and voice communication
   5. Off-line
      a) Evaluation
      b) Call review
      c) Continuing education
      d) EMT training
      e) Quality assurance
      f) Field observation
      g) Protocols **(Slide 1-21)**
   6. Discuss local medical control structure

Content

- VI. The Roles and Responsibilities of the EMT **(Slide 1-22)**
  - A. EMT work is diversified
    1. Medical
    2. Technical
    3. Social
    4. Clerical
  - B. Primary responsibilities
    1. Patient assessment
       - a) Most difficult aspect of EMT work
       - b) Requires systematic approach
       - c) Practice in clinical situations is essential
    2. Prompt and effective care
       - a) Time is one of the most important variables
       - b) Protocols should guide treatment when available
       - c) Minimal time should be spent at the scene
    3. Patient handling
       - a) Removal of patient is guided by circumstances
       - b) EMT's must be ready to adapt to varied situations
       - c) Spinal immobilization is performed early in trauma
    4. Safe and efficient transport
       - a) Little time can be saved by "fast" rides
       - b) Most patients benefit from controlled transport
    5. Transfer of responsibility to the hospital staff
       - a) Clear communication is essential
       - b) Documentation supports verbal
       - c) Systematic approach is essential
  - C. Other or secondary responsibilities **(Slide 1-23)**
    1. Extrication
       - a) Usually performed by fire, police or rescue
       - b) "Light extrication" may be performed by EMT
       - c) Some regions extrication is primary function of EMT's
    2. Communications
       - a) Clear and appropriate use of the radio is essential
       - b) The radio is a form of documentation
       - c) Notification to hospital staff is important
    3. Record keeping
       - a) Most important medical legal prevention instrument
       - b) Important to the follow-up care of the patient
       - c) Documents conditions and treatment that doctors need to guide inhospital therapy
       - d) Essential to quality control

Content

4. Vehicle and equipment maintenance
    a) Faulty equipment can injure patients
    b) The vehicle and equipment must be checked, serviced and replaced regularly

VII. Certification **(Slide 1-24)**

A. State license and certification varies
1. Written exams
2. Practical exams
3. Clinical requirements
4. Recertification every 2-3 years

B. National Registry of Emergency Medical Technicians
1. Developed to establish national standards
2. Requirements
    a) Written
    b) Practical
    c) Continuing education
3. Levels
    a) EMT-A
    b) EMT-D
    c) EMT-I
    d) EMT-P

C. National Association of Emergency Medical Technicians
1. Represents 400,00 EMT's throughout the United States. Founded in 1975
2. Maintains three societies
    a) The National Society of EMS Administrators
    b) The National Society of Instructor Coordinators
    c) The National Society of EMT - Paramedics
3. Serves several functions
    a) Legislative change
    b) Continuing education
        (1) Educational conference
        (2) Prehospital Trauma Life Support
    c) Job placement

D. The American Heart Association
1. Standards and guidelines for emergency cardiac care
    a) Inhospital and prehospital providers
    b) Updated every 4 to 5 years
    c) Basic Life Support
    d) Advanced Life Support
2. Provide the basis of practice

Chapter 1

Section 3

Ethical and Medical Legal Issues

Objectives
(Slide 1-25)

At the conclusion of the lesson the student will be able to:

1. **Discuss the following issues related to ethics:**
   - **Competence**
   - **Professionalism**
   - **Patient perception**
   - **Confidentiality**
2. **List 3 elements that comprise the standard of care.**
3. **List 4 ingredients of medical malpractice.**
4. **State the difference between informed and implied consent.**
5. **State the purpose of a "Good Samaritan Law."**
6. **Define abandonment.**
7. **List 3 criteria for withholding CPR.**
8. **List 3 principles of risk management in prehospital care.**

Instructor Preparation

Reading preparation for the lesson:

EMT Prehospital Care, pages 15-21
State laws and regulations
Local laws and regulations

Optional reading:

Morrissey JM, Hoffmann AD, and Thrope JC: Consent and Confidentiality in the Health Care of Children and Adolescents A Legal Guide. The Free Press, A Division of Macmillan, 1986

Suggested Learning Activities

Using slides or transparencies review the important areas related to ethical and legal issues.

Have the students develop and explore the key elements of ethical and legal issues through group discussion or case histories.

Content

VIII. Ethics and Medical Legal Issues
- A. Ethics **(Slide 1-26)**
  - 1. The "Golden Rule"
  - 2. Assumes a responsible and caring approach
  - 3. Competence
    - a) The knowledge/ability to provide effective care
    - b) Mastered in initial education and work
    - c) Maintained through continuing education
    - d) Requires effort and diligence to keep current
  - 4. Professionalism **(Slide 1-27)**
    - a) Webster
      - (1) "Acting requisite to the body of knowledge which defines the service and abilities of the professional"
      - (2) "According to the oath of the profession" "
      - (3) "Historical first to religious vows"
    - b) Review medical oath of Geneva
  - 5. Patient perception **(Slide 1-28)**
    - a) Appearance can evoke patient confidence
    - b) Personal attitude develops trust
      - (1) Sensitivity
      - (2) Interest in your work
      - (3) Awareness of the environment
      - (4) Accepting responsibility
  - 6. Confidentiality **(Slide 1-29)**
    - a) Patient has the right to confidentiality
    - b) Regard all information as private
    - c) Reportable incidents
      - (1) Child, spousal, elderly abuse
      - (2) Crimes
    - d) Information to friends and family
      - (1) Consult with administrator or medical control physician to confirm the appropriateness of any information before it is released to the media
- B. Medical legal considerations
  - 1. The standard of care **(Slide 1-30)**
    - a) Guidelines which provide the basis of EMT practice
    - b) Consist of many elements
      - (1) Certification and license
      - (2) Body of knowledge, e.g. textbooks
      - (3) Laws
      - (4) Comparison of similarly trained EMT's in similar circumstances
      - (5) Policies and protocols

Content

(6) Standards set forth by various organizations
(a) State health regulations
(b) American Heart Association
(c) National Research Council
(d) DOT

c) In legal actions standard of care is used as a reference point for comparison

C. Laws pertaining to prehospital care **(Slide 1-31)**

1. States have laws that define EMT practice
2. May address several issues
   a) Training standards
   b) Medical control
   c) Vehicle and equipment specifications
   d) License or certification
3. Scope of practice
   a) Parameters/limitations medical provider
   b) Defines performance standards

D. Legal principles - Four ingredients of malpractice **(Slide 1-32)**

1. Duty to treat
   a) EMT must have a duty to treat the patient
   b) EMT has duty when responding to call
   c) May have no legal duty when not at work
   d) Once treatment is performed duty is established
2. Breach of duty
   a) Negligent act/omission violating standard of care
   b) EMT must perform reasonable care
   c) Failure to do so is negligence
3. Injury
   a) Negligent performance by itself is not enough
   b) Patient must have suffered harm
4. Causal connection
   a) Connection between injury-actions taken or omitted by the EMT
   b) Plaintiff must prove injury was caused by EMT

E. Consent **(Slide 1-33)**

1. Patients have a right to consent or refuse treatment
2. May be given by patient, parent, or guardian
3. In hospitals patients may sign consent
4. Written consent is not done in prehospital care
5. Consent is not always possible
   a) Disoriented patients, altered mental states
   b) Minors with no parent or guardian available
   c) Incompetent, i.e. mentally retarded patients
6. Informed consent
   a) Patient is aware of risks, benefits, options
   b) Very important where patient refuse consent
   c) Patient must sign a release

Content

7. Implied consent
    a) Where verbal/written consent is not possible
        (1) Unconscious person
        (2) Children or retarded individuals without parent or guardian
8. Persons capable of consenting **(Slide 1-34)**
    a) Competent adult
    b) Emancipated minor
        (1) Under the legal adult age
        (2) Living independently of the parents/guardians
        (3) Self-supporting, married or parent
9. Refusal of treatment **(Slide 1-35)**
    a) Competent adult/emancipated minor has the right to refuse care
    b) Make every attempt to help patient
    c) Family and friends may help
    d) Release must be signed

F. Immunities **(Slide 1-36)**
1. Laws often provide legal immunities for
    a) Government institutions
    b) Medical professionals
    c) Laypeople
2. "Good Samaritan Laws"
    a) Designed to protect citizen functioning in a nonprofessional capacity
    b) Developed to encourage helping attitudes in emergencies
    c) Varies from state to state

G. Abandonment **(Slide 1-37)**
1. Definition
    a) The unilateral severance of a professional patient-provider relationship...
    b) Without affording the patient notice and reasonable time to find substitute and equivalent treatment
2. Premature cessation of care
3. Leaving the patient on the scene

H. High risk areas for EMT's **(Slide 1-38)**
1. Equipment related injuries
    a) Vehicle failure
    b) Equipment failure
    c) Missing equipment
2. Emotionally disturbed patients
    a) Use care when removing patient against will
    b) Law enforcement personnel should be utilized
    c) Care and empathy when using restraints

Content

3. Withholding CPR
    a) Should when any hope exists for resuscitation
    b) Obvious death must be present
    c) Time is not a good criteria
    d) Do not rely on bystanders
    e) Criteria for death
        (1) Extreme dependant lividity
        (2) Rigor mortis
        (3) Obvious death, e.g. decapitation
    f) Terminal Illness
        (1) More controversial area regarding withholding CPR
        (2) Doctor should be requested to decide
        (3) When in doubt - resuscitate
        (4) Check local standards
    g) Cardiovascular Unresponsiveness
        (1) Requires application of ALS
        (2) Some systems permit prehospital decision
4. Reporting Requirements - Potentially reportable cases **(Slide 1-39)**
    a) Child, spousal, elderly abuse
    b) Infectious diseases
    c) Violent crimes such as rape and assault
    d) Check local protocols
5. Risk Management **(Slide 1-40)**
    a) "An ounce of prevention..."
    b) Should not be apprehensive about lawsuits
    c) Adhere to certain principles
        (1) Act according to the standard of care
        (2) Document actions carefully
        (3) Act in the best interest of the patient
    d) An abusive attitude breeds lawsuits
    e) Caring, empathetic attitude prevents lawsuits

IX. Summary
  A. Questions and answers
  B. Assignments

Chapter 1

INTRODUCTION TO PREHOSPITAL EMERGENCY CARE

Examination

1. An Emergency Medical Service system is best described as:

   a. a system of ambulances that respond to injured and ill persons.
   b. a system of communications that receive the call for help.
   c. a system of resources and personnel necessary to provide immediate care to the ill and injured.
   d. hospital emergency services that deal with emergency care of the ill and injured.

2. Dr. Jonathan Letterman was a noted historical figure in the development of EMS systems during the:

   a. Civil War
   b. San Francisco Earthquake
   c. World War I
   d. Chicago Fire

3. Ambulances were first utilized to transport the wounded during the ____________________ war.

   a. Vietnam
   b. Civil
   c. Napoleonic
   d. Korean

4. Helicopters were first used for the transport of casualties during [the]:

   a. Vietnam war
   b. World War I
   c. World War II
   d. Korean

5. The first motorized ambulance is said to have been provided by ____________________________ in 1899.

   a. Michael Reese Hospital of Chicago
   b. Bellevue Hospital of New York City
   c. Cincinnati General
   d. Massachusetts General

6. Accidents cause approximately __________ deaths every year in the United States.

    a. 1,000,000
    b. 512,000
    c. 100,000
    d. 5,000

7. The National Academy of Sciences published a landmark paper entitled "Accidental Death and Disability: The Neglected Diseases of Modern Society" in:

    a. 1966
    b. 1970
    c. 1945
    d. 1973

8. Heart disease is the ________ leading cause of death in the United States.

    a. 1st
    b. 2nd
    c. 3rd
    d. 4th

9. Approximately _____________ deaths result from heart disease each year in the United States.

    a. 200,000
    b. 1,000,000
    c. 540,000
    d. 100,000

10. Lay rescuers, first responders, EMT's and paramedics, emergency departments, and intensive care units are all components of a[n]:

    a. health care agency
    b. emergency network
    c. crisis intervention team
    d. EMS system

11. The leading cause of accidental death in the United States is:

    a. drowning
    b. assaults
    c. auto accidents
    d. child abuse

12. The current EMT curriculum was developed under the guidance of the United States Department of:

    a. Health
    b. Education
    c. Transportation
    d. Safety

13. This component of an EMS system provides stabilizing measures just prior to transfer to the operating room or critical care unit.

    a. lay rescuers
    b. emergency departments
    c. emergency medical technicians
    d. intensive care units

14. This member of the EMS system is the first help the patient has in many instances. He provides critical initial life support such as CPR or bleeding control. If the cardiac arrest patient does not have the benefit of his help within 4 minutes his chances of survival significantly diminish.

    a. lay rescuer
    b. emergency physician
    c. EMT and paramedic
    d. nurse

15. This method of hospital designation according to capabilities in different areas of care (i.e. Trauma, Burns, Neonatology, Replantation) is an essential part of an EMS system.

    a. categorization
    b. standardization
    c. systemization
    d. alteration

16. This aspect of an EMS system brings to the scene individuals who may use either basic or advanced skills to support or stabilize the critical patient.

    a. lay rescuers
    b. emergency departments
    c. EMT's and paramedics
    d. intensive care units

17. This stage of an EMS system provides specialized definitive care (such as cardiac, neonatal, burn or respiratory) that is needed to stabilize the critical patient.

    a. rehabilitation unit
    b. emergency department
    c. critical care unit
    d. outpatient unit

18. The type of communication system that allows the transfer of EKG in the field to the medical control base station is called:

    a. biotransfer
    b. biotelemetry
    c. biorhythms
    d. biometrics

19. The component of the communications system that receives the call for help and sends the appropriate response vehicles to the scene is called the:

    a. telemetry system
    b. ambulance system
    c. dispatch system
    d. hospital system

20. Which of the following is <u>not</u> a role of the dispatch component of a communications system:

    a. receiving the call
    b. dispatching the call
    c. interfacing with other agencies
    d. receiving telemetry

21. Direct voice communication with EMT's in the field by a physician at a base station is an example of:

    a. on-line medical control
    b. off-line medical control
    c. fine-line medical control
    d. direct-line medical control

22. A formal educational session, provided by a physician for field personnel, where cases are reviewed and critiqued is called:

    a. field critique session
    b. case history practice
    c. call review
    d. field feedback session

23. A standardized approach to emergency care that is developed for field personnel by physicians and usually reflects regional and national guidelines is called a:

    a. procedure
    b. process
    c. protocol
    d. policy

24. Physician involvement and participation in all phases of the EMS system to assure quality care best defines the concept of:

    a. categorization
    b. standardization
    c. systemization
    d. medical control

25. Off-line medical control of prehospital care should include all of the following, except:

    a. needs assessment and evaluation of the system
    b. training and certification
    c. quality assurance
    d. equipment inventory

Match the level of certification in column B to performance standards that best describe the scope of practice in column A.

Column A	Column B
26. provides electrical therapy in cardiac arrest.	a. EMT-P
27. entry level prehospital provider, over 400,000 in U.S.	b. EMT-A
28. EKG interpretation, invasive airway skills, broader based pharmacology	c. EMT-D
29. advanced airway management, IV therapy, sometimes limited pharmacology	d. EMT-Intermediate

30. A serious effort to acquire the requisite skills taught in the initial EMT training program, as well as a continued effort to prevent deterioration of knowledge is the best way to maintain:

    a. respect
    b. competence
    c. certification
    d. analytical skills

31. "Acting requisite to the body of knowledge which defines the service and abilities of the professional...according to the oath of the profession. Historical first to religious vows...." This definition (Webster) best describes:

    a. competence
    b. professionalism
    c. ethics
    d. honorable

32. When treating an adult patient, you can routinely provide <u>specific</u> information about the condition and care of the patient to:

    a. the press
    b. friends
    c. employers
    d. none of the above

33. The <u>"four general ingredients"</u> of a malpractice case include all of the following <u>except</u>:

    a. causal connection between injury and EMT's actions
    b. injury to the patient
    c. verbal abuse of the patient
    d. a breach of duty

34. When the patient is made aware of the benefits and consequences of the care provided he is being treated under the concept of:

    a. implied consent
    b. applied consent
    c. informed consent
    d. none of the above

35. A child or mentally incompetent adult in need of emergency care, without a parent or guardian present, is treated under the concept of:

    a. implied consent
    b. applied consent
    c. informed consent
    d. emergency consent

36. The EMT's unilateral severance of a patient-provider relationship without sufficient time to find a substitute, best describes:

    a. malfeasance
    b. abandonment
    c. negligence
    d. unlawful

37. When treating an unconscious person the paramedic is functioning under the concept of ________ consent:

    a. informed
    b. presumed
    c. implied
    d. surrogate

38. A person who is under the legal adult age but who is living independent of his or her parents in some states may be considered to be a[n]:

    a. adult
    b. minor
    c. emancipated minor
    d. alienated minor

39. Specific laws designed to protect the private citizen who is functioning in a non-professional capacity and without an expectation of remuneration are often referred to as:

    a. medical practice laws
    b. EMS acts
    c. good Samaritan laws
    d. citizen protection acts

40. Which of the following is an acceptable criteria for withholding CPR?

    a. 15 minute history of cardiac arrest
    b. rigor mortis
    c. dilated pupils
    d. very cold skin

Chapter 2

ANATOMY AND PHYSIOLOGY AND PATIENT ASSESSMENT

Materials and Equipment for Lesson

1. Anatomy posters, overhead transparencies or slides
2. Live model/manikin for patient assessment demonstration
3. Human skeleton
4. Handouts
    Anatomy and physiology
    Patient assessment
5. Sphygmomanometer, stethoscope, penlight
6. Blanket to perform demonstration
7. Slide projector, overhead projector, flipchart and/or blackboard
8. Reading list

Section 1

Anatomy and Physiology

Objectives
(Slide 2-1)

At the conclusion of the lesson the student will be able to:

1. Define the following topographic and anatomical terms:

- medial	**- anterior**	**- posterior**
- lateral	**- proximal**	**- midline**
- distal	**- inferior**	**- abduction**
- superior	**- lateral**	**- adduction**
	- recumbent	

2. Identify the major anatomy and describe the general functions of the following major body systems:

- respiratory	**- nervous**	**- circulatory**
- digestive	**- muscular**	**- genitourinary**
- skeletal	**- reproductive**	

3. Explain the concept of Heart-Lung-Brain relationship.

Chapter 2

Instructor Preparation

Reading preparation for the lesson:

EMT Prehospital Care, Chapter 2, pages 22 - 47

Optional reading:

Guyton, A.C.: Textbook of Medical Physiology. 8th Edition, W.B. Saunders. Philadelphia, PA, 1991.

Solomon, E.P., Philips, G.A.: Understanding Human Anatomy and Physiology. W.B. Saunders. Philadelphia, PA, 1987.

Suggested Learning Activities

Using a lecture format with the aid of slides, overhead transparencies or charts, provide an overview of anatomy and physiology.

When appropriate, have students palpate pulses and feel surface landmarks on themselves and other students.

Content

I. Introduction to Anatomy and Physiology
- A. Anatomy: the study of structure or form of living things **(Slide 2-2)**
- B. Physiology: the study of function [activities and processes].
- C. Structural organization of the human body
  - 1. Atoms and molecules
    - a) Atoms are smallest unit of matter
    - b) Molecules consist of 2 or more atoms **(Slide 2-3)**
    - c) Element - substance with identical atoms (Oxygen)
    - d) Main body molecules are water and proteins
      - (1) Water is vital to body functions
        - (a) When it surrounds particles - solvent
        - (b) Particles are solutes **(Slide 2-4)**
  - 2. The cell **(Slide 2-5)**
    - a) Principles of cells same **(Slide 2-6)**
      - (1) Exchange of materials with immediate environment
      - (2) Obtaining energy from nutrients
      - (3) Synthesizing proteins
      - (4) Reproduction
    - b) Specialization
  - 3. Tissues **(Slide 2-7)**
    - a) Specialized cells working together
    - b) Types of tissues
      - (1) Epithelial
      - (2) Connective
      - (3) Muscle
      - (4) Nerve
    - c) Tissue fluid or interstitial fluid **(Slide 2-8)**
      - (1) Cells surrounded with interstitial fluid
      - (2) Source of nutrients and secretion of waste
      - (3) Cell membrane regulates passages of substances in and out of cell
        - (a) Diffusion - movement of substance from an area of higher to lower concentration **(Slide 2-9)**
        - (b) Osmosis - movement of solvent from an area of higher concentration to an area of lower concentration of solutes **(Slide 2-10)**
  - 4. Organs **(Slide 2-11)**
    - a) A structure comprised of several types of tissues
    - b) Work together to serve a given function
    - c) Examples of organs
      - (1) Kidney
      - (2) Lung
      - (3) Brain

Content

5. Organ systems **(Slide 2-12)**
    a) A group of organs working together to perform a complex function
    b) Examples of systems
        (1) Respiratory
        (2) Circulatory
        (3) Reproductive
6. Essential processes **(Slide 2-13)**
    a) Metabolism
    b) Nutrition
    c) Homeostasis

II. Anatomical Terms and Relationships
  A. Anatomical position **(Slide 2-14)**
    1. Body standing erect
    2. Feet together and parallel
    3. Arms at the sides
    4. Palms and the head forward
  B. Terms relating to position and movement
    1. Medial - closer to the midline
    2. Lateral - away from the midline
    3. Proximal - closer to the trunk
    4. Distal - away from the trunk
    5. Superior - closer to the head
    6. Inferior - closer to the ground or feet
    7. Anterior {ventral} - toward the front of the body
    8. Posterior {dorsal} - toward the rear of the body
    9. Midline - imagining a plane through the nose, sternum and umbilicus
    10. Erect - standing upright
    11. Supine - lying on one's back
    12. Prone - lying face down
    13. Lateral recumbant - lying on one's side
    14. Abduction - movement away from midline **(Slide 2-15)**
    15. Adduction - movement toward midline
    16. Flexion - bending of a joint **(Slide 2-16)**
    17. Extension - straightening of a joint
    18. Medial rotation - anterior surface of **(Slide 2-17)** the limb is rotated to face medially
    19. Lateral rotation - anterior surface rotates to face laterally

III. Specific Organ Systems
  A. Skeletal system and body cavities **(Slide 2-18)**
    1. Gives structure and support
    2. Protects
    3. Permits movement in conjunction with muscles
    4. Other forms of connective tissue
        a) Cartilage
        b) Ligaments
        c) Tendons
    5. Axial and appendicular **(Slide 2-19,20)**

Content

6. Skull cranium [one liter internal capacity] and facial bones
7. Spinal column 33 vertebrae
    - a) 7 cervical vertebrae
    - b) 12 thoracic vertebrae
    - c) 5 lumbar vertebrae
    - d) Sacrum - 5 fused vertebrae
    - e) Coccyx - 4 fused vertebrae
    - f) Provides support, mobility and protection for spinal cord
8. Upper extremities
9. Lower extremities
10. Thoracic cavity **(Slide 2-21)**
    - a) Below neck to diaphragm
    - b) Rib cage surrounds and attached to sternum and thoracic spine
    - c) Diaphragm attaches to xiphoid process lower six ribs, upper lumbar vertebrae
    - d) Divided into mediastinum and pleural cavities
        - (1) Mediastinum - heart great vessels, esophagus, trachea, and mainstem bronchi
        - (2) Pleural cavity - lungs, bronchi
11. Abdominal - pelvic cavity
    - a) Bounded by diaphragm and boney pelvic cavity
    - b) Lined with peritoneum
    - c) Pelvic cavity is lowermost portion
    - d) Pelvic girdle
        - (1) Sacrum
        - (2) Ilium [2]
        - (3) Ischium [2]
        - (4) Pubis [2] bones
    - e) Superior border of pelvic cavity is imaginary plane from pubic bone to sacrum
    - f) Floor is formed by muscles and connective tissue
    - g) Quadrants **(Slide 2-22)**
        - (1) Imaginary lines [horizontal and vertical] through the umbilicus
        - (2) Left Upper
        - (3) Right Upper
        - (4) Left Lower
        - (5) Right Lower
    - h) Other terms
        - (1) Epigastric [below xiphoid and costal margins]
        - (2) Periumbilical [near the umbilicus]
        - (3) Suprapubic [just above the symphysis pubis
        - (4) Flank describes posterior portion of abdomen between the ribs and the ilium

B. Muscular system **(Slide 2-23)**

1. Tissues capable of contraction or shortening

<u>Content</u>

    2. Permit body movement and functions
    3. Three types
        a) Involuntary or smooth muscle **(Slide 2-24)**
        b) Cardiac muscle
        c) Voluntary or skeletal muscles **(Slide 2-25)**

C. Respiratory system **(Slide 2-26)**
    1. Intake of oxygen and release of carbon dioxide
    2. Create voice
    3. Heat loss
    4. Anatomy
        a) Nose and mouth
        b) Pharynx
        c) Larynx
        d) Epiglottis
        e) Trachea and bronchi
        f) Bronchioles
        g) Alveoli
        h) Lungs

D. Circulatory system **(Slide 2-27)**
    1. Distribution or transport system
        a) Delivery of oxygen and nutrients
        b) Pick up of carbon dioxide and other waste products
    2. Heart
        a) Atria
        b) Ventricles
    3. Vessels - arteries, veins, capillaries
        a) Pulmonary arteries and veins
        b) Aorta and vena cavae
        c) Arterioles and venules
    4. Blood
        a) Red cells
        b) White cells
        c) Platelets
        d) Plasma
    5. Circulations
        a) Pulmonary
        b) Systemic
        c) Coronary
    6. Lymphatic system
        a) Conduction of lymph
        b) Special function tissues

E. Nervous system **(Slide 2-28)**
    1. Controlling and regulating functions
    2. Decision maker and communicator
    3. Structure
        a) Central - brain and spinal cord
        b) Peripheral
        c) Autonomic

Content

4. Function
    a) Brain
        (1) Consciousness
        (2) Regulatory center
        (3) Seat of sensations
        (4) Voluntary acts
        (5) Emotion
        (6) Higher mental processes
        (7) Complex reflex center
    b) Spinal cord
        (1) Conducting pathway
        (2) Simple reflex center
    c) Peripheral nervous system
        (1) Afferent fibers - impulses to the brain
        (2) Efferent fibers - impulses from the brain to the body
    d) Autonomic nervous system [automatic]
        (1) regulates activities of visceral organs
        (2) balances body system
        (3) Parasympathetic - in action when body at rest
        (4) Sympathetic - inaction when body in action, widespread effect

F. Endocrine system **(Slide 2-29)**
1. Regulatory system
2. Gland tissue secreting hormones
3. Help maintain homeostasis and influence growth, reproduction, and response to stress
4. Include
    a) Growth hormone [pituitary gland]
    b) Thyroxine [thyroid gland]
    c) Testosterone [testes]
    d) Estrogen [ovaries]
    e) Adrenaline [adrenals]
    f) Insulin [pancreas]

G. Digestive system **(Slide 2-30)**
1. Main source of all nutritional intake except oxygen
2. Eat, digest [breakdown and absorb], and eliminate foods
3. Anatomy
    a) Mouth and throat
    b) Esophagus
    c) Stomach
    d) Liver
    e) Gallbladder
    f) Pancreas
    g) Small and large intestines
    h) Rectum and anus

Content

H. Urinary system **(Slide 2-31)**
  1. Elimination of waste materials filtered from the blood
  2. Controls production and elimination of urine
  3. Maintains salt, water and acid base balance. Organs include kidneys, ureters, bladder, urethra

I. Reproductive system
  1. Male **(Slide 2-32)**
    a) Testes [in scrotum]
    b) Vas deferens
    c) Prostate
    d) Urethra
  2. Female **(Slide 2-33)**
    a) Ovaries
    b) Fallopian tubes
    c) Uterus
    d) Vagina

J. Integumentary system (skin) **(Slide 2-34)**
  1. Largest organ in body
  2. Protects, barrier to bacteria, prevents water loss, insulates, regulates heat, allows for sensation

IV. Heart - Lung - Brain relationship **(Slide 2-35)**

A. Failure of any one organ can lead to collapse of the other two
  1. Cardiac arrest
    a) Hypoxia to brain
    b) Respiratory arrest
    c) Brain death
  2. Respiratory arrest
    a) Hypoxia to heart
    b) Cardiac arrest
    c) Brain death
  3. Brain injury
    a) Respiratory arrest
    b) Hypoxia to heart
    c) Cardiac Arrest
    d) Brain death

B. Clinical death = no pulse and no respirations. Biological death = begins after brain deprived of oxygen for 4-6 minutes.

C. Sudden and unexpected death
  1. CPR
  2. ALS

Section 2

Patient Assessment

Objectives
(Slide 2-36)

At the conclusion of the lesson the student will be able to:
1. List four patient vital signs and their normal range.
2. List the four phases of patient assessment.
3. Given a programmed patient, demonstrate the patient assessment approach.
4. Given a programmed patient, present a history in the correct order.

Instructor Preparation

Reading preparation for the lesson:

EMT Prehospital Care, Chapter 2, pages 47 - 79

Patient assessment critical performance sheet.

Optional reading:

Bates, B.: A Pocket Guide to Physical Examination and History Taking. J.B. Lippincott Co. Philadelphia, PA, 1991

Prehospital Trauma Life Support Committee of The National Association of EMT'ss: Pre-Hospital Trauma Life Support. 2nd Edition. Emergency Training. Akron, Ohio, 1990

Suggested Learning Activities
Using a lecture format with the aid of slides, overhead transparencies or charts, provide an overview of patient assessment.
Using a programmed patient, demonstrate the patient assessment process.
Using a tape cassette, present a patient history and analyze the presentation with the class.

Content

V. Patient Assessment **(Slide 2-37)**
- A. Foundation of all decisions related to treatment, triage and transportation
- B. Includes environmental clues, mechanism of injury, history and physical exam
- C. Systematic approach is essential
    1. Prioritize treatment
    2. Transport decision
    3. Assure a comprehensive survey
- D. Divided into 4 distinct phases
    1. Dispatch review
    2. Scene survey
    3. Primary survey
    4. Secondary survey

VI. The Dispatch Review **(Slide 2-38)**
- A. Information is provided by the dispatcher
- B. Varies from region to region
- C. Some systems may have the EMT receiving the call directly
- D. Allows the EMT to anticipate the worst possible conditions, for example
    1. "Cardiac" - cardiac arrest
    2. "Pedestrian Struck" - multiple trauma
    3. "Overdose" - respiratory arrest
- E. Allows strategy development between you and your partner
- F. Plan your route carefully to shorten the response
    1. Distance
    2. Traffic conditions
    3. Time of day

VII. The Scene Survey **(Slide 2-39)**
- A. Series of observations should be made upon arrival at scene
- B. Consider clues to the underlying problem
    1. Medications
    2. Evidence of trauma
    3. Position of the patient
    4. Track marks or other evidence of drug abuse
    5. Information from bystanders
- C. Mechanism of injury
- D. Hazards - secure scene
- E. Need for additional units or specialized rescue

VIII. The Primary Survey **(Slide 2-40)**
- A. Search for life threatening conditions
- B. Evaluates three major body systems: nervous, respiratory, circulatory
- C. Positive findings are treated immediately

Content

D. A - Airway **(Slide 2-41)**
- 1. Establishing responsiveness **(Slide 2-42)**
  - a) In trauma patients cervical spine is **(Slide 2-43)** immobilized **(Slide 2-44)**
  - b) Provide verbal and tactile stimuli
  - c) If the patient is not supine, roll **(Slide 2-45)** patient as a unit in order to proceed
- 2. Open the airway **(Slide 2-46)**
  - a) Tongue may fall against pharynx and block the airway
  - b) Head tilt - chin lift (non-traumatic) **(Slide 2-47)**
    - (1) Tilt head
    - (2) Lift jaw with index and middle fingers
  - c) Jaw thrust - without head tilt (trauma **(Slide 2-48)** patients)
    - (1) Fingers at angle of jaw
    - (2) Thumbs on maxilla
    - (3) Lift mandible
  - d) Check for signs of obstruction or secretions
    - (1) Suction, if necessary
    - (2) Obstructed airway maneuvers, if necessary

E. B - Breathing **(Slide 2-49)**
- 1. Look, listen and feel method
  - a) Look for chest rise
  - b) Listen for air exchange
  - c) Feel for air exchange
- 2. Evaluate the adequacy of breathing **(Slide 2-50)**
  - a) Chest wall injury
  - b) Respiratory rate and depth
  - c) Shortness of breath
  - d) Cyanosis
  - e) Accessory muscle use
  - f) Breath sounds **(Slide 2-51)**
  - g) Distended neck veins **(Slide 2-52)**
  - h) Deviated trachea **(Slide 2-53)**
  - i) Altered mental state
- 3. Consider need for
  - a) Supplemental oxygen
  - b) Positive pressure ventilation

F. C - Circulation **(Slide 2-54)**
- 1. Check for a pulse **(Slide 2-55)**
  - a) Carotid artery
    - (1) Groove between the larynx and muscle in the neck
    - (2) Same side as the evaluator
  - b) Check for 5 - 10 seconds
  - c) No pulse - begin cardiac compressions
  - d) Check for obvious hemorrhage

e) Evaluate adequacy of circulation **(Slide 2-56)**
(1) Pale, cool and sweaty skin
(2) Rapid pulse
(3) Delayed capillary refill
(4) Altered mental state
(5) Vomiting blood
(6) Rectal bleeding
(7) Hypotension
(a) Major pulses as rapid method for determining BP
i) Carotid = 60 systolic **(Slide 2-57)**
ii) Femoral = 70 systolic
iii) Radial = 80 systolic
(b) If necessary - auscultation
f) Provide essential treatment **(Slide 2-58)**
(1) CPR
(2) Pneumatic Antishock Garment
(3) Position
(4) Shock treatment
G. D - Disability **(Slide 2-59)**
1. Signs of central nervous system problems
a) Altered mental state
(1) AVPU
(a) Alert
(b) Responds to verbal stimuli
(c) Responds to painful stimuli
(d) Unresponsive
b) Pupillary changes
c) Motor
d) Sensory
H. E - Expose **(Slide 2-60)**
1. Expose and examine trunk
2. Pulsatile masses in abdomen
I. Critical or unstable - provide essential treatment and transport rapidly
J. Stable - proceed with the secondary survey
IX. Secondary Survey **(Slide 2-61)**
A. History, vital signs, head to toe survey and neurological exam
B. Performed on the scene or during transport
C. Should almost <u>never</u> be performed entirely on scene
1. Essential data collected on scene
2. Transport
3. Other information gathered enroute to hospital
4. One EMT - collect history, other vital signs
D. The patient history **(Slide 2-62)**
1. Medical patients often diagnosed primarily on the basis of history

Content

2. Several principles **(Slide 2-63)**
    a) Use open ended questions = objective history
    b) Direct the interview and do not allow the patient drift into non-essential areas
    c) Do not delay urgent treatment
        (1) Collect the essential data to establish a "working diagnosis"
        (2) Collect the remainder of information enroute to the hospital
    d) Whenever possible do not allow bystanders to answer for the patient
3. Components of the history **(Slide 2-64)**
    a) The Chief Complaint
        (1) Expression of the patient's main problem <u>in his or her own words</u>
        (2) Do not direct or suggest adjectives
        (3) If unclear, request clarifying adjectives
    b) History of present illness **(Slide 2-65)**
        (1) Expands upon the chief complaint
        (2) Several standard questions
            (a) The sequence of events
            (b) Activity at the onset of the problem
            (c) Location and radiation of pain
            (d) Aggravating and relieving factors
            (e) Similar past experiences
            (f) Associated signs and symptoms
            (g) Description of pain or other symptoms
        (3) Other questions (depending on the chief complaint)
            (a) Abdominal pain (examples)
                i) Vomiting
                ii) Antacids
                iii) Rectal bleeding
                iv) Orthostatic dizziness
            (b) Dyspnea (examples)
                i) Paroxysmal nocturnal dyspnea
                ii) Orthopnea
                iii) Edema
                iv) Productive cough
            (c) Seizures
                i) Focal or general
                ii) Length of seizure
                iii) Tongue biting
    c) The past history **(Slide 2-66)**
        (1) Clarifies or reinforces the diagnosis
        (2) Major illness and hospitalizations

Content

(3) Always question about four major in illness adults
(a) Heart disease
(b) Diabetes
(c) Chronic pulmonary disease
(d) High blood pressure
(4) Other inquiries depend on chief complaint, i.e.
(a) Vomiting blood - GI history
(b) Altered M.S. - seizures, stroke
d) Medications and allergies **(Slide 2-67)**
(1) Identify preexisting disease
(2) Essential part of the history
(3) When possible, bring medications to hospital
(4) An allergy history prevents inappropriate drug administration
e) Medic alert tags may provide **(Slide 2-68)** information
4. Technique for history taking requires a great practice under the supervision
5. Confidential information
E. Physical assessment **(Slide 2-69)**
1. Auditory, tactile and visual senses to elicit information
2. Principles of physical assessment
a) Utilize manpower - One EMT take vital signs, other performs head to toe survey
b) Maintain the systematic approach
c) Do not lose focus with obvious injuries
d) Perform gentle palpation to avoid aggravating injuries, i.e. skull fractures
e) Examine the dependent areas of the body
f) Consider the mechanism of injury
g) Do not spend excessive time on the scene
3. Vital signs **(Slide 2-70)**
a) Objective measure of assessment - good intra-observer reliability
b) Respirations, pulse, blood pressure and temperature
c) Basis for implementing certain protocols, i.e. PASG
d) Evaluated on the basis of "norms"
(1) Norms are averages of large groups
(2) Provide a frame of reference to identify abnormal variations
(3) Should be considered in light of the patient's overall condition

Content

e) Respirations **(Slide 2-71)**
- (1) Evaluated by rate, depth, pattern and abnormal sounds
  - (a) Rate is 12-20 in an adult patient
  - (b) Count the number of breaths in 15 seconds and multiply by 4
  - (c) Evaluate depth by observing chest excursion
  - (d) Abnormal patterns caused by certain diseases or central nervous system injury (Cheynne-Stokes)
  - (e) Sounds associated with obstruction of the airway
    - i) Gurgling = fluid in the airway
    - ii) Wheezing = narrowed lower airways
    - iii) Stridor = narrowed upper airway
    - iv) Snoring = partial obstruction, usually by tongue

f) Pulse **(Slide 2-72)**
- (1) Evaluated by rate, quality and rhythm
  - (a) Radial artery is most commonly used
  - (b) Normal rate for an adult at rest is approximately 60-80 per minute
  - (c) Average is 72 beats per minute in adult
    - i) Pulse is counted for 15 seconds and multiplied times 4
    - ii) Note irregularity
  - (d) Quality is expressed as normal, bounding or thready
    - i) Shock states - pulse may be nonpalpable
    - ii) A central artery may be used to monitor the pulse
  - (e) Rhythm may be regular, regularly irregular or irregularly irregular

g) Blood pressure **(Slide 2-73)**
- (1) The force exerted on the wall of the artery
  - (a) Determined by cardiac output and the resistance of vessels (PVR)
  - (b) Changes in either parameter may increase or decrease the pressure
- (2) Blood pressure is measured with a sphygmomanometer
- (3) There are two techniques for measuring blood pressure

Content

(a) Auscultation **(Slide 2-74)**
i) Sounds created by turbulent blood flow through an artery
ii) Bladder is placed just **(Slide 2-75)** above the elbow
iii) The brachial artery is **(Slide 2-76)** palpated
iv) Stethoscope is placed **(Slide 2-77)** over the artery
v) Cuff is pumped up until **(Slide 2-78)** the dial or mercury stops undulating
vi) Air is released while **(Slide 2-79)** listening for sounds
i) First sound = systolic
ii) Sound disappears or decreases = diastolic
vii) Normal values are: **(Slide 2-80)**
i) Systolic: 100 plus the age of the patient up to 140 mm/hg
ii) Diastolic: 65-90 mm/hg
(b) Sizes of cuffs **(Slide 2-81)**
i) Important to accurate reading
ii) Width of cuff should be 40% of the arm's circumference
(c) Palpation **(Slide 2-82)**
i) Used when there is extraneous noise or time is limited
ii) Cuff in the same position as auscultation
iii) Distal pulse [radial or brachial] is palpated
iv) Inflated until pulse is obliterated
v) Pressure released noting point of pulse return
vi) Only a systolic reading is documented

h) Temperature **(Slide 2-83)**
(1) Temperature
(a) EMT's are interested in significant changes in temperature
(b) Thermometer rarely needed
(c) Skin is palpated on the patient's face with back of your hand
(d) Moisture is also noted

4. Head to toe survey **(Slide 2-84)**
a) Systematic search for injuries and diagnostic signs
b) Relies upon working knowledge of topographic anatomy

Content

c) Systematic approach is essential in order to not overlook critical signs
d) Four techniques are utilized:
  (1) Observe for visual signs of injury or illness
  (2) Listen for auditory evidence, i.e. snoring or abnormal conditions
  (3) Palpate gently for evidence of injury, swelling, crepitus and other signs
  (4) Smell for evidence of disease or toxic substances
e) Mental status **(Slide 2-85)**
  (1) Responsiveness is again in the secondary survey
  (2) Terms that describe consciousness
    (a) Alert - able to express clearly and maintain normal conversation
    (b) Confused - refers to inability to provide correct answers
    (c) Lethargy - a term used to describe a sleepy state
    (d) Coma - a state characterized by total unresponsiveness
  (3) Orientation as a measurement **(Slide 2-86)**
    (a) The degree is noted according to person, place and time
    (b) Oriented X's 1, 2 or 3 relative to knowing name, location and date/time
  (4) The Glasgow Coma Score **(Slide 2-87)**
    (a) A score is given for each response with ranges from 1-6
    (b) Scores are then totaled to determine the GCS ranging from 3-15
      i) Eye opening
        i) 4 - Opened spontaneously
        ii) 3 - Opens to verbal stimuli
        iii) 2 - Opens to painful stimuli
        iv) 1 - Does not open
      ii) Verbal response **(Slide 2-88)**
        i) 5 - Alert and oriented
        ii) 4 - Confused
        iii) 3 - Inappropriate [confused] cannot maintain continuous conversation
        iv) 2 - Moans incomprehensibly
        v) 1 - No response

Content

iii) Motor response **(Slide 2-89)**
i) 6 - Obeys commands
ii) 5 - Localizes to pain
iii) 4 - Withdraws from pain
iv) 3 - Abnormal flexion **(Slide 2-90)**
v) 2 - Abnormal extension
vi) 1 - No response

(5) The Glasgow should be noted early and repeated as circumstances permit

(6) Specific responses should be **(Slide 2-91)** described in history and total score

f) Examination of the head

(1) Observe and palpate for cuts, **(Slide 2-92)** bruises, swelling and deformity **(Slide 2-93)**

(2) Observe facial area for signs of **(Slide 2-94)** wounds or fractures

(3) Note secretions from the nose or **(Slide 2-95)**

(4) Gentle palpation to avoid further injury

(5) Specific signs to be noted include "Battle's signs" and "raccoon's eyes" **(Slide 2-96)**

(6) The oral cavity should be **(Slide 2-97)** inspected for foreign bodies or fluid

(7) Pupils should be inspected for **(Slide 2-97)** diameter, reactivity and equality

(a) Can be expressed as pinpointed, midpositional or dilated

(b) Specific diameter may be **(Slide 2-98)** expressed in millimeters

g) Examination of the neck **(Slide 2-99)**

(1) Examined circumstantially for **(Slide 2-100)** wounds and signs of fractures to the spine

(2) Observe accessory muscles **(Slide 2-101)** [respiratory distress]

(3) Observe neck veins for distension

(4) Palpate larynx and trachea for fractures or deviation from midline

(5) Note subcutaneous emphysema [air beneath the skin] evidenced by crepitus

h) Chest examination

(1) Examine thorax anterior, **(Slide 2-102)** posterior and lateral **(Slide 2-103)**

(2) Seal open wounds with an airtight dressing

(3) Note symmetrical expansion and paradoxical breathing

Content

(4) Auscultate breath sounds
(5) Observe for abnormal shape of thorax (i.e. barrel chested)

i) Abdominal examination
(1) Observe for wounds, contusions **(Slide 2-104)** and abdominal distension
(2) Perform gentle palpation and **(Slide 2-105)** note tenderness, rigidity and pulsatile masses
(3) Palpate away from the area of pain first

j) Examination of the pelvic girdle **(Slide 2-106)**
(1) Gently compress on iliac **(Slide 2-107)** crests toward midline and the pubic **(Slide 2-108)** symphysis
(2) Observe for wounds and contusions circumstantially
(3) Check for sacral edema

k) Check back if circumstances permit **(Slide 2-109)**

l) Extremity examination **(Slide 2-110)**
(1) Check for ankle edema **(Slide 2-111)**
(2) Check distal pulses
(a) Dorsalis pedis **(Slide 2-112)**
(b) Posterior tibial **(Slide 2-113)**
(c) Disparity of pulses
(3) Capillary refill **(Slide 2-114)**
(4) Neurological exam
(a) Sensory **(Slide 2-115)**
i) Lower extremities
ii) Upper extremities **(Slide 2-116)**
(b) Motor **(Slide 2-117)**
i) Lower extremities
ii) Upper extremities **(Slide 2-118)**
(c) Dermatome chart **(Slide 2-119)**

F. Presenting your history **(Slide 2-120)**
1. Primary survey
2. Chief complaint
3. History of present illness
4. Past medical history
5. Medications and allergies
6. Vital signs
7. Physical exam finding
8. Treatment
9. Changes in the patient status

X. Summary **(Slide 2-121)**
A. Foundation of all decisions
B. Systematic approach is essential
C. Prioritize treatment
D. Transport decision
E. Continue assessment enroute
F. Assure a comprehensive survey
G. Practice to master techniques

ANATOMY AND PHYSIOLOGY AND PATIENT ASSESSMENT

Examination

1. The term that describes "toward the center of the body" is:

    a. lateral
    b. proximal
    c. medial
    d. abduction

2. The term that describes "lying face down" is:

    a. supine
    b. prone
    c. recumbent
    d. Fowler's

3. The study of <u>processes and activities</u> of living organisms is called:

    a. anatomy
    b. physics
    c. biology
    d. physiology

4. Arms extended, and palms and head facing forward, describes the ____________________ position.

    a. decerebrate
    b. normal anatomical
    c. flexed
    d. decorticate

5. The human body has _______ spinal vertebrae:

    a. 30
    b. 33
    c. 36
    d. 39

6. There are ___ cervical vertebrae.

    a. 4
    b. 5
    c. 7
    d. 12

7. All of the following structures are located in the mediastinum <u>except the</u>:

   a. heart
   b. esophagus
   c. lungs
   d. great vessels

8. The pelvic girdle is made up of all of the following bones, <u>except the</u>:

   a. ilium
   b. ischium
   c. pubis
   d. pons

9. Two intersecting lines that meet at the umbilicus form the:

   a. level of the diaphragm
   b. abdominal quadrants
   c. left and right flank
   d. pelvic girdle

10. Voluntary or skeletal muscles are responsible for:

   a. movement of the arms
   b. pumping of blood
   c. digestion
   d. reflexes

11. Involuntary or smooth muscles are responsible for:

   a. movement of the arms
   b. pumping of blood
   c. digestion
   d. eye movement

12. Cardiac muscle is responsible for:

   a. movement of the arms
   b. pumping of blood
   c. digestion
   d. reflexes

13. The epiglottis is responsible for:

   a. producing sound
   b. protecting the esophagus from gastric distention
   c. preventing aspiration of food and other materials into the airway
   d. production of surfactant

14. The passageway for air from the larynx to the bronchi is called the:

    a. esophagus
    b. alveolar duct
    c. bronchioles
    d. trachea

15. The air sacs in the lungs where the exchange of oxygen from the lungs to the blood occurs are called:

    a. bronchioles
    b. alveoli
    c. trachea
    d. papules

16. The functions of the nose, nasopharynx, and oropharynx are all of the following except:

    a. filter the air
    b. moisten the air
    c. regulate ventilation
    d. warm the air

17. The "pumping" chambers of the heart that pump blood to the lungs and rest of the body are called:

    a. septums
    b. sinuses
    c. atria
    d. ventricles

18. The major vein that receives blood from the body or systemic circulation is called the:

    a. aorta
    b. pulmonary vein
    c. coronary vein
    d. vena cava

19. The capillary level is where:

    a. oxygen passes from the blood cells and plasma to the tissue cells
    b. carbon dioxide passes from the blood cells and plasma to the tissue cells
    c. blood under high pressure leaves the left ventricle
    d. blood under low pressure enters the right atrium

20. The white blood cells are responsible for:

    a. plasma production
    b. carrying oxygen
    c. combating infection
    d. clotting

21. Hemoglobin is responsible for the:

    a. transport of oxygen and carbon dioxide
    b. clotting of blood
    c. combating of infection
    d. maintenance of body temperature

22. The spinal cord is part of the:

    a. peripheral nervous system
    b. caudal nervous system
    c. central nervous system
    d. posterior nervous system

23. The body system concerned with all nutritional intake except for oxygen is called the:

    a. digestive system
    b. circulatory system
    c. endocrine system
    d. lymphatic system

24. The organ responsible for the storage and secretion of bile to aid in fat absorption is the:

    a. kidney
    b. gallbladder
    c. pancreas
    d. spleen

25. The part of the digestive tract, where <u>absorption</u> of excess water occurs is called the:

    a. esophagus
    b. liver
    c. large intestine
    d. rectum

26. The part of the urinary system which filters the blood and reabsorbs essential ingredients while excreting excesses and waste products is called the:

    a. ureter
    b. urethra
    c. kidney
    d. urinary bladder

27. The respiratory, circulatory and nervous system are dependent upon one another to maintain vital functions. Which of the following reasons best explains why a patient experiences cardiac arrest following prolonged respiratory arrest:

 a. hypoxia to the heart
 b. toxicity of blood
 c. damage to the cerebrum
 b. loss of voluntary breathing control

28. Biological death is defined as:

 a. lack of oxygen blood flow to the brain as evidenced by no pulse and no respirations
 b. sustained oxygen deprivation after which recovery without brain damage is unlikely
 c. biological death of the heart
 d. sudden cardiac death

29. The evaluation of the mechanism of injury is part of the:

 a. primary survey
 b. dispatch review
 c. secondary survey
 d. scene survey

30. The "D" of the primary survey relates to the evaluation of the:

 a. heart
 b. central nervous system
 c. respiratory system
 d. digestive system

31. Determining the adequacy of breathing, evaluating the pupils, and determining the patients AVPU status are all components of the:

 a. Primary survey
 b. Scene survey
 c. Secondary survey
 d. Dispatch review

32. You arrive at the scene of a patient struck by a car. The patient is lying on his left side. After establishing <u>unresponsiveness</u> you should:

 a. Logroll the patient in the supine position and continue with your survey
 b. Leave the patient in the prone position and transport immediately
 c. Leave the patient in the prone position and continue with your survey
 d. Logroll the patient in the lateral recumbent position and continue with your survey

33. Placing both thumbs on the patient's maxilla and your index and middle fingers on both sides of the mandible where it angles toward the ear and applying upward pressure with your fingers best describes the:

 a. jaw thrust-without head tilt
 b. chin pull maneuver
 c. head tilt-neck lift
 d. head tilt-chin lift

34. Observing the chest rise is:

 a. a poor indication of the adequacy of ventilation
 b. useful for evaluating ventilation if used in conjunction with a mirror
 c. an excellent method for evaluating the adequacy of ventilation
 d. an indication that the patient is perfusing properly

35. Checking a peripheral pulse and looking for arterial bleeding are all part of the _______________ assessment within the primary survey

 a. circulatory
 b. neurological
 c. respiratory
 d. secondary

36. The groove between the trachea and muscle in the neck is the correct location for palpating the ___________ pulse.

 a. cerebral
 b. popliteal
 c. carotid
 d. cervical

37. Compressing the patient's nail surface with your finger and then releasing the pressure best describes the method for:

 a. checking capillary refill
 b. providing painful stimuli to the patient
 c. checking for sensation in the upper extremities
 d. ensuring a full range of motion in the injured extremity

38. The presence of a femoral pulse suggests a minimum systolic blood pressure of:

 a. 50
 b. 60
 c. 70
 d. 90

39. The presence of a radial pulse suggests a minimum systolic blood pressure of:

    a. 50
    b. 60
    c. 70
    d. 80

40. The "P" of the AVPU evaluation of mental state refers to a patient's ability to respond to:

    a. pupillary stimulation with a penlight
    b. psychological stimulation
    c. painful stimulation
    d. positive pressure ventilation

41. When taking a medical history all of the following are general principles to maximize the validity and reliability of information gathered <u>except</u>:

    a. use open ended questions
    b. direct the interview to avoid unnecessary information
    c. obtain a complete history prior to initiating any care
    d. do not allow bystanders to answer for the patient

42. The patient tells you that his head hurts and that he is dizzy. This is called the patient's:

    a. history of present illness
    b. primary problem
    c. primary complaint
    d. chief complaint

43. The patient tells you that he was shoveling snow when his chest pain began. He goes on to say that the pain is in the middle of his chest, radiates to his left arm and was not relieved by taking two nitroglycerine tablets. The second part of his information is an example of the:

    a. history of present illness
    b. past medical history
    c. primary survey
    d. chief complaint

44. The four major diseases (The Big Four) that are routinely inquired about during the past medical history with older adult patients include all of the following <u>except</u>:

    a. high blood pressure
    b. stroke
    c. diabetes
    d. chronic obstructive pulmonary disease (COPD)

45. The normal range of respiratory rate in the adult is approximately:

    a. 5-15
    b. 10-15
    c. 12-20
    d. 15-25

46. A high pitched whistling sound created by narrowed bronchioles best describes:

    a. gurgling
    b. snoring
    c. wheezing
    d. stridor

47. A sound created by air moving through fluid in the upper airway best describes:

    a. gurgling
    b. snoring
    c. wheezing
    d. stridor

48. Stridor is caused by:

    a. obstruction by the tongue
    b. fluid in the airway
    c. a narrowed lower airway
    d. a narrowed upper airway

49. Snoring is commonly caused by:

    a. obstruction by the tongue
    b. fluid in the airway
    c. a narrowed lower airway
    d. a narrowed trachea

50. The radial artery is:

    a. monitored to ensure adequate CPR compressions
    b. the easiest pulse to monitor in patients suffering from shock
    c. located in the wrist on the pinky side of the hand
    d. utilized to monitor the rate, regularity and quality of the pulse

51. The normal range of pulse rate for an adult at rest is approximately _____ per minute.

    a. 40-60
    b. 50-70
    c. 60-80
    d. 80-100

52. The amount of blood ejected from the heart each minute and the space within the arteries determines:

    a. stroke volume
    b. cardiac output
    c. pulse pressure
    d. blood pressure

53. All of the following may alter the blood pressure <u>except</u>:

    a. changes in heart function
    b. blood vessel diameter
    c. ratio of white to red blood cells
    d. total blood volume

54. Blood pressure determined by feeling a radial or brachial pulse during cuff deflation is called blood pressure by:

    a. auscultation
    b. palpation
    c. oscillation
    d. vibration

55. The point when the sounds disappear or significantly diminish in volume when listening for a blood pressure that reflects the relaxation phase of the heart is called the __________ pressure.

    a. diastolic
    d. systolic
    c. pulse
    d. contractile

56. A disadvantage of a blood pressure taken by palpation is that you can only obtain the ______________________ pressure.

    a. pulse
    d. systolic
    c. diastolic
    d. contractile

57. A patient who was struck by a car does not open his eyes, does not move in response to pain, and emits no sound has a score on the Glasgow Coma Scale of:

    a. 1
    b. 3
    c. 5
    d. 7

58. All of the following are signs of a potential skull fracture <u>except</u>:

    a. raccoon's eyes
    b. Battle's sign
    c. subcutaneous emphysema
    d. blood and/or CSF from the nose

59. The four techniques utilized during the head to toe survey are:

    a. observe, listen, palpate and question
    b. observe, listen, palpate and smell
    c. palpate, listen, measure and question
    d. palpate, measure, listen and smell

60. Subcutaneous emphysema is defined as:

    a. air beneath the skin that is characterized by a "crackling sensation" during palpation
    b. air in the pleural space compressing against one or both lungs producing progressively increased difficulty in breathing
    c. fluid beneath the skin, generally resembling a purplish bruise, caused by blunt trauma
    d. fluid in the pleural space compressing against one or both lungs producing progressively increased difficulty in breathing

61. The structure that can be palpated midline just above the suprasternal notch is called the:

    a. esophagus
    b. pharynx
    c. glottis
    d. trachea

62. An airtight dressing should be used to cover:

    a. an impaled object in the thigh whether or not there are signs of vascular compromise
    b. either eye if the patient has suffered a chemical burn to the eye
    c. an open wound to the chest
    d. an open wound to the abdomen

63. Paradoxical breathing is characterized by:

    a. the use of accessory muscles in the neck for ventilation
    b. the rhythmic pattern of gradually increasing and then decreasing rates of respiration
    c. a shift of the trachea away from the injured side of the thorax
    d. sections of the chest wall moving in the opposite direction of the rest of the thorax during ventilation

64. Decreased movement on one side of the chest suggestive of underlying chest injury is called:

a. splinting
b. immobilization
c. paradoxical breathing
d. Cheyne-Stokes breathing

65. Examination of the abdomen should begin with:

a. palpation
b. auscultation
c. observation
d. measurement

66. The bone of the pelvis that is palpated in the pubic region is the:

a. ilium
b. pubis
c. femur
d. ischium

67. The pulse located halfway between the iliac crest and the pubic symphysis is the ______________ pulse.

a. umbilical
b. femoral
c. pubic
d. popliteal

68. The tibia can be palpated on the:

a. anterior surface of the lower leg
b. anterior surface of the upper leg
c. posterior surface of the lower leg
d. posterior surface of the upper leg

69. A patient with paralysis of the upper and lower extremities has most likely injured his or her:

a. cervical spine
b. cerebrum
c. lumbar spine
d. brain stem

70. Inflammation of the meninges due to meningitis is suggested by the presence of:

a. neck stiffness
b. one sided paralysis
c. sensory loss in the lower extremities
d. pinpointed pupils

Skill Performance Sheet

Patient Assessment

Student's Name ______________________________ Date __________

Performance Standard	Perform	Failed
PRIMARY SURVEY		
One EMT maintains in-line immobilization (if trauma patient)		
Checks responsiveness		
Opens airway with appropriate maneuver (head tilt-chin lift or jaw thrust)		
Corrects problems with airway i.e. suction		
Checks adequacy of breathing		
Corrects problems with breathing i.e. positive pressure ventilation		
Checks pulse and adequacy of circulation		
Corrects problems with circulation i.e. bleeding control		
Evaluates disability (AVPU, pupils motor and sensory)		
Exposes (removes clothing)		
SECONDARY SURVEY		
Checks radial pulse		
Takes blood pressure		
Checks respiratory rate		
Checks skin color and moisture		

CONTINUED ON NEXT PAGE

Chapter 2

Skill Performance Sheet

Patient Assessment (continued)

Performance Standard	Perform	Failed
HISTORY		
Chief complaint		
History of present illness		
Past medical history		
Medications		
Allergies		
HEAD TO TOE SURVEY (Observes, Palpates, Listens)		
Head (scalp, face, pupils, ears, nose mouth, Battle's sign)		
Neck (vertebrae, trachea, neck veins, soft tissues)		
Chest (anterior, lateral, posterior)		
Breath sounds		
Abdomen (anterior, lateral, posterior)		
Pelvis (medial, posterior and pubic symphysis palpation)		
Buttocks		
Extremities		

Comments ____

____

____

____

Instructor ________________ Circle One: Pass Fail

Chapter 3

RESPIRATORY EMERGENCIES

Materials and Equipment for Lesson

1. Anatomy slides, overhead transparencies, drawings or flipcharts
2. Bottle with balloon to demonstrate negative pressure
3. Spirometer to demonstrate respiratory volumes available
4. Handouts
   - Anatomy and physiology
   - Patient assessment
   - Breath sounds
   - Airway obstruction
   - Specific respiratory emergencies
   - Performance sheets for respiratory skills
5. Slide projector, overhead projector, flipchart and/or blackboard
6. Slides or transparencies
7. Breath sound tape
8. Tape recorder
9. Male subject for respiratory assessment
10. CPR manikin with lights or other indicator
11. Airway, ventilation and oxygen equipment

Section 1

Anatomy and Physiology

Objectives
(Slide 3-1)

At the conclusion of the chapter the student will be able to:

1. **State the significance of oxygen to body tissues, particularly the brain.**
2. **Given an anatomy diagram, label the major structures of the respiratory system.**
3. **Given a respiratory structure, define its function.**
4. **Define diffusion.**
5. **Define the following respiratory volumes:**
   - **Tidal volume**
   - **Minute volume**
   - **Residual volume**
   - **Vital capacity**
   - **Total lung capacity**

Instructor Preparation

Reading preparation for the lesson:

EMT Prehospital Care, Chapter 3, pages 81-94
Local respiratory protocols
Performance sheets for respiratory skills

Optional reading:

Guyton, A.C.: Textbook of Medical Physiology. 8th Edition, W.B. Saunders. Philadelphia, PA. 1991

Solomon, E.P., Phillips G.A.: Understanding Human Anatomy and Physiology. W.B. Saunders. Philadelphia, PA, 1987

Suggested Learning Activities

Using a lecture format with the aid of slides, overhead transparencies or charts, provide an overview of respiratory system anatomy and physiology.

Using a balloon in a bottle illustrate the concept of "relative negative pressure" with the pleural space.

Have the student breathe into a spirometer to measure his or her own respiratory volumes (if available).

Content

I. Introduction
- A. Overview **(Slide 3-2)**
    - 1. Humans are oxygen dependent
        - a) Cells will die without oxygen
        - b) Brain cells will die within 4-6 minutes
        - c) Three systems most involved in 0_2 delivery
            - (1) Respiratory
            - (2) Cardiovascular
            - (3) Central nervous system
    - 2. Heart-Lung-Brain relationship **(Slide 3-3)**
        - a) Each system depends on the other to survive
            - (1) Lungs deliver oxygen
            - (2) Heart circulates oxygen
            - (3) Brain regulates both
        - b) Emphasize importance of management of these systems in prehospital care (ABC's)
            - (1) A - Airway
            - (2) B - Breathing
            - (3) C - Circulation
            - (4) ABC's directed toward assuring brain viability

II. Anatomy and Physiology
- A. Respiration **(Slide 3-4)**
    - 1. Define - uptake and delivery of 0_2 to cells
    - 2. Four phases of respiration
        - a) Ventilation - Delivery of air from atmosphere to the alveoli
        - b) Diffusion - Movement of gases from the alveoli to the blood and the blood to the tissues
        - c) Transport - The delivery of oxygen and removal of carbon dioxide in blood via hemoglobin
        - d) Regulation - The control of respiration based on the needs of the cells through the brain stem
- B. Overview of respiratory function **(Slide 3-5)**
    - 1. Delivery of oxygen
    - 2. Removal of carbon dioxide
    - 3. Voice
    - 4. Function dependent on working parts
        - a) Airways
        - b) Clear alveoli
        - c) Respiratory nerves and muscles
        - d) Brain
- C. Airway (Upper) **(Slide 3-6)**
    - 1. A series of "tubes" which lead to alveoli
    - 2. Must retain adequate diameter for effectiveness
    - 3. Nasal passage **(Slide 3-7)**
        - a) External and internal nose
        - b) Nares
        - c) Cartilage and bone

Content

d) Nasal septum - two separate compartments
e) Functions: filtering, warming, moisturizing air and smell
f) Injuries can compress patency of airway
g) Bleeding can cause airway blockage

4. Pharynx
   a) Nasal, oral laryngeal
   b) Can obstruct with tongue or anaphylaxis
   c) Emphasize importance of airway maneuvers
   d) Explain gag reflex
5. Larynx (voice Box) **(Slide 3-8)**
   a) Formed by cartilage, bone and ligament
   b) Contains vocal cords **(Slide 3-9)**
   c) Functions: protects airway, voice
   d) Thyroid, cricoid cartilage, border cricothyroid
   e) Explain cricothyroidotomy **(Slide 3-10)**
   f) Explain how vocal cords "spasm"
   g) Dry drowning example of laryngospasm
6. Epiglottis
   a) Cartilaginous fluid
   b) Extends up from anterior larynx
   c) Swallowing mechanism
   d) Protects airway
   e) Epiglottitis can lead to complete obstruction
7. Trachea **(Slide 3-11)**
   a) Horseshoe -shaped rings
   b) Muscular posterior wall
   c) Strong but flexible; permits food passage and neck movement
   d) Tracheostomy is a common surgical intervention for obstruction
   e) Carina - dividing point
   f) Palpate your own tracheal rings
8. Bronchi **(Slide 3-12)**
   a) Main stem bronchi
      (1) First Division
      (2) Cartilage and muscle
      (3) Left is at greater angle to trachea
      (4) Objects tend to lodge in right main stem
   b) Bronchi and bronchioles
      (1) Subdivide and become less cartilaginous
      (2) Fifteenth division loses cartilage and are muscular bronchioles
      (3) Bronchiole can change diameter - main component of bronchial asthma
      (4) Aminophylline and adrenalin are bronchodilators

D. Alveoli **(Slide 3-13)**
1. Microscopic air sacs where gas exchange takes place
2. One cell thick which permits gas exchange
3. Interface with microscopic vessels (capillaries)
4. Function is dependent upon surface area
   a) 50 sq meters normal alveolar surface

Content

E. Surfactant **(Slide 3-14)**
  1. Contributes to elasticity of lung
  2. Surface tension property
  3. Give soap bubble analogy
    a) Smaller bubbles - increased strength
    b) Prevents atelectasis
  4. Premature babies have atelectasis due to surfactant deficiencies
  5. Drowning victims also suffer from loss of surfactant

F. Mucous membrane **(Slide 3-15)**
  1. Provides filtering, warming and moisture to inhaled air
  2. Consists of mucous cells which produce mucus
  3. Cilia are hair - like projections
    a) Push particles up toward the pharynx to be swallowed
    b) Can be destroyed by cigarette smoking and other pollutants
  4. Excessive mucus production results in sputum
    a) Caused by irritation, such as smoke inhalation
    b) Results in productive cough
  5. Also provides moisture for dry incoming air (give example of breath in cold weather)
  6. Warms air to maintain core temperature

G. Lungs, thorax, and muscles
  1. Lungs **(Slide 3-16)**
    a) Bronchi, bronchioles, alveoli form lungs
    b) Two cone -shaped organs in each side of chest
    c) Two lobes on left, three lobes on right
    d) Lobes or lungs may be removed due to disease
      (1) Only small amount of lung is needed to survive
      (2) Lobes may removed due to cancer
    e) Lungs are suspended in chest cavity and are only attached at hilum
    f) Mediastinum
      (1) Separates right and left pleural space
      (2) Contains heart, great vessels, esophagus, trachea, nerves
    g) Chest cavity
      (1) Anterior - sternum, ribs, muscles
      (2) Posterior - spine, scapula, muscles, ribs
      (3) Superior - clavicle, neck
      (4) Inferior - diaphragm (primary muscle of respiration)
  2. Pleura
    a) Line chest cavity - parietal pleura
    b) Line lung - visceral pleura
    c) Pleural space in between contains fluid to reduce friction
    d) Inflammation, pleurisy, results in pleuritic pain
  3. Negative pressure **(Slide 3-17)**
    a) Lungs stay expanded by negative pressure (less than atmospheric pressure)
    b) Lungs have natural tendency to collapse
    c) Give balloon in bottle example (see text)
    d) Pneumothorax disturbs relationship; lungs collapse due to elasticity

Content

H. Muscles of breathing **(Slide 3-18)**
1. Cause chest movement that results in air exchange (bellows effect)
2. Quiet breathing involves two muscles:
    a) The diaphragm is dome-shaped muscle which separates chest and abdomen, responsible for two-thirds of quiet breathing
    b) External intercostals between ribs, responsible for one third of quiet breathing
3. Inspiration (quiet)
    a) Diaphragm flattens, increases inferior-superior diameter of chest
    b) External intercostals pull ribs up, increase anterior-posterior, lateral dimensions
    c) Increase in size - more volume, less gas, decrease in pressure, air rushes in
    d) Inspiration continues until pressure between lung and atmosphere equalizes, end of inspiration
4. Expiration (quiet)
    a) Elastic recoil of lungs plus muscle relaxation
    b) Passive process
    c) Chest cavity decreases in size = less volume, more gas, air rushes out to atmosphere
    d) Expiration continues until atmosphere and chest pressure are equal
    e) End of expiration
5. Accessory muscles **(Slide 3-19)**
    a) Intercostals and diaphragm enough for quiet breathing. Accessories needed for forceful breathing.
    b) Accessory muscles of inspiration: increase the size of chest cavity by lifting rib cage and increasing diameter
    c) Inspiratory muscles: scalene, sternocleidomastoids, parasternal
    d) Accessory muscles of expiration; assist in evacuating trapped air
    e) They pull down on ribs and compress abdominal contents into diaphragm
    f) Expiratory muscles; internal intercostals and abdominal muscles
    g) Active accessories indicate respiratory distress, signs include bulging neck muscles, retraction between ribs, abdominal distension
6. Physiology **(Slide 3-20)**
    a) Respiratory volumes
        (1) Parameters to quantify respiration function
        (2) Measured by special in-hospital equipment but important to EMT's in understanding function
        (3) Define and explain the following parameters:
            (a) Tidal volume - Amount of air taken with each breath
            (b) Minute volume - Tidal volume x Respiratory rate
            (c) Residual volume - Amount of air remaining in the lung after a forceful exhalation
            (d) Vital capacity - Maximum amount of air that can be exhaled after a maximum inhalation

Content

(e) Total lung capacity - Amount of air in the lungs after a maximum inhalation
(4) Describe factors about values
(a) C.O.P.D. - increases residual volume
(b) Minute volume - decreased in respiratory failure
b) Nervous system regulation of breathing **(Slide 3-21)**
(1) The body has a "thermostat" that monitors respiratory function
(2) Messages are sent to the muscles
(3) Unconscious controls regulate breathing most of the time
(a) Consist of regulators, connecting sensors with a feedback mechanism
(b) Respiratory centers in the pons and medulla
(c) Receptors in carotid arteries, aorta and brain
i) Aorta and carotid arteries monitor oxygen and carbon dioxide levels
ii) Brain receptors monitor the pH of the fluid surrounding the brain
(d) Carbon dioxide is the main stimulus to breath
(4) Conscious controls permit us to slow down, speed up, increase and decrease breathing at will **(Slide 3-22)**
(a) Conscious stimulus arises from the higher brain centers in the frontal lobe
(b) Communicate through the unconscious control centers
(c) Conscious controls may alter assessment of respiratory rate
(5) Review sequence of regulation with class
c) Special considerations during oxygen therapy **(Slide 3-23)**
(1) Patients exposed to high CO_2 over a long period (COPD) causes changes in neuroreceptors
(2) Become insensitive to increases in CO_2
(3) Switch over to hypoxic drive
(a) Low O_2 will become the dominant force
(b) Excessive oxygen administration may result in loss of stimulation: Respiratory arrest
(c) When treating C.O.P.D. patients, oxygen must be administered with caution
d) Diffusion **(Slide 3-24)**
(1) Definition - the movement of gases or particles from an area of higher concentration to an area of lower concentration
(2) The primary force contributing to gas exchange
(a) In the lungs oxygen is in higher concentration in the alveoli and moves toward blood
(b) Carbon dioxide is higher in the blood and moves toward alveoli
(c) At the tissues the reverse is true
(3) Diffusion can be impaired by fluids or other obstructions in the alveoli

Section 2

Patient Assessment

Objectives
(Slide 3-25)

At the conclusion of the chapter the student will be able to:

1. **List four signs of respiratory distress.**
2. **State three mental state changes that may occur with hypoxia.**
3. **Define the following signs and symptoms:**

Hemoptysis	**Retractions**
Cyanosis	**Paradoxical breathing**
Hypoventilation	**Subcutaneous emphysema**
Hyperventilation	**Tracheal shift**
Tachypnea	

4. **Describe the normal character and locations of the following breath sounds:**
   - **Tracheal**
   - **Bronchial**
   - **Bronchovesicular**
   - **Vesicular**
5. **Given a tape recording, identify the following adventitious breath sounds and list one possible cause:**
   - **Crackles (rales)**
   - **Rhonchi**
   - **Wheezes**
   - **Friction rubs**
   - **Stridor**

Instructor Preparation

Reading preparation for the lesson:

EMT Prehospital Care, Chapter 3, pages 94-100
Review breath sound tape

Optional reading:

Bates, B.: A Pocket Guide to Physical Examination and History Taking. J.B. Lippincott Co. Philadelphia, PA, 1991

Schwartz, G.R., Safer, P., Stone, J.H., Storey, P.B., Wagner, D.K.: Principles and Practices of Emergency Medicine. 2nd Edition. W.B. Saunders. Philadelphia, PA, 1986

Suggested Learning Activities

Using lecture format with handouts, provide overview of respiratory assessment.

Using a male subject, demonstrate the key landmarks, breath sound locations and other respiratory signs.

Using a breath sound tape, review the common normal and adventitious breath sounds.

Content

III. Patient Assessment
- A. Dyspnea **(Slide 3-26)**
  1. Unpleasant sensation, difficulty in breathing
  2. Dyspnea is the most common symptom of respiratory failure, except related to CNS depression
  3. May be due to several factors
     - a) Increased minute volume may produce a sensation of dyspnea (i.e. during exercise)
     - b) Respiratory muscle fatigue may initiate a dyspneic response
     - c) Increased effort to initiate a breath will produce the sensation of dyspnea
     - d) Dyspnea may be precipitated by exertion or occur at rest
- B. Pleuritic chest pain **(Slide 3 -27)**
  1. Chest pain associated with movement of the chest wall
  2. Irritation to the pleura or chest wall muscles may precipitate
  3. Should inquire if pain increases with breathing
- C. Central nervous system signs **(Slide 3-28)**
  1. Mental State may change with hypoxia or dyspnea
  2. Type of alteration may be associated with the degree of hypoxia or patient perception
     - a) Agitation
     - b) Restlessness
     - c) Lethargy
     - d) Coma
  3. Pupils
     - a) Hypoxia may cause dilated or sluggishly reactive pupils
     - b) Consider other causes of pupil change
  4. Hypoxic seizures
     - a) Severe hypoxia may be heralded by an hypoxic seizure
     - b) Will usually dissipate with prolonged anoxia or restoring oxygenation
- D. Cyanosis **(Slide 3-29)**
  1. Cyanosis appears when approximately 5 gm. of hemoglobin/100ml of blood is unsaturated with oxygen
  2. Some studies have shown that lower levels are needed before cyanosis becomes evident
  3. The base of the tongue is a good site for early detection of cyanosis
- E. Hemoptysis **(Slide 3-30)**
  1. Coughing up blood
  2. May be stained sputum or frank blood
  3. May be caused by several respiratory conditions
     - a) Pulmonary edema
     - b) Pulmonary lacerations
     - c) Tracheal or bronchial injury

Content

F. Accessory muscle use **(Slide 3-31)**
   1. Muscles of inspiration include the sternocleidomastoids and scalenes (neck)
   2. Muscles of expiration are abdominal and internal intercostals
   3. Accessory muscle use is visible during forced inspiration or expiration
   4. This increased work of breathing contributes to the exhaustion of the patient

G. Ventilation
   1. Hypoventilation **(Slide 3-32)**
      a) Decreased minute volume
      b) May be caused by decreased tidal volume or decreased rate
         (1) Respiratory rate below 10 or above 30 is generally inadequate
         (2) Decreased tidal volumes are noted by shallow chest wall movement
      c) Most often caused by depression of neuro-stimulation mechanisms
   2. Hyperventilation
      a) Increased minute volume
      b) May be caused by increased tidal volume or increased rate
      c) Normal compensatory mechanism to hypoxia
   3. Tachypnea
      a) Rapid breathing
      b) Does not imply hyperventilation may be rapid but shallow

H. Respiratory muscle fatigue **(Slide 3-33)**
   1. Tachypnea represents an early sign of fatigue
   2. Abdominal paradox (abdominal muscles moving in during inspiration)
   3. Respiratory alternans (alternate use of chest and abdominal muscles)
   4. Sign of respiratory failure

I. Retractions **(Slide 3-34)**
   1. Suprasternal and intercostal retractions
   2. Increased negative intrathoracic pressure
   3. Increased work of inspiration
   4. Common sign in children

J. Inspection of the neck and chest **(Slide 3-35)**
   1. Paradoxical breathing
      a) Movement of a section of the chest wall in opposite direction during breathing
      b) May suggest a flail chest
   2. Tracheal shift
      a) Important sign of pneumothorax and tension pneumothorax
      b) Caused by increased pressure in pleural space
   3. Subcutaneous emphysema
      a) Air beneath the skin noted by "crackling" sensation on palpation
      b) May result from tracheal, bronchial or lung injury

Pulse oximetry
   Device designed to evaluate the saturation of hemoglobin
   Attached to the fingers or ear lobe
   Uses

Content

IV. Auscultation of Breath Sounds
   A. Overview **(Slide 3-36)**
      1. One of the most difficult procedures performed by the EMT
      2. Requires patience, technique, good hearing and knowledge of various sounds
      3. In order to retrieve reliable and valid information you must:
         a) Know the locations for auscultation
         b) Listen for a sufficient period of time
         c) Control for extraneous noises
         d) Be familiar with the variants in breath sounds
   B. Stick grams **(Slide 3-37)**
      1. Provide a visual presentation of breath sounds
      2. Components:
         a) Angle - the pitch of the sound
         b) Thickness of the line the relative amplitude of the sound
         c) Length - the duration of the sound
   C. Types of breath sounds
      1. There are three primary findings **(Slide 3-38)**
         a) The character of the basic sounds
            (1) Length of inspiration and expiration
            (2) Pitch of sound and the amplitude
         b) Sounds that are superimposed over the basic sounds, such as rales (crackles), wheezing, rhonchi and friction rubs
         c) Breath sounds heard in areas other than normal may suggest underlying pathophysiology
      2. Specific sounds
         a) Locations **(Slide 3-39)**
            (1) Tracheal - directly over the trachea
            (2) Bronchial - at top of sternum and between scapulas (posteriorly)
            (3) Bronchovesicular - over the upper/middle sternum and its left and right borders
            (4) Vesicular - in all other areas of the chest
         b) Tracheal **(Slide 3-40)**
            (1) Relatively loud, high pitched sounds
            (2) Have a relatively equal inspiratory and expiratory phase
            (3) A break between the inspiratory and expiratory phase
            (4) Created by turbulent flow in the trachea
         c) Bronchial **(Slide 3-41)**
            (1) Loud and high pitched
            (2) Created by turbulent flow of air in the large bronchi
         d) Bronchovesicular **(Slide 3-42)**
            (1) High pitched but a lower pitch, and softer than tracheal
            (2) A combination of air through the central airways where there is smoother flow of air
            (3) There is no break between inspiration and expiration

Content

e) Vesicular **(Slide 3-43)**
(1) The most common areas listened to by EMT's
(2) Most auscultation limited to bronchovesicular and vesicular areas
(3) Lower pitched, softer sounds
(4) Have a longer inspiratory phase
(5) Created by air flow through smaller bronchioles and alveoli

f) Abnormal and adventitious breath sounds **(Slide 3-44)**
(1) Sounds may be superimposed or change in character
(2) Types of adventitious sounds:
(a) Absent or diminished sounds
i) Collapse of a lung (pneumothorax)
ii) Blood in the chest cavity (hemothorax)
iii) COPD or asthma
iv) Obesity
v) Any cause of hypoventilation
vi) Consolidation in the on pleura or lung
vii) Comparisons should be noted by auscultating equivalent regions on each side of the chest wall
(b) Rales (crackles) **(Slide 3-45)**
i) Crackling discontinuous sounds that are
ii) Usually caused by:
i) The presence of fluid the lungs
ii) Opening of collapsed airways
iii) May occur throughout inspiratory cycle of breath sound
iv) Intensity and duration is affected by the degree of fluid build-up
i) Excessive fluid buildup = coarse, loud rales (crackles)
ii) Rales (crackles) will first appear at bases and evolve to the upper lobe due to the effects of gravity
(c) Rhonchi **(Slide 3-46)**
i) Low-pitched continuous sounds
ii) Created by obstruction in the larger airways
iii) Mucus plugs, tumors and other sources of obstruction may cause rhonchi
iv) May occur in the inspiratory or expiratory phase
(d) Wheezes **(Slide 3-47)**
i) A high-pitched continuous sound
ii) High-pitched whistling noise which may lengthen expiratory phase
iii) Occur on inspiration or expiration
iv) Result of narrowed bronchioles
v) Inspiratory phase wheezes tend to be more severe and of a greater intensity

vi) Commonly associated with asthma and COPD or other cause of bronchiole constriction
vii) Pulmonary edema may present with wheezing
i) Expiratory phase is usually not lengthened as in asthma
ii) Patient's history will help you to differentiate

(e) Friction rub **(Slide 3-48)**
i) Coarse, grating sound created by inflamed pleura rubbing against each other
ii) Described as "creaking" sound of old leather
iii) Will usually be found in painful local areas on the chest
iv) Auscultate areas of pleuritic pain to determine the presence of a friction rub

(f) Stridor **(Slide 3-49)**
i) High-pitched continuous sound arising from the upper airway
ii) Usually occurs on inspiration
iii) Caused by narrowing of the upper airway
iv) Commonly occurs in croup or epiglottitis
v) May be accompanied by a "barking" cough
vi) May be caused by foreign body or swelling of upper airway

g) Sounds in relation to problems
(1) Must evaluate the basic breath sound and adventitious sounds
(2) Examples of sounds and conditions **(Slide 3-50)**
(a) Patient with pneumonia
i) Bronchial sounds in vesicular areas
ii) Rales (crackles)
(b) Patient with pulmonary edema
i) Diminished sounds
ii) Rales (crackles)
(c) Patient with asthma
i) Diminished sounds
ii) Wheezes
(d) Pneumothorax **(Slide 3-51)**
i) Diminished or absent
ii) Compare both sides
(e) COPD
i) Diminished
ii) Bronchial sounds in vesicular areas
iii) Wheezes
iv) Prolonged expiratory phase

D. Technique for auscultation
1. Auscultate anterior, posterior and lateral aspects of chest wall **(Slide 3-52)**
2. Patient should be sitting upright when possible **(Slide 3-53)**

Content

3. May not always be possible to auscultate all areas
    a) Trauma patients can often not be moved
    b) Some patients cannot tolerate the sitting position
4. Diaphragm portion of stethoscope should be placed firmly on chest wall
5. Avoid extraneous noise
    a) Chest hair can be moisturized to reduce noise
    b) Keep stethoscope tube from touching objects
    c) Quiet the scene when possible
6. Avoid a prolonged examination of the chest **(Slide 3-54)**
    a) May not be necessary to establish a "working diagnosis"
    b) May contribute negatively to patient care by extending time
7. Have the patient open his mouth and take deep breaths
    a) In confused patients, demonstrate the desired breathing pattern
    b) Patient should breath faster than usual respiratory rate
    c) Be careful not to allow your patient to hyperventilate
        (1) Dizziness, tingling or a feeling of faintness signal hyperventilation
        (2) Patient should rest before further auscultation
8. Listen carefully at each location and note abnormalities
    a) One breath cycle at each location is usually enough
    b) Vague abnormality you should listen longer to clarify your findings

E. Switch to audio cassette to sample actual breath sounds

F. Summary **(Slide 3-55)**

1. Breath sounds are essential diagnostic skill to prehospital personnel
2. Positive findings may provide the basis for critical patient decisions
3. Effective technique includes several factors
    a) Preparing the environment by controlling for extraneous noise
    b) Programming the patient to breath properly during auscultation
    c) Listening at the correct locations
    d) Being familiar with the various normal and abnormal findings
    e) Evaluating your findings in the context of the entire assessment
    f) Reporting your findings clearly to in-hospital personnel
4. To become effective at auscultation of breath sounds, you must:
    a) Exercise the principles of effective technique
    b) Validate your findings with a physician, nurse or clinical EMT instructor
    c) Tapes are an excellent source of learning
    d) Listen to breath sounds of friends and family members to acquire your listening skill

Chapter 3

Section 3

Airway, Ventilation and Oxygen Therapy

Objectives
(Slide 3-56)

At the conclusion of the chapter the student will be able to:

1. Describe two infection control measures that should be used during the performance of airway and ventilation.

2. Demonstrate the following airway maneuvers on a training manikin:
- **head tilt-chin lift**
- **jaw thrust without head tilt**
- **chin pull**

3. Demonstrate the following airway techniques on a manikin:
- **oropharyngeal airway**
- **nasopharyngeal airway**
- **esophageal gastric tube airway (optional)**
- **endotracheal intubation (optional)**

4. Demonstrate the following positive pressure ventilation techniques on a manikin, achieving a minimum tidal volume of 800 mls and a maximum tidal volume of 1200 ml.
- **mouth to mouth**
- **pocket mask**
- **bag valve mask**
- **manually triggered demand valve resuscitator**

5. Demonstrate the assembly and disassembly of an oxygen cylinder regulator.

6. List the delivered oxygen percentages for the following administration devices:
- **nasal cannula**
- **nonrebreather**
- **simple face mask**
- **Venturi mask**

Instructor Preparation

Reading preparation for the lesson:

EMT Prehospital Care, Chapter 3, pages 100-127

Optional reading:

American Heart Association: Standards and Guidelines for Cardiopulmonary Resuscitation and Emergency Cardiac Care. JAMA 255(21):2841-3044. June 1986

Roberts, J.R., Hedges, J.R.: Clinical Procedures in Emergency Medicine. W.B. Saunders. Philadelphia, PA, 1985

Suggested Learning Activities
Using lecture format with handouts, provide overview of airway, ventilation and oxygen therapy. **Using a manikin, demonstrate the use of the various airway, ventilation and oxygen devices.**

Content

V. Airway, Ventilation and Oxygen Therapy **(Slide 3-57)**
A. The primary management in all emergencies includes three essential steps
1. Establish and maintain a patent airway
2. Assure adequate ventilation
3. Assure adequate oxygenation
B. Airway management
1. Overview
a) Includes both manual and mechanical methods
b) Gloves and goggles should be worn during airway maintenance to avoid splash
c) Advanced airway skills
(1) Prevent aspiration of secretions into the lungs
(2) Allow direct access to the tracheal-bronchial tree for suctioning
(3) Reduce chances for gastric distension
2. Manual methods **(Slide 3-58)**
a) Lift the tongue away from the pharynx
b) Head tilt-chin lift is the most effective manual procedure **(Slide 3-59)**
(1) Hyperextending the head while lifting the jaw
(2) Teeth should be almost touching but the mouth should not be closed
c) Jaw thrust-without head tilt should be used in suspected spinal injury **(Slide 3-60)**
(1) Fingers lift the jaw from behind the mandible
(2) Thumbs provide counter pressure on the maxilla
d) Chin pull is utilized during airway obstruction procedures or to displace a fractured or dislocated mandible
(1) The thumb grasps the lower jaw and tongue
(2) Jaw is pulled anterior
(3) Use caution in semi-responsive patients
3. Mechanical airway techniques
a) Oropharyngeal airway **(Slide 3-61)**
(1) Displaces the tongue away from pharynx
(2) May be used in unconscious patients to maintain an open airway
(3) Should never be used in patient with gag reflex
(4) Insertion may result in tongue being pushed into airway
(5) Proper technique avoids this complication
(6) Insertion techniques
(a) Measure the airway center of mouth to angle of the jaw **(Slide 3-62)**
(b) Grasp jaw with chin pull procedure **(Slide 3-63)**
(c) Place airway initially with point toward roof of mouth **(Slide 3-64)**
(d) Rotate airway into pharynx when safely past tongue **(Slide 3-65)**
(e) May also be inserted using tongue blade to secure tongue **(Slide 3-66)**

Content

b) Nasopharyngeal airway **(Slide 3-67)**
- (1) Serves same purpose as oropharyngeal airway
- (2) Less likely to produce gag reflex
- (3) Can be used when oral access is not possible
- (4) May result in nasopharyngeal bleeding
- (5) Proper technique reduces chances of bleeding
- (6) Insertion technique
    - (a) Lubricate the airway prior to insertion **(Slide 3-68)**
    - (b) Listen to air exchange in each nostril to determine best access route
    - (c) Most quiet nostril is best choice
    - (d) Tilt back tip of nostril **(Slide 3-69)**
    - (e) Gently advance airway following the normal anatomical curvature **(Slide 3-70)**
    - (f) Do not force the airway
    - (g) If obstruction is encountered, try other nostril

c) Esophageal Gastric Tube Airway (EGTA) **(Slide 3-71)**
- (1) Gastric tube prevents aspiration and directs airflow into trachea
- (2) Allows access to esophagus for suctioning
- (3) Can be inserted with head in neutral position in suspected spinal injury
- (4) Certain contraindications must be observed **(Slide 3-72)**
    - (a) Should not be used in persons less than 5' or more than 7' tall
    - (b) Should not be used in caustic ingestions
    - (c) Should not be used in responsive patients
    - (d) Should not be used in patients with known esophageal disease
- (5) Insertion technique
    - (a) Ventilate with other methods prior to insertion
    - (b) Lift the jaw with the head in the neutral or flexed position **(Slide 3-73)**
    - (c) Insert the device along the natural curvature of the airway **(Slide 3-74)**
    - (d) Attempt to ventilate and confirm placement with stethoscope **(Slide 3-75)**
    - (e) Inflate cuff with 30 ml of air **(Slide 3-76)**
    - (f) Recheck placement
- (6) Removal technique
    - (a) Ideally should have endotracheal tube inserted prior to removal
    - (b) Suction should be at the ready and the head turned to the side **(Slide 3-77)**
    - (c) Deflate cuff and remove device

Content

d) Endotracheal intubation **(Slide 3-78)**
(1) Most effective method of airway management
(2) Most EMT's are not trained in this procedure
(3) May be used in many systems at the EMT-I or EMT-P level
(4) Necessary equipment
(a) Bag-valve-mask
(b) Proper oropharyngeal airway
(c) Laryngoscope handle
(d) Laryngoscope blades (3 or 4)
i) Straight
ii) Curved
(e) Endotracheal tubes (7, 8 or 9)
(f) Stylet
(g) 20 cc syringe
(h) Tape
(i) Gloves
(j) Goggles
(5) Insertion technique
(a) Test laryngoscope blade light
(b) Test endotracheal tube cuff **(Slide 3-79)**
(c) Assure adequate ventilation **(Slide 3-80)**
(d) Place head in the "sniffing" position **(Slide 3-81)**
(e) Engage laryngoscope blade and bring blade to a right angle with handle
(f) Laryngoscope with left hand
(g) Endotracheal tube (with stylet recessed 1/2 inch) in right hand
(h) Enter patient's mouth with blade **(Slide 3-82)**
(i) With curved blade place in vallecula **(Slide 3-83)**
(j) With straight blade place directly under epiglottis
(k) Visualize the vocal cords without pressure on teeth **(Slide 3-84)**
(l) Insert endotracheal tube until the cuff passes the vocal cords **(Slide 3-85)**
(m) Remove the laryngoscope
(n) Attach bag-valve-mask **(Slide 3-86)**
(o) Ventilated once every 5 seconds
(p) Auscultate lung field (anterior and lateral) and stomach **(Slide 3-87)**
(q) Inflate tube cuff **(Slide 3-88)**
(r) Palpate pilot balloon, and check for leaks around
(s) Insert oropharyngeal airway and secure endotracheal tube **(Slide 3-89)**
(t) Auscultate lung field

C. Positive pressure ventilation **(Slide 3-90)**
1. Positive pressure ventilation is a method of supporting inadequate or absent ventilation
2. May be performed by manual or mechanical means
3. Chest excursion is the best measurement of adequate volume

Content

4. Several methods of positive pressure
   a) Mouth to mouth **(Slide 3-91)**
      (1) The most reliable form of positive pressure
      (2) Exhaled air contains 16% oxygen and can provide adequate oxygenation
      (3) Advantages
         (a) Sense of airway compliance
         (b) Can easily observe chest excursion
         (c) Adequate tidal volume
      (4) Disadvantages
         (a) Potential for disease transmission
         (b) Aesthetic factors
         (c) Low oxygen delivery
      (5) Technique **(Slide 3-92)**
         (a) Perform head tilt-chin lift procedure to open airway
         (b) Determine need via look, listen, feel
         (c) Seal your mouth around victim's mouth
         (d) Provide two initial slow breaths (1-1.5 seconds)
            i) 800 ml minimum and 1200 ml maximum
            ii) One breath every five seconds (adult)
            iii) Every four seconds child
            iv) Every 3 seconds infant
         (e) Observe chest rise to confirm adequacy
   b) Pocket mask **(Slide 3-93)**
      (1) Mask with ventilation port and one way valve, direct ventilation via mouth
      (2) May have oxygen port
      (3) Allows up to 50% oxygen delivery
      (4) Advantages
         (a) Feel lung compliance
         (b) Two hands allow for superior mask seal
         (c) Increased oxygen delivery over mouth to mouth
         (d) Readily available for immediate use
         (e) Position to easily observe chest rise
         (f) Decreases the aesthetic factor
      (5) Disadvantages
         (a) Lower oxygen delivery than other mechanical aids
         (b) Does not eliminate disease transmission potential to rescuer
      (6) Technique **(Slide 3-94)**
         (a) Position mask over bridge of nose and above lower margin of mandible
         (b) Seal with the heel of both hands on mask
         (c) Ventilate while observing chest rise
         (d) Attach oxygen delivery tube
   c) Bag-valve-mask **(Slide 3-95)**
      (1) Most commonly used emergency device
      (2) Consists of self inflatable bag, nonrebreather valve and mask
      (3) Allows for oxygen delivery

(4) Advantages
(a) A sense of compliance by the rescuer
(b) Aesthetic concerns and disease transmission minimized
(c) High concentration oxygen delivery (90-100%)
(d) Relatively portable and can be used with room air
(5) Disadvantages
(a) Low tidal volumes when used improperly
(b) Requires practice to master technique
(6) Technique
(a) Position mask as above **(Slide 3-96)**
(b) "C" clamp hand position
(c) Squeeze bag against body or face to maximize collapse
(d) Observe chest rise
(e) Two handed technique when possible **(Slide 3-97)**
d) Manually triggered demand valve resuscitator **(Slide 3-98)**
(1) Oxygen powered ventilation device
(2) Delivers 100% oxygen
(3) 40 liter/minute flow
(4) Powered by portable or central oxygen source
(5) Triggered by patient demand or manual button or lever
(6) Advantages
(a) 100% oxygen delivery
(b) High tidal volumes result in more adequate ventilation
(7) Disadvantages
(a) Need oxygen tanks, less portable
(b) No sense of compliance by rescuer
(c) Create high airway pressure which increase chances of gastric distension
(8) Technique **(Slide 3-99)**
(a) Position mask as above
(b) "C" clamp hand position
(c) Squeeze button or lever
(d) Observe chest rise
(e) Two handed technique when personnel available
(f) Be alert to gastric distention
D. Oxygen therapy **(Slide 3-100)**
1. Increase the percentage of delivered oxygen to body tissues
a) Increased inspired O_2
b) Increased alveolar O_2
c) Increased arterial O_2
d) Increased hemoglobin saturation
e) 97% of oxygen is transported via hemoglobin
2. Selection of delivery system depends on several factors **(Slide 3-101)**
a) Degree of hypoxia, hypoperfusion and or ischemia
(1) Severe hypoxia, ischemia or shock should receive high concentration oxygen

Content

(2) Hypoxic COPD should be well oxygenated and observed for signs of respiratory depression

b) The ventilatory status of the patient

(1) Patients demonstrating signs of respiratory failure should receive positive pressure

(2) Key signs of respiratory failure include

(a) Little or no evidence of chest excursion

(b) Decreased level of consciousness

(c) Signs of exhaustion

(d) Cyanosis

(e) Pupil dilation

(f) Accessory muscle use

c) Chronic Obstructive Pulmonary Disease

(1) Generally, patients with COPD should receive 24-28% oxygen

(2) Hypoxic conditions oxygen can be increased accordingly

d) The ability of the patient to tolerate a face mask

(1) Severely hypoxic patients may not tolerate a face mask device

(2) Nasal cannula (even though it delivers lower concentration) should be considered

(3) Patients forced on a face mask may increase oxygen consumption causing no net benefit

3. Oxygen delivery systems **(Slide 3-102)**

a) Oxygen bottle identification

(1) The standard tank pressure of oxygen is 2000 lbs./sq. in.

(2) Green is the standard color of oxygen cylinders

(3) The cylinder should be labeled, indicating its contents and its status, i.e. full, empty

(4) The pin index safety system prevents inappropriate use of gas **(Slide 3-103)**

(5) Larger cylinders use thread system

(a) Oxygen is identified by two parallel holes beneath the opening

(b) A washer should be used to avoid leakage

(6) Cylinder sizes **(Slide 3-104)**

(a) The volume of gas varies from tank to tank

(b) C or D are portable cylinders and bring oxygen to patient's side

(c) M or H cylinders are used for inboard supplies

b) Oxygen regulators **(Slide 3-105)**

(1) Reduces the tank pressure from 2000 lbs. to a safe delivery pressure (approx 50 psi)

(2) A typical regulator consists of a pressure gauge, flowmeter and a yoke

(3) Single staged

(a) The most common type

(b) Reduces pressure to 40-70 PSI in single step

Content

(4) Double stage
(a) Reduces pressure in two stage process
(b) 700 than to 40-70 at liter flow gauge
(c) Saves wear and tear on regulator
(d) Additional safety net if part fails
(5) Flowmeter types
(a) Pressure compensated **(Slide 3-106)**
i) Tube with a ball that rises and falls according to flow rates
ii) More accurately records delivered flow rates
iii) Gravity dependent and can only be positioned upright
iv) Usually attached to the inboard system
(b) Bourdon gauge flowmeter **(Slide 3-107)**
i) Dial on a printed calibrated face
ii) Obstructions to flow may result in high false readings
iii) Gravity will not affect the reading
iv) Should be calibrated regularly for accuracy
(c) Constant flow selector **(Slide 3-108)**
i) Flow rates marked on dial
ii) More durable than other flowmeters
iii) Obstructions to flow may result in high false readings
(6) Tank pressure and flow rates **(Slide 3-109)**
(a) Tank pressures should never drop below 200 PSI
(b) To predict amount of time apply formula
i) Tank pressure (-200) x Constant
ii) Liter flow
iii) Constants
i) D - 0.16
ii) E - 0.28
iii) M - 1.56
iv) H - 3.14
(c) Pressures should be monitored closely
c) Humidifiers **(Slide 3-110)**
(1) Used to moisturize delivered oxygen
(2) Serves two major functions in prehospital care
(a) Prevents damage to the mucosa caused by long term oxygen administration
(b) Loosens dry encrustations within the airway
(3) Not essential in most patients due to the short-term nature of prehospital therapy
(4) Important for epiglottitis, croup and smoke inhalation
(5) Should be changed after each use

Content

d) Setting up and removing regulator
 (1) Setting up
  (a) Identify the contents of the cylinder **(Slide 3-111)**
  (b) Check for rubber washer on cylinder or regulator
  (c) Check the valve opening for foreign matter
  (d) Open main valve to clear particles **(Slide 3-112)**
  (e) Connect regulator, taking care to line up pin index system **(Slide 3-113)**
  (f) Tighten clamp with hand pressure **(Slide 3-114)**
  (g) Open main valve a minimum of 2 full turns and observe pressure gauge (approx 2000 psi)
  (h) Check flowmeter to desired rate of flow
  (i) Attach device to regulator **(Slide 3-115)**
  (j) Apply device to patient **(Slide 3-116)**
 (2) Removing
  (a) Remove device from patient **(Slide 3-117)**
  (b) Turn off main valve **(Slide 3-118)**
  (c) Bleed regulator with flowmeter control **(Slide 3-119)**
  (d) Return flowmeter to off position
  (e) Carefully remove regulator from cylinder **(Slide 3-120)**
  (f) Mark tag on cylinder as empty **(Slide 3-121)**
  (g) Place empty cylinder in appropriate storage area

e) Specific delivery devices **(Slide 3-122)**
 (1) Two types of devices
  (a) Low flow cannot meet the minute volume needs of the patient
  (b) High flow can meet the minute volume needs
 (2) Nasal cannula consists of two prongs placed in the nasal opening **(Slide 3-123)**
  (a) Nasal cannulas can deliver 24%-40% at 2-6 liters/min)
  (b) They do not cover the face and are well tolerated by the patient
  (c) Can be used for COPD patients or patients who cannot tolerate a mask
  (d) Flow rates should never exceed 6 liters per minute
 (3) Venturi masks are used to provided high flow/low concentration oxygen **(Slide 3-124)**
  (a) It consists of a mask with large lateral ports and an opening at the base **(Slide 3-125)**
  (b) Generally, the larger the opening, the higher the air mix, the lower the O_2
  (c) Venturi masks are adjustable by changing base piece or rotating opening
  (d) It is the device of choice for COPD patients who are not severely hypoxic
  (e) Capable of 24-40% at 4-8 liters/minute **(Slide 3-126)**

(4) A simple face mask consists of a mask with open ports on the lateral sides **(Slide 3-127)**

(a) It delivers moderate concentrations of oxygen (50-60%) at flow rates of 8-12 liters per minute

(b) It is useful in the treatment of stable ischemic and hypoxic conditions, i.e. MI

(c) It is contraindicated in COPD patients who are not severely hypoxic

(5) Partial rebreather **(Slide 3-128)**

(a) Delivers medium concentration oxygen

(b) Reservoir attached

(c) Patient exhales first 1/3 of air into bag

(d) Slight amount of carbon dioxide is inhaled

(e) Carbon dioxide can be reduced by increasing oxygen flow

(6) A nonrebreather mask is used to administer high concentration oxygen **(Slide 3-129)**

(a) Consists of

i) Face mask

ii) Partially covered lateral ports

iii) Reservoir bag

iv) Valve preventing exhalation into the bag

(b) It permits the highest oxygen delivery among free flow devices

(c) Approximately 90% at flow rates of 10-12 liters per minute

(d) Flow rates are adjusted according to the patient's tidal volume

(e) The bag should not completely deflate (a minimum of 1/3 full) during inspiration

(f) Device of choice for severely hypoxic, ischemic and hypoperfused patients

E. Suctioning **(Slide 3-130)**

1. Needed to clear secretions or prevent aspiration
2. Should be able to generate in excess of -300 mmHg of pressure
3. May be portable or inboard on ambulance **(Slide 3-131)**
4. Different varieties of suction catheters

a) Rigid curved suction catheters (Yankauer) are useful for upper airway suctioning **(Slide 3-132)**

b) Tracheobronchial catheters have soft tubes with proximal ports to apply intermittent suction

(1) Theses catheters must be sterile to avoid infectious complications

(2) They must be long enough to reach the tip of an endotracheal tube

(3) Not reliable for thick secretions

Content

5. Upper airway suctioning
    a) Assure adequate ventilation
    b) Test equipment
    c) Measure catheter from ear lobe to corner of mouth **(Slide 3-133)**
    d) Place suction catheter into oral cavity **(Slide 3-134)**
    e) Apply suction
    f) Suction for less than 10 seconds
6. Endotracheal suctioning
    a) Place the catheter into the tube using sterile technique
    b) Apply suction by covering opening at the proximal end of the catheter
    c) Suction for no more than 10 seconds

Chapter 3

Section 4

Airway Obstruction

Objectives
(Slide 3-135)

At the conclusion of the chapter the student will be able to:

1. **List 3 categories of airway obstruction and provide 1 example of each.**

2. **Describe the management techniques for the following types of airway obstruction:**
   - **Partial with good air exchange**
   - **Partial with poor air exchange**
   - **Complete**

3. **Demonstrate the following techniques for a complete foreign body airway obstruction on a manikin according to AHA/ARC standards:**
   - **Conscious adult**
   - **Unconscious adult**
   - **Conscious to unconscious adult**
   - **Conscious child**
   - **Unconscious child**
   - **Conscious to unconscious child**
   - **Conscious infant**
   - **Unconscious infant**
   - **Conscious to unconscious infant**

4. **Given a scenario, differentiate between a foreign body vs. a pathologic obstruction of the airway.**

5. **List the signs and symptoms and treatments for the following diseases:**
   - **Bronchitis**
   - **Emphysema**
   - **Asthma**

Instructor Preparation

Reading preparation for the lesson:

EMT Prehospital Care, Chapter 3, pages 127-141

Optional reading:

American Heart Association: Standards and Guidelines for Cardiopulmonary Resuscitation and Emergency Cardiac Care. JAMA 255(21):2841-3044. June 1986

Safer P., Bircher N.: Cardiopulmonary Cerebral Resuscitation. 3rd Edition, W.B. Saunders. Philadelphia, PA, 1988

Suggested Learning Activities

Using lecture format with handouts, provide overview of airway obstruction.

Using a manikin and a human subject, demonstrate the adult, child and infant airway techniques.

Provide case histories to illustrate the different types of patients using class participation.

Content

VI. Upper airway obstruction
- A. Overview **(Slide 3-136)**
  - 1. Foreign body airway obstruction kills 3000 people per year
  - 2. Accident victims often die due to airway obstruction secondary to the tongue or injury to the tracheal bronchial tree
  - 3. Patients may also obstruct the airway due to severe allergic reactions
  - 4. Airway obstructions may be partial or complete
  - 5. EMT must recognize and treat airway obstruction quickly since death occurs within minutes
- B. Anatomical airway obstruction **(Slide 3-137)**
  - 1. Most common cause of airway obstruction is the tongue
    - a) In unconscious states the tongue may obstruct the airway
    - b) Tongue, which is attached to the lower jaw, may block the pharynx due to relaxation of jaw muscles and neck flexion
    - c) Tongue may also block airway in maxillofacial trauma due to fracture dislocation of the jaw
    - d) Airflow may be partially or totally obstructed
      - (1) Partial obstruction may be characterized by snoring
      - (2) Complete obstruction is identified by total absence of air movement
  - 2. Management of anatomical obstruction includes basic and adjunctive airway maneuvers
    - a) Head tilt-chin lift is primary and most effective airway maneuver
    - b) Jaw thrust without head tilt is maneuver utilized in suspected spinal injury victims
    - c) Chin pull may be necessary in maxillofacial trauma
    - d) Oropharyngeal or nasopharyngeal airways may be used to maintain tongue away from pharynx
- C. Foreign body airway obstruction **(Slide 3-138)**
  - 1. Food is the most common cause of <u>foreign body</u> airway obstruction
  - 2. Toys and other objects may result in foreign body obstruction in children
  - 3. There are several predisposing factors for adult airway obstruction
    - a) Poorly chewed food may result in obstruction due to large pieces of meat becoming lodged in the upper airway
    - b) Patients with dentures or no teeth are at increased risk
    - c) Alcohol ingestion and laughing and talking during eating cause an increased risk
  - 4. Prevention **(Slide 3-139)**
    - a) Cut food into small pieces
    - b) Do not talk or laugh while eating
    - c) Avoid excessive alcohol before and during meals
    - d) Do not allow small children to run while eating
    - e) Keep small objects away from small children
  - 5. Recognition and management of airway obstruction
    - a) Foreign body airway obstruction may be partial or complete
      - (1) Partial airway obstruction with good air exchange **(Slide 3-140)**

Content

(a) May be characterized by forceful coughing and wheezing
(b) Patient should be encouraged to cough to expel foreign object
(c) Back blows and thrusts should be avoided

(2) Partial airway obstruction with poor air exchange **(Slide 3-141)**
(a) May occur initially or good air exchange may evolve to poor
(b) Recognized by weak, ineffective cough and/or stridor
(c) Accessory muscle use and cyanosis may also be present
(d) Treated by administration of Heimlich maneuver (abdominal thrusts)

(3) Complete airway obstruction **(Slide 3-142)**
(a) Recognized by inability to speak in the conscious patient and inability to ventilate in the unconscious patient
(b) Universal choking sign **(Slide 3-143)**
(c) Treated the same as partial obstruction with poor air exchange

b) Techniques for relieving obstruction
(1) Abdominal thrusts force objects out by applying pressure from within **(Slide 3-144)**
(a) Standing
i) Locate umbilicus
ii) Place fist just above umbilicus and well below xiphoid
iii) Apply a forceful upward thrust
(b) Sitting or lying position
(c) Can be self administered with hand or blunt object (chair)

(2) Chest thrusts **(Slide 3-145)**
(a) Standing
(b) Supine

(3) Finger sweep **(Slide 3-146)**
(a) Can be used in unconscious patient
(b) Perform chin pull and sweep the pharynx
(c) Hooking action is used
(d) Should only be used in infants and small children unless object is visualized
(e) Be careful not to push object further

6. Specific sequence for airway obstruction relief
a) Conscious patient **(Slide 3-147)**
(1) Assess by asking, "Are you choking?"
(2) Administer Heimlich maneuver just above the umbilicus and well below xiphoid process

Content

(3) Thrusts are directed inward and upward
(4) Each thrust is given with the intent of dislodging the obstruction
(5) Thrusts are continued until obstruction is removed or patient becomes unconscious

b) Conscious patient who becomes unconscious **(Slide 3-148)**
(1) Perform finger sweep while maintaining chin pull maneuver
(2) Attempt to ventilate using head tilt-chin lift maneuver
(3) Administer 6 to 10 abdominal thrusts with heel of hand followed by finger sweep
(4) Attempt to ventilate
(5) If ventilations are effective, assess pulse and breathing and administer CPR if needed

c) Unconscious airway obstruction **(Slide 3-149)**
(1) Recognized by inability to ventilate the unconscious patient
(2) Reopen airway and attempt to ventilate
(3) If unable to ventilate, proceed with 6-10 abdominal thrusts, finger sweep and ventilation sequence

D. Airway obstruction in infants and children **(Slide 3-150)**
1. More common in infants and children than in adults
2. Infant - less than 1 year
3. Child - 1-8 years
4. Infectious causes must be considered in infants and children
a) History of a cold, barking cough or fever may suggest croup or epiglottitis
b) If infectious cause, rapid transport with ventilation enroute
c) If partial obstruction, administer humidified oxygen
5. Foreign body obstruction
a) Child is same as adult except finger can only be performed with visualization
b) Infants - Conscious **(Slide 3-151)**
(1) Determine the need by the inability to speak, cry or cough
(2) Support the infant on one arm, keeping the head lower that the upper torso
(3) Arm can rest on your thigh for further support
(4) Face of the infant cupped in your hand
(5) Administer 4 back blows, forcefully between the shoulder blades with heel of other hand
(6) Rotate the infant, face up
(7) Deliver 4 chest thrust on the breastbone (1 finger breadth below nipple line) **(Slide 3-152)**
(8) Continue back blows and thrusts until object is removed or the victim becomes unconscious
c) If the victim becomes unconscious **(Slide 3-153)**
(1) Lay victim on his back
(2) Lift the jaw and visualize the airway for a foreign body
(3) Sweep the airway if the foreign body is visualized

Content

(4) Open the airway and attempt to ventilate
(5) Deliver 4 back blows
(6) Perform 4 chest thrusts
(7) Repeat sequence of back blows, thrusts, finger sweep, ventilation until successful

d) If the infant is found unconscious **(Slide 3-154)**
(1) Establish unresponsiveness
(2) Call for help (if alone)
(3) Open the airway
(4) Attempt to ventilate
(5) If you cannot ventilate, reposition head and try again
(6) If unsuccessful, deliver 4 back blows
(7) Apply 4 manual chest thrusts
(8) Perform the finger sweep, if you visualize an object
(9) Open the airway, attempt to ventilate
(10) If the victim cannot be ventilated repeat thrusts, finger sweep, ventilate until effective

E. Pathological airway obstruction **(Slide 3-155)**

1. The airway may obstruct secondary to swelling
a) Severe allergic reactions cause swelling due to histamine release and related tissue edema
b) Infectious airway diseases, i.e. croup and epiglottis, may cause obstructions in infants and children
c) Obstruction may be partial or complete
(1) Partial obstruction may be characterized by stridor, wheezing, accessory muscle use, intercostal retraction and signs of allergic reaction, e.g. hives, itching, swelling of face
(2) Complete obstruction may be recognized by an inability to speak in the conscious patient and an inability to ventilate in the unconscious patient

2. Management of the pathological obstruction **(Slide 3-156)**
a) Early recognition and access to life saving drugs such as epinephrine is essential
b) For partial obstruction with good air exchange, high concentration free-flow oxygen should be administered
c) If ventilatory efforts are ineffective, positive pressure ventilation should be instituted
d) If airway obstruction is complete, perform needle cricothyroidotomy
e) If needle cricothyroidotomy fails to secure the airway, rapid transport is essential
f) Epinephrine is an essential prehospital intervention of anaphylaxis

Content

VII. Lower Airway Obstruction
- A. Chronic Obstructive Pulmonary Disease **(Slide 3-157)**
  - 1. Overview
    - a) A common respiratory disorder
    - b) Results in obstruction and air trapping
    - c) Due to narrowing of bronchioles or loss of alveoli
    - d) Most commonly the result of smoking
    - e) Consists of two diseases: bronchitis and emphysema
      - (1) Although discussed separately often patients have both diseases
      - (2) May lead to severe distress and death
      - (3) Management directed at assuring adequate ventilation and oxygenation
  - 2. Bronchitis **(Slide 3-158)**
    - a) Caused by smoking and environmental pollution
    - b) Results in a number of physiologic changes
      - (1) Cilia are destroyed
      - (2) Mucous secreting glands enlarge causing excessive mucous production
        - (a) Phlegm producing cough prevalent in the morning
        - (b) Bronchiole narrowing may cause wheezing
        - (c) Rales and rhonchi are possible due to heart failure
        - (d) Impairs oxygen delivery/removal of carbon dioxide
        - (e) Shunting of blood results in tissue hypoxia
      - (3) Long term effects result in pulmonary hypertension and right sided heart failure **(Slide 3-159)**
        - (a) Swelling of abdomen, hips and ankles
        - (b) Distended neck veins
      - (4) Cyanotic due to poor saturation of hemoglobin
      - (5) Cyanosis and tissue edema lead to the term "Blue Bloater"
  - 3. Emphysema **(Slide 3-160)**
    - a) Caused by destruction of alveoli and loss of elastic recoil of lung tissue
    - b) Emphysema causes loss of alveoli
      - (1) Less surface area = less ability to diffuse oxygen and carbon dioxide
      - (2) Tissue hypoxia results
    - c) Loss of elasticity in lung tissue

Content

d) Loss of muscular nature of bronchioles
- (1) Bronchioles can collapse during exhalation
  - (a) Results in "air trapping"
  - (b) Patients use accessory muscles in the chest and abdomen to force air past obstruction **(Slide 3-161)**
    - i) Key sign in emergency
    - ii) Chronic use causes a "barrel chested" appearance
  - (c) Patients breathe through "pursed lips" to keep bronchioles open
  - (d) Increased red blood cell count increases to improve oxygen transport
  - (e) Combination of pursed lip breathing and pink appearance created the term "pink puffer"
  - (f) Patients may also have "clubbing of finger tips"

4. Oxygen therapy for the COPD patient **(Slide 3-162)**
   - a) COPD patient develops alterations in monitoring and regulation of oxygen needs
     - (1) Carbon dioxide primary force for respiratory drive
     - (2) Chronically elevated CO_2 levels cause switch "hypoxic drive"
     - (3) Increases in blood oxygen may eliminate respiratory drive
   - b) Oxygen therapy must be performed cautiously with these patients
     - (1) Patients who are not severely hypoxic should receive 24% via Venturi or nasal cannula
     - (2) Hypoxic patients should receive increased oxygen concentration and be observed
     - (3) Oxygen should be adjusted as needed
     - (4) Consult local protocols
5. Management of COPD patients **(Slide 3-163)**
   - a) Patients with COPD cannot tolerate further compromise of respiratory function
     - (1) Respiratory infections can lead to severe respiratory problems
     - (2) Little or no ability to compensate

Content

b) Signs of respiratory distress develop
(1) Dyspnea aggravated by exertion
(2) Accessory muscle use
(3) Wheezing and asthmatic breath sounds
(4) Cyanosis
(5) Tachypnea and tachycardia are common
c) Treatment **(Slide 3-164)**
(1) Compensated patients
(a) Low concentration oxygen
(b) Position of comfort (usually upright)
(c) Reassure to reduce oxygen demand
(d) Transport quietly to reduce anxiety
(2) Patients in respiratory failure
(a) Patients may decompensate due to extreme exhaustion
(b) Positive pressure ventilation
(c) If the patient cannot tolerate positive pressure a nonrebreather can be utilized

B. Asthma **(Slide 3-165)**
1. Acute respiratory disease precipitated by several factors
a) Allergies, infection and stress
b) Bronchiole spasm causes narrowed airways
c) Increased secretion of mucus
d) Air trapping occurs
e) Wheezing and asthmatic breath sounds
f) Attacks may be transient or prolonged
2. Recognition **(Slide 3-166)**
a) Sudden onset of dyspnea
b) History of asthma
c) Accessory muscle use
d) Tachypnea and bolt upright posture
e) Binding chest pain
f) May be taking inhalants or oral medication (i.e. aminophylline, theophylline, Theodor)
3. Management **(Slide 3-167)**
a) Most patients are well compensated
b) Patients in respiratory failure
(1) Exhaustion may lead to failure
(2) Positive pressure ventilation should instituted immediately

Section 5

Specific Respiratory Emergencies

Objectives
(Slide 3-168)

At the conclusion of the chapter the student will be able to:

1. **List 3 signs and symptoms and describe the prehospital treatment for pneumonia.**
2. **Describe the sequence of near drowning and discuss the differences between salt and fresh water drowning.**
3. **Given a scenario, describe the management of a patient in respiratory arrest.**
4. **List 3 signs and symptoms and describe the prehospital treatment for hyperventilation syndrome.**
5. **Provide 1 condition that may result from each of the following mechanisms of injury to the thoracic cage:**
   - **Deceleration**
   - **Compression**
   - **Penetrating: Knife vs. Missile**
6. **Given a scenario, recognize and provide the appropriate treatment for the following types of chest trauma:**
   - **Rib fracture**
   - **Flail chest**
   - **Hemothorax**
   - **Pneumothorax**
   - **Tension pneumothorax**

Instructor Preparation

Reading preparation for the lesson:

EMT Prehospital Care, Chapter 3, pages 141-154

Optional reading:

Prehospital Trauma Life Support Committee of The National Association of EMT's: Pre-Hospital Trauma Life Support. 2nd Edition, Emergency Training. Akron, Ohio, 1990

Safer P., Bircher N.: Cardiopulmonary Cerebral Resuscitation. 3rd Edition, W.B. Saunders. Philadelphia, PA, 1988

Suggested Learning Activities
Using lecture format with handouts, provide overview of specific respiratory emergencies. **Summarize the session with case histories using an interactive approach with the students.**

Content

VIII. Disease Affecting the Alveoli and Diffusion of Oxygen
- A. Pneumonia **(Slide 3-169)**
    1. Inflammation of alveolar spaces
    2. Caused by various types of infecting organisms or by aspiration of fluid
    3. Collection of fluid reduces the diffusion surface
    4. Assessment
        - a) History
            - (1) Respiratory infection
            - (2) Fever and productive cough (containing pus)
            - (3) Dyspnea
            - (4) Chills
            - (5) Headache
            - (6) Local pleuritic chest pain on the affected side
        - b) Physical
            - (1) Fever as high as 105 degrees
            - (2) Profuse sweating
            - (3) Severe episodes, cyanosis
            - (4) Lethargic or confused
            - (5) Vital signs might include a rapid pulse and increased respiratory rate
            - (6) Breath sounds present with rales and diminished sounds in local areas
    5. Management **(Slide 3-170)**
        - a) Patient is hypoxic but ventilating adequately
            - (1) High concentrations oxygen via nonrebreather
            - (2) Sitting position
        - b) Signs of respiratory failure including lethargy, hypoventilation or cyanosis
            - (1) Positive pressure ventilation
            - (2) High concentrations of oxygen should be started
- B. Near drowning **(Slide 3-171)**
    1. 6,500 people die from drowning each year in U.S.
    2. Factors leading to drowning
        - a) Overestimated his or her endurance
        - b) Intoxicated
        - c) Fallen in the water and is unable to swim
    3. Sequence of events **(Slide 3-172)**
        - a) Panic
        - b) Water swallowing and aspiration
        - c) Laryngospasm may occur
            - (1) Closes the glottic opening
            - (2) Prevents water from entering airway
            - (3) Dry drowning may occur (10-20%)

Content

d) Salt water drowning
(1) Pulmonary edema due to the salt pulling water from the pulmonary circulation
(2) Massive shunt
(3) Unconscious due to poor brain oxygenation
e) Fresh water
(1) Water is absorbed into the pulmonary circulation, destroys red blood cells
(2) Washing away surfactant results in the collapse of alveoli
(3) Massive shunting
4. Time to cardiac arrest and brain death **(Slide 3-173)**
a) Time may vary, particularly in cold water
b) "Mammalian Diving Reflex" slows down metabolism
(1) Decreased oxygen consumption
(2) Redistribution of blood to vital organs
(3) Prolongs time to biological death
(4) Always give drowning victims benefit of the doubt
5. Management of near drowning **(Slide 3-174)**
a) Airway should be established as soon as possible (in the water)
b) Positive pressure ventilation
c) High concentration oxygen
d) Clearing lungs is usually not needed
(1) Some physicians recommend abdominal thrusts
(2) Suctioning may be needed as fluids are expelled
e) Water may be aspirated into the stomach
(1) May interfere with ventilation efforts
(2) Characterized by difficulty in delivery of positive pressure
(3) Abdominal thrust can be applied in this instance
(4) Suction should be on standby
f) Spinal injury suspected- removed while maintaining spine immobilization
(1) Backboard or other floatable surface (i.e. surf board)
(2) Jaw thrust - without head tilt maneuver should be utilized

IX. Respiratory Depression and Arrest **(Slide 3-175)**
A. Overview
1. Respiratory depression and arrest may be caused by a variety of factors
2. Mechanisms for loss of neural control affecting the pons and medulla
a) Electric shock may cause paralysis of respiratory muscles or direct dysfunction of brain stem respiratory centers
b) Head trauma or stroke may result in damage to respiratory centers
c) Drugs may depress respiratory centers
3. Drug depressant causes may result in gradual loss of respiration, depression followed by arrest
4. Trauma, electric shock or circulatory failure may result in direct respiratory arrest

Content

B. Assessment **(Slide 3-176)**

1. Adequacy of respiratory function is assessed by several factors
   - a) Look, listen and feel to assess adequate ventilation
   - b) Tidal volume is evaluated by observing chest excursion (700 ml of air)
   - c) Respiratory rate below 10 or above 30 is generally inadequate
   - d) Mental state, cyanosis, and pupillary response are other indicators of hypoxia
2. Patients in respiratory distress who show signs of lethargy or hypoventilation should be ventilated, i.e. asthma or COPD

C. Management **(Slide 3-177)**

1. Airway should be established utilizing manual or adjunctive measures
2. Positive pressure ventilation should be instituted without delay via mouth to mouth or with adjunctive equipment
3. Suctioning should be on standby should secretions develop
4. Supplemental high concentration oxygen should be added as soon as possible
5. Specific technique
   - a) Patient should initially receive two breaths followed by one breath every five seconds in the adult, one breath every four seconds in the child, and one breath every three seconds in the infant
   - b) Chest excursion is the prime indicator of effective positive pressure ventilation
   - c) Breaths should be given slowly (1 to 1.5 seconds per breath) to reduce chances of gastric distension
   - d) Minimum breath of 800 ml; maximum breath 1200 ml
   - e) Cricoid pressure can be utilized to reduce gastric distension
6. Observe for signs of improved oxygenation
   - a) Pink skin and mucous membranes
   - b) Small, reactive pupils
   - c) Improved mental state
7. Gastric distension should be left alone unless it interferes with adequate ventilation
   - a) Gastric distension is relieved by turning the patient on his side and gently compressing the epigastric region
   - b) Suction should be at standby in the event of vomiting and head should be positioned to promote drainage

D. Hyperventilation syndrome **(Slide 3-178)**

1. A common respiratory problem
2. Precipitated by some emotional event
3. Patient overrides the normal respiratory stimulus and begins to breathe rapidly and forcefully
4. Causes a depletion of carbon dioxide in the blood
5. Assessment
   - a) Chief complaint of shortness of breath
   - b) History of present illness may reveal no other significant respiratory complaints

Content

c) "Tingling" about the mouth or fingers
d) Nausea and a feeling of dizziness
e) Question about a precipitating emotional event

6. Physical exam **(Slide 3-179)**
a) Pronounced tachypnea
b) Using accessory muscles
c) Rapid pulse rate
d) Possibly an elevated blood pressure
e) Carpopedal spasm (fingers in a rigid flexed state)

7. Treatment **(Slide 3-180)**
a) Check first for serious underlying cause
b) Have the patient take slower breaths
c) Calm reassurance is needed
d) Supplemental oxygen
(1) Won't harm the hyperventilating patient
(2) Should be given if there is any question of the diagnosis
e) Breathing into a paper bag is sometimes used
(1) Blood carbon dioxide concentration returns to normal more quickly
(2) However, one investigator found that rebreathing from a paper bag caused hypoxia
(3) Check local protocols

X. Chest Trauma
A. Mechanism of injury **(Slide 3-181)**
1. Blunt
a) Sudden arrest of chest against a fixed object
(1) Compression
(a) Thoracic cage
i) Rib fractures
ii) Sternum fractures
iii) Flail chest
(b) Intrathoracic injuries
i) Cardiac compression
i) Contusion
ii) Pericardial tamponade
ii) Pneumothorax
i) Brown bag effect
ii) Penetrating bone injuries
(2) Deceleration
(a) Aortic tears
i) Aortic arch most frequent
ii) High mortality
(3) Penetrating **(Slide 3-182)**
(a) Knife
i) Low velocity
ii) Damage by sharp point
iii) Relative to location

Content

iv) Pneumothorax
v) Hemorrhage, hemothorax
vi) Cardiac injuries
vii) Pericardial tamponade
(b) Missile
i) Medium velocity
i) 2-3 times diameter of missile
ii) Results in permanent injury
ii) High velocity
i) 2-3 times diameter of missile
ii) Variable area of hemorrhage
iii) Wound exit versus entrance
i) Entrance - implosion, small wound carries tissue and bone
ii) Exit - explosion, ragged wound edges, larger than entrance
iv) Common injuries
i) Pneumothorax
ii) Cardiac
iii) Vascular

B. Specific Problems and Management
1. Pneumothorax **(Slide 3-183)**
a) Physiologic effects
(1) Air in pleural space
(a) Lung rupture
(b) Penetration of chest wall and/or lung
(c) Compression versus - penetration
(2) Loss of negative pressure
(3) Mediastinal shift
(4) Loss of alveolar surface (atelectasis)
b) Types **(Slide 3-184)**
(1) Spontaneous
(a) Due to rupture of bleb
(b) Young muscular males and COPD patients
(2) Traumatic
(a) Penetrating wounds through chest wall and/or lung
(b) Rib fracture and puncture of lung
(c) Brown bag
c) Assessment and recognition **(Slide 3-185)**
(1) Sucking wound
(2) Dyspnea
(3) Pleuritic chest pain
(4) Absent or diminished breath sounds on affected side
(5) Signs of respiratory distress
(6) Historical profile (COPD, young muscular male)
(7) Subcutaneous emphysema
(8) Mechanism of injury

Content

d) Management **(Slide 3-186)**
(1) ABC's
(2) Seal wound, airtight dressing on 3 sides
(3) Oxygen
(4) Transport on affected side (except spinal injury/ventilation patients)
(5) Positive pressure ventilation, if needed

2. Tension pneumothorax **(Slide 3-187)**
a) Physiologic effects
(1) Air trapping due to one-way valve
(2) Increased intrathoracic pressure
(3) Pressure effects
(a) Diaphragm domes downward
(b) Mediastinal shift
(c) Pressure collapses venous system
(d) Decreased venous return (obstructive shock)
(e) Impedes "good lung" function
(4) Assessment and recognition **(Slide 3-188)**
(a) Increasing respiratory distress and cyanosis
(b) Distended neck veins
(c) Tracheal shift
(d) Signs of shock
(5) Management **(Slide 3-189)**
(a) Remove dressing
(b) MAST trousers
(c) Transport rapidly
(d) Decompression with a needle is the definitive treatment at hospital

3. Hemothorax **(Slide 3-190)**
a) Blood within the pleural space
b) Thorax has the capacity for massive blood loss
c) Physiologic effects
(1) Primary effect is hypovolemic shock
(2) May exist with or without an associated pneumothorax
(3) May occur due to penetrating injuries or to rib fractures
d) Assessment and recognition **(Slide 3-191)**
(1) Signs of hypovolemic shock
(a) Delayed or absent capillary refill
(b) Pale, cool, sweaty skin
(c) Tachycardia
(d) Rapid and shallow breathing
(e) Hypotension (late sign)
(f) Altered mental state (late sign)
(g) Cardiovascular collapse (cardiac arrest)
(2) Dyspnea
(3) Breath sounds absent on the affected side
(4) Hemoptysis (coughing blood)
e) Management **(Slide 3-192)**
(1) Establish a patent airway
(2) Suction available to deal with hemoptysis

Content

(3) High concentration oxygen via nonrebreather
(4) Positive pressure if needed
(5) MAST trousers
(6) Rapid transport
(7) Notification of emergency department
(8) Intravenous therapy is done enroute

4. Rib Fractures **(Slide 3-193)**
   a) Most common 5-9
   b) Assessment and recognition
      (1) Pain
      (2) Deformity
      (3) Swelling
      (4) Crepitus
      (5) Splinting of chest wall
      (6) Tenderness
      (7) Ecchymosis
   c) Treatment **(Slide 3-194)**
      (1) Sling/swathe
      (2) Do not restrict ventilation
5. Flail Chest **(Slide 3-195)**
   a) Physiologic effects
      (1) Two or more ribs fractured in two or more places
      (2) Loss of structural "bellows system"
      (3) Pulmonary contusion
   b) Assessment and recognition **(Slide 3-196)**
      (1) Same as rib fractures
      (2) Paradoxical chest wall movement
      (3) Mechanism of injury
      (4) Signs of respiratory distress
   c) Management **(Slide 3-197)**
      (1) Splint chest wall
         (a) Blanket or sheet
         (b) Rigid splint
      (2) Positive pressure ventilation
         (a) When hypoventilating, and can tolerate
         (b) Restores adequate ventilation
         (c) Otherwise nonrebreather device
6. Traumatic asphyxia **(Slide 3-198)**
   a) Results from high velocity injury
   b) Thorax compressed with severe force (steering wheel)
   c) Blood driven through veins to thorax and neck
      (1) Diffuse ecchymosis
      (2) Swelling
   d) Ecchymosis and swelling not life threatening
   e) Severe injury may be caused by pulmonary contusion

XI. Summary **(Slide 3-199)**
   A. Respiratory emergencies are among most life threatening problems
   B. Attention to ABCs is essential
   C. Rapid transport may be needed
   D. Review respiratory protocols

RESPIRATORY EMERGENCIES

Examination

1. The structure just above the trachea which is the only complete cartilaginous ring on the trachea or larynx is the:

   a. pharynx
   b. epiglottis
   c. thyroid cartilage
   d. cricoid cartilage

2. The muscles between the ribs that lift during normal resting breathing are called the:

   a. diaphragm
   b. intercostals
   c. abdominis recti
   d. sternocleidomastoids

3. The alveoli is the portion of the lung where the force of __________ moves oxygen into blood:

   a. diffusion
   b. osmosis
   c. active transport
   d. hydrostatic pressure

4. When the diaphragm relaxes and decreases the size of thoracic cavity, the pressure within the thoracic cavity _______________, causing air to rush out.

   a. increases
   b. decreases
   c. remains the same
   d. none of the above

5. The "hairlike" structures that line the tracheobronchial tree that trap and facilitate the removal of foreign material are called:

   a. pleura
   b. surfactant
   c. cilia
   d. fimbrae

6. The maximum amount of air that can be expired after the maximum inspiration is called the:

   a. tidal volume
   b. vital capacity
   c. expiratory reserve
   d. total lung capacity

7. Normal exhaled air contains approximately _____% oxygen.

   a. 16%
   b. 21%
   c. 28%
   d. 50%

8. The portion of the brain responsible for regulation of breathing is called the:

   a. cerebrum
   b. cerebellum
   c. hypothalamus
   d. brainstem

9. Tachypnea is the medical term for:

   a. difficulty breathing
   b. inability to speak
   c. rapid breathing
   d. noisy breathing

10. Pleuritic chest pain is chest pain that:

    a. is squeezing in nature
    b. radiates to the arm
    c. increases with chest movement
    d. increases while lying down

11. Cyanosis reflects poor oxygen saturation of:

    a. white blood cells
    b. platelets
    c. hemoglobin
    d. plasma

12. The term "hemoptysis" refers to:

    a. vomiting blood
    b. coughing up blood
    c. bloody stools
    d. bloody urine

12. The accessory muscles of <u>expiration</u> are primarily noted by observing the:

    a. chest wall
    b. neck
    c. abdominal wall
    d. back

14. Normal bronchovesicular breath sounds are found at the:

    a. lateral aspect of the chest
    b. at the upper outer margin of the chest
    c. upper and middle sternum
    d. above the suprasternal notch

15. Stridor is associated with a narrowed:

    a. lower airway
    b. bronchi
    c. alveoli
    d. upper airway

16. During positive pressure ventilation, effective tidal volume is evaluated primarily on the basis of:

    a. chest excursion
    b. skin color
    c. pupil response
    d. mental state

17. Gastric distention is a common complication of:

    a. underventilation
    b. slow ventilation
    c. forceful ventilation
    d. endotracheal ventilation

18. Which of the following administration devices results in approximately 90% oxygen delivery to the patient?

    a. nasal cannula
    b. Venturi mask
    c. nonrebreather mask
    d. simple face mask

19. The jaw thrust without head tilt is the primary airway maneuver used for:

    a. all children
    b. medical patients
    c. suspected spinal injury
    d. relieving airway obstruction

20. The maximum tidal volume needed to effectively ventilate an adult respiratory arrest victim is _____ ml of air.

    a. 500
    b. 1000
    c. 1200
    d. 3000

21. The correct ventilation rate for a non-breathing adult patient is approximately _____ breaths per minute.

    a. 5
    b. 8
    c. 12
    d. 20

22. In medical patients (with no suspected spinal injury), the airway maneuver of choice is the:

    a. jaw thrust without head tilt
    b. head tilt-neck lift
    c. head tilt-chin lift
    d. tongue pull

23. To assure proper sizing, an oropharyngeal airway is measured from the angle of the jaw to the:

    a. center of the patient's mouth
    b. tip of the nose
    c. cheek bone on the same side
    d. chin on the same side

24. Which of the following devices is least reliable in delivering adequate tidal volumes to the patient:

    a. bag-valve-mask
    b. pocket mask
    c. manually triggered demand valve resuscitator
    d. mouth to mouth

25. A bag-valve-mask used with oxygen tubing and no reservoir is capable of achieving a maximum of approximately _____% oxygen delivery to the patient's airway.

    a. 20
    b. 50
    c. 75
    d. 90

26. Which of the following cylinders is likely to be used for the <u>inboard</u> supply of oxygen feeding the wall mounted devices within the ambulance?

    a. D cylinder
    b. E cylinder
    c. M cylinder
    d. A cylinder

27. The pin index safety system is used to:

    a. secure the regulator in place on portable oxygen cylinders
    b. avoid using the wrong gas on portable oxygen cylinders
    c. avoid fires when using oxygen devices
    d. properly align regulators in place

28. A pressure compensated flowmeter uses a _______________ to measure the liter flow rates to the delivery device.

    a. dial
    b. digital readout
    c. gravity fed ball
    d. mercury manometer

29. A patient who is exhibiting cyanosis and has an inability to speak or cough is probably suffering from a:

    a. complete airway obstruction
    b. partial airway obstruction with good air exchange
    c. partial airway obstruction with poor air exchange
    d. none of the above

30. The proper hand position for administering a chest thrust for relieving foreign body airway obstruction in an adult is:

    a. the upper end sternum
    b. the lower half of the sternum
    c. the middle of the sternum
    d. one finger below nipple line

31. If the initial attempt at ventilation is unsuccessful in an unconscious patient, you should next:

    a. deliver four back blows
    b. deliver four abdominal thrusts
    c. reopen the airway and attempt ventilation
    d. perform a finger sweep

32. When attempting to clear a complete airway obstruction in the unconscious patient, you should administer ____ abdominal thrusts.

    a. 2-4
    b. 4-6
    c. 6-10
    d. 2-15

33. A finger sweep should only be used in a child or infant with a complete airway obstruction, if:

    a. they are conscious
    b. they are larger than 15 kg.
    c. ventilations are unsuccessful
    d. you can visualize the object

34. Back blows used in the treatment of a complete airway obstruction in infants should be administered:

    a. in the lumbar region
    b. medial to the kidneys
    c. between the scapulas
    d. below the scapulas

35. All of the following are possible signs of anaphylaxis, <u>except</u>:

    a. wheezing
    b. stridor
    c. hives
    d. rales

36. Cyanotic skin, ankle edema, ascites and dyspnea best describe the signs and symptoms of what form of chronic obstructive pulmonary disease (COPD)?

    a. asthma
    b. chronic bronchitis
    c. emphysema
    d. croup

37. Respiratory arrest is a possible complication of ______________ for a chronic obstructive pulmonary disease patient.

    a. suctioning of the lower airway
    b. airway insertion
    c. endotracheal intubation
    d. high concentration oxygen administration

38. Dilution of blood and hemolysis (rupture) of blood cells is most common in which type of drowning:

    a. fresh water
    b. salt water
    c. dry drowning
    d. both a and c

39. Respiratory arrest is most often due to injury or depressant effects upon the:

    a. cerebrum
    b. medulla and pons
    c. cerebellum
    d. hypothalamus

40. A patient with hives, wheezing and stridor following a bee sting is probably suffering from:

    a. foreign body obstruction
    b. anaphylaxis
    c. epiglottitis
    d. croup

41. If the patient in the previous question were to develop a complete airway obstruction, what would be your immediate action:

    a. deliver abdominal thrusts and attempt to ventilate
    b. perform a finger sweep and abdominal thrusts
    c. initiate rapid transport while attempting to ventilate
    d. insert a nasal pharyngeal airway to clear the obstruction.

42. The major problem caused by an asthmatic attack is:

    a. fluid collecting in the alveoli
    b. narrowing of the bronchioles
    c. swelling of the vocal cords
    d. inflammation of the pleura

43. The management of a patient with asthma who becomes lethargic and cyanotic should include:

    a. positive pressure ventilation
    b. administration of oxygen via a nasal cannula
    c. sitting the patient up and suctioning the airway
    d. administering oxygen via a simple face mask

44. A chest injury characterized by dyspnea and paradoxical movement of the chest wall is:

    a. pericardial tamponade
    b. tension pneumothorax
    c. flail chest
    d. traumatic asphyxia

45. Which of the following treatments should be provided to stabilize the condition described in the previous question?

    a. splint the chest wall with a towel or blanket
    b. lay the patient on the non-injured side
    c. oxygen via nasal cannula
    d. a sling and swathe

46. A patient with deviated trachea, neck vein distention, subcutaneous emphysema and breath sounds which are decreased on one side is probably related to:

    a. tension pneumothorax
    b. flail chest
    c. pericardial tamponade
    d. pulmonary embolus

47. The prehospital treatment for the patient described in the previous question would include:

    a. rapid transport to definitive surgical care
    b. oxygen via nasal cannula
    c. splinting the chest wall
    d. transport in the prone position

48. What definitive intervention is needed at the hospital to temporarily stabilize the patient described in the previous two questions?

    a. tracheostomy to secure an airway
    b. needle decompression of the chest
    c. needle decompression of the heart
    d. cricothyroidotomy to secure an airway

49. After applying an airtight dressing to a open chest wound the patient develops signs of increasing respiratory distress, agitation, neck vein distension and tracheal deviation. What would your next immediate action be?

    a. turn the patient on the non-injured side
    b. begin positive pressure ventilation
    c. temporarily remove the dressing
    d. insert an oropharyngeal airway

50. Upon removing a 4 year old child victim of near drowning from a pool you note respirations 3/minute. What breathing rate would you use on this patient?

    a. 1 breath every 3 seconds
    b. 1 breath every 4 seconds
    c. 1 breath every 5 seconds
    d. 1 breath every 7 seconds

51. You open the airway of an adult patient and attempt to ventilate but encounter resistance and observe no chest rise. Your <u>first</u> action should be:

    a. reopen the airway and attempt to ventilate
    b. perform a finger sweep maneuver
    c. apply 6-10 abdominal thrusts
    d. rapidly transport the patient to the hospital

52. The correct <u>rescuer position</u> for administering an abdominal thrust to an adult patient is:

    a. kneeling adjacent but parallel to the patient
    b. straddling the thighs of the patient
    c. straddling the umbilicus of the patient
    d. straddling the lower leg of the patient

53. A patient who is found breathing deeply and forcefully following an argument with his or her boss and complains of tingling around the mouth and "crampy" fingers is probably suffering from:

    a. asthma
    b. COPD
    c. emphysema
    d. hyperventilation syndrome

Skill Performance Sheet

Inserting Oropharyngeal Airway

Student's Name ______________________________ Date __________

Performance Standard	Performed	Failed
Universal precautions (gloves, goggles)		
Measure airway from mouth to angle of jaw		
Opens mouth with cross finger or tongue-jaw lift		
Inserts airway with point toward roof of mouth		
Rotates when safely past tongue		
Flange rests on outer lips		
Removes if gag reflex is noted		

Comments ____

____

____

____

Instructor ____________________ Circle One: Pass Fail

Skill Performance Sheet

Inserting Nasopharyngeal Airway

Student's Name ____________________________ Date __________

Performance Standard	Performed	Failed
Universal precautions (gloves, goggles)		
Measure airway from nares to tip of the ear		
Lubricates airway with surgical jelly		
Inserts airway into nasal opening until flange touches opening of nares		
If resistance is encountered, try other nostril		

Comments ____

____

____

____

Instructor __________________ Circle One: Pass Fail

Skill Performance Sheet

Inserting a Esophageal Gastric Tube Airway

Student's Name ____________________________ Date _________

Performance Standard	**Performed**	**Failed**
Universal precautions (gloves, goggles)		
Check equipment		
Assure adequate ventilation with other method prior to insertion		
Place head in neutral or slightly flexed position		
Perform tongue-jaw lift		
Insert tube into posterior pharynx until face mask contacts face		
Seal mask against face and attempt ventilation		
Observe chest rise and auscultate chest and epigastric region		
Inflate cuff with approximately 35 ml of air		
Recheck ventilation		

Comments ____

____

____

____

Instructor _________________ Circle One: Pass Fail

Skill Performance Sheet

Endotracheal Intubation

Student's Name ______________________________ Date __________

Performance Standard	**Performed**	**Failed**
Universal precautions (gloves, goggles)		
Check equipment		
Assure adequate ventilation with other method prior to insertion		
Place head in "sniffing" position		
Hold laryngoscope in left hand		
Insert blade in mouth carefully		
Curved blade - place blade in vallecula, view epiglottis and view glottic opening		
Straight blade - place blade beyond epiglottis and view glottic opening		
Insert tube cuff slightly beyond vocal cords		
Inflate cuff as appropriate		
Ventilate and auscultate chest and epigastric region		
Insert oropharyngeal airway		
Tape airway and ET tube in place		

Comments ____

____

____

____

Instructor ___________________ Circle One: Pass Fail

Skill Performance Sheet

Mouth to Mouth Breathing

Student's Name ____________________________ Date _________

Performance Standard	Performed	Failed
Open airway with appropriate maneuver (head tilt-chin lift or jaw thrust)		
Assess breathing (look, listen and feel)		
Seal mouth around the patient's mouth and pinch nose		
Give two smooth breaths while observing chest rise (1-1.5 seconds per breath)		
Take mouth away between breaths		
Check carotid pulse (pulse is present)		
Give one breath every 5 seconds for adult (every 4 for child)		

Comments ____

____

____

____

Instructor __________________ Circle One: Pass Fail

Skill Performance Sheet

Mouth to Nose Breathing

Student's Name ______________________ Date _________

Performance Standard	Performed	Failed
Open airway with appropriate maneuver (head tilt-chin lift or jaw thrust)		
Assess breathing (look, listen and feel)		
Seal mouth around the patient's nose and seal mouth		
Give two smooth breaths while observing chest rise (1-1.5 seconds per breath)		
Open mouth to allow for exhalation		
Check carotid pulse (pulse is present)		
Give one breath every 5 seconds for an adult (every 4 for child)		

Comments ____

____

____

____

Instructor ______________ Circle One: Pass Fail

Skill Performance Sheet

Infant Mouth to Mouth and Nose Breathing

Student's Name ____________________________ Date _________

Performance Standard	**Performed**	**Failed**
Open airway with appropriate maneuver (head tilt-chin lift or jaw thrust)		
Assess breathing (look, listen and feel)		
Seal mouth around the patient's mouth and nose		
Give two smooth breaths while observing chest rise (1-1.5 seconds per breath)		
Take mouth away between breaths		
Check brachial pulse (pulse is present)		
Give one breath every 3 seconds (adult)		

Comments ____

____

____

____

Instructor __________________ Circle One: Pass Fail

Skill Performance Sheet

Pocket Mask Breathing

Student's Name ____________________________ Date _________

Performance Standard	Performed	Failed
Universal precautions (gloves, goggles)		
Check pocket mask before use		
Assess breathing (look, listen and feel)		
Seal mask around patient's mouth with nose portion placed on the bridge of nose		
Maintain seal with two hands and maintain head tilt with fingers along the jaw line		
Give two smooth breaths while observing chest rise		
Give one breath every 5 seconds		

Comments ____

____

____

____

Instructor __________________ Circle One: Pass Fail

Skill Performance Sheet

Bag-Valve-Mask Breathing

Student's Name ______________________________ Date __________

Performance Standard	**Performed**	**Failed**
Universal precautions (gloves, goggles)		
Connects reservoir and oxygen		
Checks oxygen flow rate		
Check bag-valve-mask before use		
Assess breathing (look, listen and feel)		
Seal mask around patient's mouth with nose portion placed on the bridge of nose		
Maintain seal with "C clamp" maintain head tilt with fingers along the jaw line		
Squeeze the bag against the patient's head or your body while observing chest rise		
Give one breath every 5 seconds		

Comments ____

____

____

____

Instructor ____________________ Circle One: Pass Fail

Skill Performance Sheet

Manually Triggered Resuscitator

Student's Name ______________________________ Date __________

Performance Standard	**Performed**	**Failed**
Universal precautions (gloves, goggles)		
Check resuscitator before use		
Assess breathing (look, listen and feel)		
Seal mask around patient's mouth with nose portion placed on the bridge of nose		
Maintain seal with "C clamp" maintain head tilt with fingers along the jaw line		
Push button or squeeze lever while observing chest rise		
Give one breath every 5 seconds		

Comments ____

____

____

____

Instructor __________________ Circle One: Pass Fail

Skill Performance Sheet

Setting Up an Oxygen System

Student's Name ______________________________ Date __________

Performance Standard	**Performed**	**Failed**
Confirms that gas is oxygen		
Checks for rubber washer		
Opens main valve to clear opening		
Immediately closes valve		
Attaches regulator (carefully aligning pin index system)		
Tightens regulator with hand pressure		
Opens main valves two full turns		
Checks pressure gauge		
Attaches delivery device to regulator		
Adjusts flow rate		
Attaches delivery device to patient		

Comments ____

____

____

____

Instructor ____________________ Circle One: Pass Fail

Chapter 3

Skill Performance Sheet

Detaching a Regulator from an Oxygen Cylinder

Student's Name ______________________________ Date __________

Performance Standard	Performed	Failed
Turn off main valve		
Bleed regulator		
Loosen clamp and detach regulator		
Store in appropriate area		

Comments ____

____

____

____

Instructor ____________________ Circle One: Pass Fail

Skill Performance Sheet

Oropharyngeal Suctioning

Student's Name ______________________ Date ________

Performance Standard	**Perform**	**Failed**
Universal precautions (gloves, goggles)		
Tests suction device		
Measures catheter from mouth to ear		
Inserts catheter or rigid tip into posterior pharynx		
Applies suction during removal		
Does not exceed 10 seconds		

Comments ____

____

____

____

Instructor ________________ Circle One: Pass Fail

Chapter 3

Skill Performance Sheet

Conscious Complete Airway Obstruction

Student's Name ______________________________ Date __________

Performance Standard	**Performed**	**Failed**
Confirm obstruction by asking, "Are you choking?"		
Apply manual abdominal thrusts (chest thrusts for pregnant or obese patient)		
Repeat thrusts until effective or until the patient becomes unconscious		

Comments ____

____

____

____

Instructor ____________________ Circle One: Pass Fail

Skill Performance Sheet

Conscious Complete Airway Obstruction that becomes Unconscious

Student's Name ______________________________ Date __________

Performance Standard	Performed	Failed
Perform finger sweep (in child only if object is visible		
Open airway and attempt to ventilate		
Apply 6 to 10 abdominal thrusts		
Perform finger sweep		
Attempt to ventilate		
Repeat sequence of thrusts, finger sweeps and ventilation until effective		

Comments ____

____

____

____

Instructor __________________ Circle One: Pass Fail

Skill Performance Sheet

Unconscious Complete Airway Obstruction

Student's Name ______________________________ Date __________

Performance Standard	**Performed**	**Failed**
Check for unresponsiveness		
Position the patient supine		
Open airway		
Attempt to ventilate (obstructive)		
Perform 6 to 10 abdominal thrusts		
Perform finger sweep		
Attempt to ventilate		
Repeat sequence of thrusts, sweeps and ventilation until effective		

Comments ____

____

____

____

Instructor ____________________ Circle One: Pass Fail

Chapter 4

CARDIOVASCULAR SYSTEM

Materials and Equipment for Lesson

1. Anatomy slides, overhead transparencies, drawings or flipcharts
2. Model of the heart to show chambers, valves, etc.
3. Handout on anatomy and physiology
4. Slide projector, overhead projector, flipchart and/or blackboard

Anatomy and Physiology

Objectives
(Slide 4-1)

At the conclusion of the section, the student will be able to:

1. **List three functions of the circulatory system.**
2. **List the three components of the circulatory system.**
3. **Describe the components of blood and explain their function.**
4. **Given an anatomical chart, identify the major parts of the circulatory system.**
5. **Explain how valves control blood flow within the circulatory system.**
6. **Describe the function of the conduction system within the heart.**
7. **Explain the following concepts relating to circulatory physiology:**
   - **Cardiac output**
   - **Starling's law**
   - **Autonomic control**
   - **Pulse pressure**
   - **Blood pressure**
   - **Diffusion**
   - **Osmosis**

Instructor Preparation

Reading preparation for the lesson:

EMT Prehospital Care, Chapter 4, pages 157-185

Optional reading:

Guyton, AC: Textbook of Medical Physiology. 8th Edition, WB Saunders. Philadelphia, PA, 1990

Solomon, EP, Phillips, GA: Understanding Human Anatomy and Physiology. WB Saunders. Philadelphia, PA, 1987

Suggested Learning Activities
Using a lecture format with the aid of slides, overhead transparencies or charts, provide an overview of circulatory system anatomy and physiology. **Pass the heart model throughout the class and have the students examine the key anatomical features.** **When appropriate, have the students observe and palpate surface landmarks (pulses, veins and so forth).**

Content

I. Anatomy and Physiology of the Circulatory System
   A. Functions **(Slide 4-2)**
      1. Delivers oxygen and nutrients
      2. Removes carbon dioxide and other waste
      3. Repairs damaged tissue
      4. Combats infections
      5. Controls bleeding
      6. Maintains body temperature
   B. Components **(Slide 4-3)**
      1. Blood - Fluid in which oxygen and nutrients are transported
      2. Vessels - Pathways that deliver blood throughout system
      3. Heart - Provides the driving force to pump blood

II. Anatomy and Physiology of Blood **(Slide 4-4)**
   A. Overview of function
      1. Oxygen transport medium
      2. 5-6 liters in average adult (70 ml/kg of weight)
      3. Has liquid and solid components
   B. Plasma **(Slide 4-5)**
      1. Liquid component of blood
      2. Constitutes 55-65%
      3. Consists of water in which particles are dissolved (glucose, fats, proteins, etc.)
      4. Proteins aid in bleeding control and hold plasma in vessels
   C. Blood Cells **(Slide 4-6)**
      1. Constitutes 35-45% of blood volume
      2. Red blood cells:
         a) Largest cellular component
         b) Contain hemoglobin to transport oxygen
         c) Oxyhemoglobin is bright red, causes pink skin appearance
         d) Poorly oxygenated blood is blue or purple, accounts for cyanosis
         e) Life of red blood cell is approximately 120 days
      3. Oxygen transport **(Slide 4-7)**
         a) 98% of oxygen bound to hemoglobin (2% dissolved in plasma)
         b) Without hemoglobin, a sufficient amount of oxygen could not be transported
         c) Increased oxygen delivery can increase saturation of hemoglobin and dissolve oxygen content
      4. White blood cells **(Slide 4-8)**
         a) Combat infection
         b) Fewer in number than red blood cells and have shorter life span
         c) Accumulate at site of infection and consume bacteria and other organisms
         d) Pus is by-product of process
         e) White blood cells increase in number during infectious diseases (guides physician in diagnosis)

Content

5. Platelets **(Slide 4-9)**
    a) Necessary for clotting
    b) Forms thrombus (blood clot) with proteins
    c) Clotting time is usually 5 to 6 minutes
    d) Platelet deficiency results in tendency to bleed and bruise easily
    e) Proteins aid in clotting; deficiency (i.e., hemophiliacs) can cause excessive bleeding

III. Anatomy and Physiology of the Heart
  A. Overview **(Slide 4-10)**
    1. A muscular pump for the entire circulatory system
    2. Provides the force to open the vessels throughout the system - Perfusion
  B. Location **(Slide 4-11)**
    1. Between the sternum and the spine
    2. Size of one's fist
    3. Mediastinum - space containing the heart
    4. Superior part is the base at the right second rib
    5. Inferior portion is the apex at the left 5th-6th rib
  C. Pericardium **(Slide 4-12)**
    1. Visceral layer covers heart
    2. Parietal layer separates from mediastinum
    3. Fluid between layer provides lubrication
  D. Layers of the heart **(Slide 4-13)**
    1. Epicardium - outermost layer (visceral pericardium)
    2. Myocardium - muscular portion provides pumping force
    3. Endocardium - smooth inner lining that continues throughout vessels
      a) Smooth surface prevents clotting
      b) Diseased arteries may cause clotting
  E. Chambers and septums **(Slide 4-14)**
    1. Two receiving chambers, atria (upper heart)
      a) Left receives blood from the lungs
      b) Right receives blood from body
    2. Two pumping chambers, ventricles (lower heart)
      a) Right pumps blood to lungs
      b) Left pumps blood to body
    3. Septum divides left and right chambers (interatrial and interventricular)
      a) Atria (beat simultaneously) then ventricles
      b) Septum creates two circuits; pulmonary (right) and systemic (left)
  F. Right and left circulation **(Slide 4-15)**
    1. Two distinct circulations
    2. Pulmonary circulation - right
      a) Right atria receives deoxygenated blood from body
      b) Right ventricle pumps blood to lungs
      c) Blood receives oxygenation within lungs
      d) Blood pumped back to left heart

Content

3. Systemic circulation - left
   a) Left atria receives blood from lungs
   b) Left ventricle pumps oxygen-rich blood to body cells
   c) Blood pumped back to right heart

G. Valves - one way flow **(Slide 4-16)**
1. Unidirectional flow is maintained by valves
   a) During ventricular contraction (systole), blood is ejected to lungs and body
   b) During ventricle relaxation (diastole), blood is ejected from the atria to the ventricles
2. Atrioventricular valves (inlet valves) **(Slide 4-17)**
   a) Separate atria from ventricles
   b) Mitral (bicuspid) valve left side
   c) Tricuspid valve right side
   d) Directs blood from atria to ventricles
   e) Prevents backflow during ventricular systole
3. Semilunar valves (outlet valves) **(Slide 4-18)**
   a) Separate ventricle from outlet arteries
      (1) Aortic valve - aorta on left side
      (2) Pulmonary valve - pulmonary artery on right side
   b) Directs blood from ventricle to artery during ventricular systole
   c) Prevents backflow during ventricular diastole
4. Heart Sounds
   a) Valves closing create heart sound
   b) Diseased valves may result in heart murmurs

H. Conduction system **(Slide 4-19)**
1. Cells that initiate and control the contraction and relaxation of heart tissue
2. Spreads throughout heart to reach all cells
3. Sinoatrial node (SA node) is the pacemaker
   a) Discharges 60-80 times per minute
   b) Located in the right atrium
4. Sequence of electrical firing and conduction
   a) SA Node fires and spreads impulse through atria
   b) Impulse travels to AV node (atrioventricular node)
      (1) Travels slowly
      (2) Allow the atria to empty
   c) Bundle of His
   d) Divides into left and right branches
   e) Branches deliver impulse to Purkinje fibers
   f) Stimulate ventricular muscle
   g) Electrocardiogram (EKG) records and amplifies electrical events

I. Cardiac output **(Slide 4-20)**
1. The volume of blood pumped by the heart in one minute

Content

2. Stroke volume x heart rate
    a) Stroke volume
        (1) Amount of blood ejected with each contraction
        (2) Normal stroke volume - approximately 70 ml
    b) Heart rate
        (1) Number of contractions per minute
        (2) Heart rate approximately 70 per minute
    c) Give examples of changes in variables

J. Control of cardiac output **(Slide 4-21)**
1. The autonomic nervous system controls cardiac output
2. Intrinsic properties - heart rate
    a) Pacemaker normal rate of 60-80 times/minute
    b) Rate is altered by autonomic control
3. Intrinsic properties - force of contraction
    a) Can be increased by stretching myocardial cells **(Slide 4-22)**
    b) Frank Starling's law
        (1) Increased stretch =
        (2) Increased force of contraction =
        (3) Increased stroke volume
4. Autonomic nervous system has two divisions
    a) Sympathetic **(Slide 4-23)**
        (1) Increases heart rate
        (2) Increases force of contraction
        (3) Mediated by epinephrine
        (4) Sympathetic nerves travel down thoracic spine and out nerve pathways
    b) Parasympathetic **(Slide 4-24)**
        (1) Decreases heart rate
        (2) No effect on force of contraction
        (3) Parasympathetic nerves travel through vagus nerve
    c) Severance of sympathetic tone will prevent heart from speeding up (spinal cord injury)

K. Changes in cardiac output **(Slide 4-25)**
1. Exercise can increase C.O. several times
2. Heart beats stronger and faster
3. Cardiac output increases to meet needs of muscle
4. When one sleeps cardiac output will decrease
    a) Decrease in stroke volume
    b) Decrease in heart rate
5. Give examples of changes in cardiac output
6. Examples of factors affecting cardiac output
    a) Heart rate decreases
        (1) Pacemaker damage
        (2) Increased parasympathetic activity
        (3) Rest or sleep

Content

- b) Heart rate increases
  - (1) Increased sympathetic activity
  - (2) Epinephrine released
  - (3) Exercise
  - (4) Fever
  - (5) Fear and anxiety
- c) Stroke volume decreases
  - (1) Heart damage
  - (2) Rest or sleep
  - (3) Blood loss
- d) Stroke volume increases
  - (1) Exercise
  - (2) Pregnancy (late)

IV. Anatomy and Physiology of the Vessels
- A. Overview
  - 1. Three types of vessels **(Slide 4-26)**
    - a) Arteries - direct blood away from heart
    - b) Veins - direct blood back to heart
    - c) Capillaries
      - (1) Microscopic vessels
      - (2) Location of gas and nutrient exchange
- B. Blood volume and vascular space **(Slide 4-27)**
  - 1. Blood volume cannot fill entire vasculature space
  - 2. Blood directed to areas of need at a given time
    - a) Muscle during exercise
    - b) Digestive tract following eating
    - c) Discuss examples
  - 3. Controlled at level of arteriole
- C. Arteries **(Slide 4-28)**
  - 1. Comprised of three layers
    - a) Outer layer of connective (elastic) tissue
    - b) Middle muscular layer
    - c) Inner smooth layer to prevent clotting
    - d) Expand during systole and recoil during diastole
  - 2. Arterioles **(Slide 4-29)**
    - a) Terminal branches of arteries
    - b) Middle wall contains smooth muscle
      - (1) Constricts and dilates vessel
      - (2) Under direction of the autonomic nervous system
      - (3) Vasoconstriction results from contraction
      - (4) Vasodilation results from relaxation
- D. Capillaries **(Slide 4-30)**
  - 1. Microscopic (one cell thick) vessel
  - 2. Allows gas exchange with alveoli and tissue cells
  - 3. Diffusion can only occur at this level

Content

E. Veins
1. Similar structure to arteries **(Slide 4-31)**
2. Thinner middle layer due to low pressures
3. Can expand and contract with changes in blood volume
4. Capacitance vessels - hold 56% of the blood volume
    a) Heart/lungs 25%
    b) Arteries 15%
    c) Capillaries 4%
    d) Veins 56%
5. Contract in response to blood loss to maintain pressure
6. Expand with increased blood volume
7. Venous flow and pressure **(Slide 4-32)**
    a) Blood moves slowly due to low pressure
    b) Factors affecting flow
        (1) Muscular contraction
        (2) Valves (prevent backflow)
        (3) Intrathoracic pressure
        (4) Gravity and body position (have the students view their hand veins while elevating and lowering their arm)

F. Blood pressure **(Slide 4-33)**
1. Definition - The force exerted by the blood volume on the walls of the vessels
2. Vascular space
    a) Peripheral vascular resistance is determined by diameter of vessels
    b) Size can vary through constriction and dilation
    c) Decreased size will cause an increase in pressure
    d) Increased size will cause a decrease in pressure
3. Determinants **(Slide 4-34)**
    a) Blood pressure = cardiac output x peripheral vascular resistance
    b) A change in either variable will cause a change in pressure
4. Pressure and flow **(Slide 4-35)**
    a) Valves and vessels enable pressure to result in forward movement of blood
    b) Systolic and diastolic pressure
        (1) Blood is pumped into arteries during systole
        (2) Amount of blood volume in vascular space increases, pressure rises = <u>systolic pressure</u>
        (3) The vessels recoil and blood moves forward, pressure decreases = <u>diastolic pressure</u>
        (4) Normal values **(Slide 4-36)**
            (a) Adult systolic - 100+ age, up to 140
            (b) Adult diastolic - 65-90 mm Hg
            (c) 8-10 mm Hg lower in women

Content

- c) Pulse pressure **(Slide 4-37)**
  - (1) Difference between systolic and diastolic pressure
  - (2) Normal - about 40 mm Hg (greater than 50 and lower than 30 is abnormal)
  - (3) Determines subjective quality of palpated pulse
    - (a) Increased pulse pressure = stronger pulse, Decreased pulse pressure = weaker pulse
  - (4) Main determinants are stroke volume and tone of large arteries
  - (5) Stroke volume decrease = pulse pressure decrease
  - (6) Arteriosclerosis will cause an increase in pulse pressure
  - (7) Intense vasoconstriction will dampen pulse pressure

5. Reduction of pressure and flow **(Slide 4-38)**
   - a) Pressure highest leaving left ventricle (aorta)
   - b) Reduced throughout system
     - (1) Flow becomes continuous rather than pulsatile
     - (2) Continuous flow through capillaries and veins

G. Major arteries - review and have students palpate more superficial arteries

1. Pulmonary artery **(Slide 4-39)**
2. Aorta
3. Coronary arteries
4. Arteries to head **(Slide 4-40)**
   - a) Brachiocephalic
   - b) Subclavian
   - c) Common carotids **(Slide 4-41)**
   - d) Internal carotids **(Slide 4-42)**
   - e) External carotids
   - f) Temporal **(Slide 4-43)**
   - g) Internal maxillary
   - h) Superficial temporal
   - i) Facial
5. Arteries to the upper extremities
   - a) Axillary **(Slide 4-44)**
   - b) Brachial
   - c) Radial
   - d) Ulnar
6. Arteries to thorax, abdomen and lower **(Slide 4-45)** extremities
   - a) Aorta
   - b) Common iliac
   - c) Internal iliac
   - d) External iliac
   - e) Femoral **(Slide 4-46)**
   - f) Popliteal
   - g) Anterior tibial
   - h) Posterior tibial
   - i) Dorsalis pedis

Content

H. Major veins - review and have students observe more superficial veins
  1. Vein from head, neck and upper extremities **(Slide 4-47)**
    a) Venous sinuses
    b) Internal jugular **(Slide 4-48)**
    c) External jugular
    d) Subclavian
    e) Basilic
    f) Cephalic
    g) Superior vena cava
  2. Vein from thorax, abdomen and lower extremities **(Slide 4-49)**
    a) Vena cava
    b) Portal veins
    c) Esophageal veins

V. The Microcirculation **(Slide 4-50)**
  A. Delivery of oxygen, nutrients and removal of waste is the primary function of the circulatory system
    1. Capillaries are in close proximity to cells
    2. Red blood cells pass through one at a time due to thinness of capillary
    3. Pores in capillary allow fluid and particles to pass through to <u>interstitial fluid</u>
  B. Diffusion **(Slide 4-51)**
    1. The flow of a solute or particle from an area of higher to lower concentration **(Slide 4-52)**
    2. Oxygen and carbon dioxide diffuse across capillary membrane into tissues or alveoli
  C. Capillary pressure, osmosis **(Slide 4-53)**
    1. Continuous movement of fluid and particles across membranes is called microcirculation
    2. Blood pressure tends to move fluid and solute out of capillary at the arteriole end
    3. Fluid is brought back to capillary primarily by pulling force of particles, (i.e., proteins)
    4. Osmosis is the movement of fluid to an area of <u>lower</u> concentration to an area of <u>higher concentration</u>
    5. Plasma protein provides <u>osmotic force</u> needed to move fluid back into capillaries
    6. Plasma proteins are found primarily in blood
    7. Balance of forces **(Slide 4-54)**
      a) Blood pressure into capillary approximately 32 mm Hg in and 15 mm Hg out
      b) Plasma proteins exert a "pulling pressure" of approximately 25 mm Hg
      c) Arterial end of capillary = 32 mm Hg (pushing out of capillary), 25 mm Hg (pulling in) or 7 mm Hg out. Fluid tends to move out at arterial end

Content

d) Venous end of capillar - 15 mm Hg (pushing out of capillary), 25 mm Hg (pulling in) or 10 mm Hg in. Fluid tends to move in at venous end

e) Liver disease reduces plasma proteins **(Slide 4-55)**

(1) Reduces pulling force

(2) Results in edema

(3) Provide number on blackboard

f) Heart failure increases venous side pressure **(Slide 4-56)**

(1) Increases pushing force on venous end

(2) Results in edema

(3) Provide numbers on blackboard

g) Dehydration results in water loss and more concentrated blood **(Slide 4-57)**

(1) Increases pulling force

(2) Results in dehydrated tissues

h) Blood loss results in decreased pressure at arterial end **(Slide 4-58)**

(1) Decreases pushing at arterial end

(2) Results in fluid movement from tissues

D. Lymphatics **(Slide 4-59)**

1. Lymphatic vessels retrieve components of interstitial fluid (i.e., proteins) and return them to circulation
2. Also contain lymph nodes which filter bacteria and foreign material
3. Swollen lymph nodes are often a sign of infection
4. Help contain infection
5. Spleen contains lymphatic tissue, it filters blood and produces lymphatic cells
6. Spleen is often injured in blunt trauma and is highly vascular

VI. Summary **(Slide 4-60)**

A. Function of the circulatory system is dependant on three major components

1. Adequate blood volume and blood cells
2. Functional heart and conduction system
3. Intact and functional vessels

B. Conceptual understanding of anatomy and physiology "lays the foundation" for patient assessment and rationales of treatment

C. Review the relevant anatomy, physiology and surface anatomy to better appreciate

Chapter 4

CARDIOVASCULAR SYSTEM

Examination

1. The average adult has approximately ____ of blood/kg of body weight.

    a. 50 ml
    b. 70 ml
    c. 100 ml
    d. 120ml

2. The liquid portion of the blood is called _________.

    a. protoplasm
    b. platelets
    c. plasma
    d. hemoglobin

3. The portion of the blood which is responsible for carrying oxygen and carbon dioxide and contains the protein called hemoglobin is called _________.

    a. platelets
    b. red blood cells
    c. white blood cells
    d. plasma

4. Platelets are the portion of the blood responsible for:

    a. combating infection
    b. clotting
    c. carrying oxygen
    d. carrying carbon dioxide

5. White blood cells are the portion of the blood responsible for:

    a. combating infection
    b. clotting
    c. carrying oxygen
    d. carrying carbon dioxide

6. The left ventricle is:

    a. the portion of the heart that receives blood returning to the heart from the vena cava
    b. the portion of the heart that pumps blood to the body
    c. the portion of the heart that receives blood returning from the lungs
    d. the portion of the heart that pumps blood to the lungs

7. The right ventricle is:

   a. the portion of the heart that receives blood returning to the heart from the vena cava
   b. the portion of the heart that pumps blood to the body
   c. the portion of the heart that receives blood returning from the lungs
   d. the portion of the heart that pumps blood to the lungs

8. The left atrium is:

   a. the portion of the heart that receives blood returning to the heart from the vena cava
   b. the portion of the heart that pumps blood to the body
   c. the portion of the heart that receives blood returning from the lungs
   d. the portion of the heart that pumps blood to the lungs

9. The right atrium is:

   a. the portion of the heart that receives blood returning to the heart from the vena cava
   b. the portion of the heart that pumps blood to the body
   c. the portion of the heart that receives blood returning from the lungs
   d. the portion of the heart that pumps blood to the lungs

10. The valve that directs blood into the aorta during systole and prevents backflow into the ventricle during diastole is called the:

    a. aortic valve
    b. pulmonary semilunar valve
    c. tricuspid valve
    d. mitral valve

11. The proper sequence of electrical conduction in the heart is:

    a. SA node, Purkinje fibers, bundle of His, AV node
    b. SA node, bundle of His, SA node, Purkinje fibers
    c. SA node, AV node, bundle of His, Purkinje fibers
    d. SA node AV node, Purkinje fibers, bundle of HIS

12. Cardiac output is:

    a. the amount of blood ejected from the heart with each contraction
    b. the volume of blood pumped by the heart in one minute
    c. the difference between systolic and diastolic blood pressure
    d. the force of blood ejected from the left ventricle

13. An increase in cardiac output that occurs as a result of an increase in venous return and an increased stretch of the ventricle is a direct result of:

    a. osmosis
    b. Starling's law
    c. oncotic pressure
    d. diffusion

14. Heart rate x stroke volume is the formula that determines:

    a. systolic blood pressure
    b. cardiac output
    c. blood volume
    d. vital capacity

15. Blood is rich in oxygen and poor in carbon dioxide in all of the following structures <u>except</u>:

    a. pulmonary artery
    b. left ventricle
    c. aorta
    d. pulmonary vein

16. Which of the following vessels are thin walled permitting the exchange of oxygen, nutrients, and waste products between the blood and cell:

    a. arteries
    b. veins
    c. capillaries
    d. venules

17. The diastolic pressure best reflects the ____________ phase of the cardiac cycle.

    a. contraction
    b. relaxation
    c. intermediate
    d. recovery

18. The portion of the circulatory system which contains more than half of the blood volume is the:

    a. arteries
    b. veins
    c. capillaries
    d. arterioles

19. The axillary, brachial and radial arteries are all located in the:

    a. head
    b. lower extremities
    c. upper extremities
    d. trunk

20. The systolic pressure best reflects the ___________ phase of the cardiac cycle.

    a. contraction
    b. relaxation
    c. intermediate
    d. rapid firing

21. If the cardiac output remained the same and the arteries dilated, the blood pressure would:

    a. remain the same
    b. increase
    c. decrease
    d. none of the above

22. The most oxygen dependent organ is the __________.

    a. heart
    b. intestine
    c. brain
    d. kidney

23. If cardiac output remained the same and the peripheral vascular resistance increased, the blood pressure would:

    a. remain the same
    b. increase
    c. decrease
    d. none of the above

24. The thin covering of the heart that contains a lubricating fluid is called the:

    a. pleura
    b. peritoneum
    c. mediastinum
    d. pericardium

25. Oxyhemoglobin, which accounts for the pink appearance of the lips and nail beds, is:

    a. pale
    b. pink
    c. blue or purple
    d. bright red

26. Patients with a low supply of hemoglobin and red blood cells are said to be:

    a. anemic
    b. hypoperfused
    c. cyanotic
    d. hypoxic

27. The superior portion of the heart is located in the upper right chest at level of the second rib and is called the _______.

    a. apex
    b. base
    c. precordium
    d. apical region

28. The inferior portion of the heart is located in the left lower chest at level of 5th or 6th rib at mid-clavicular line and is called the:

    a. apex
    b. base
    c. precordium
    d. apical region

29. The lower pumping chambers of the heart are called the:

    a. ventricles
    b. septum
    c. atria
    d. pleura

30. The septum is the:

    a. wall that separates the left atrium from the left ventricle
    b. the wall that separates the left and right heart
    c. the wall that separates the right atrium from the right ventricle
    d. the wall that separates the vena cava from the aorta

31. The systemic circulation is also referred to as the:

    a. left circulation
    b. pulmonary circulation
    c. venous circulation
    d. right circulation

32. The pulmonary circulation is also referred to as the:

    a. left circulation
    b. systemic circulation
    c. venous circulation
    d. right circulation

33. The valve that controls blood flow from the right atrium to the right ventricle is the:

    a. tricuspid valve
    b. mitral valve
    c. aortic valve
    d. pulmonary valve

34. The valve that controls blood flow from the right ventricle is the:

    a. tricuspid valve
    b. mitral valve
    c. aortic valve
    d. pulmonary valve

35. The amount of blood ejected from the ventricle with each contraction x the heart rate per minute is called the ________.

    a. stroke volume
    b. cardiac output
    c. pulmonary flow
    d. tidal volume

36. The pulse pressure is:

    a. the difference between systolic and diastolic blood pressure
    b. stroke volume x beats per minute
    c. cardiac output x peripheral vascular resistance
    d. cardiac output x stroke volume

37. The artery that leaves the right ventricle and goes to the lungs is the:

    a. pulmonary artery
    b. pulmonary vein
    c. coronary artery
    d. coronary vein

38. The capillaries are:

    a. designed to withstand high pressure
    b. the smallest vessels in the arterial network
    c. the area where gas exchange occurs
    d. the body's blood reservoir containing more than half of the blood volume

39. Diffusion can best be described as the:

    a. movement of particles from an area of higher concentration to an area of lower concentration
    b. movement of water from an area of lower concentration of particles to an area of higher concentration of particles
    c. pressure exerted by a fluid on the cell membrane
    d. relationship between stroke volume, cardiac output, and blood pressure

40. Osmosis can best be described as the:

    a. movement of particles from an area of higher concentration to an area of lower concentration
    b. movement of water from an area of lower concentration of particles to an area of higher concentration of particles
    c. pressure exerted by a fluid on the cell membrane
    d. relationship between stroke volume, cardiac output, and blood pressure

41. The rate and force of contraction of the heart is regulated through the autonomic nervous system and __________.

    a. the hormone epinephrine
    b. the electrical conduction system in the heart
    c. the voluntary nervous system
    d. the osmotic pressure in the arteries

42. An increase in sympathetic tone within the nervous system will result in which of the following responses:

    a. the pulse will increase
    b. the pulse will remain the same
    c. the pulse will slow
    d. the force of contraction will decrease

43. The average adult has approximately ______ liters of blood volume.

    a. 1-2
    b. 3-4
    c. 5-6
    d. 7-8

44. The cellular portion of the blood that is responsible for combating infection is the:

    a. platelets
    b. red blood cells
    c. white blood cells
    d. hemoglobin

45. The portion of blood responsible for clotting is called:

    a. platelets
    b. red blood cells
    c. white blood cells
    d. plasma

46. Which of the following blood cells are likely to increase in number during an infection?

    a. platelets
    b. red blood cells
    c. white blood cells
    d. plasma

47. The valve that directs blood into the pulmonary artery during systole and prevents backflow into the ventricle during diastole is called the:

    a. aortic valve
    b. pulmonary semilunar valve
    c. tricuspid valve
    d. mitral valve

48. Cardiac output times peripheral vascular resistance (the diameter and tone of the vessels) is the formula that determines:

    a. stroke volume
    b. blood pressure
    c. blood volume
    d. vital capacity

49. Which of the following vessels are most muscular?

    a. arteries
    b. veins
    c. capillaries
    d. venules

50. The femoral, popliteal and dorsalis pedis arteries are all located in the:

    a. head
    b. lower extremities
    c. upper extremities
    d. trunk

51. The diastolic pressure best reflects the ___________ phase of the cardiac cycle.

    a. contraction
    b. relaxation
    c. intermediate
    d. rapid firing

52. If the cardiac output remained the same and the arteries constricted, the blood pressure would:

    a. remain the same
    b. increase
    c. decrease
    d. none of the above

53. Which of the following is a function of the cardiovascular system?

    a. delivering oxygen and transporting waste for excretion
    b. bringing oxygen into the body from the environment
    c. preparing glucose to enter cells
    d. producing and secreting hormones to regulate body activities

54. The most oxygen dependent organ is the:

    a. heart
    b. intestine
    c. brain
    d. kidney

55. Blood transports most of the body's oxygen via:

    a. plasma
    b. white blood cells
    c. red blood cells
    d. platelets

56. The thin covering of the heart that contains a lubricating fluid is called the:

    a. pleura
    b. peritoneum
    c. mediastinum
    d. pericardium

57. Blood that is poorly saturated with oxygen gives a ________ color to the lips and nailbeds.

    a. pale
    b. pink
    c. blue
    d. cherry red

58. At room air, hemoglobin transports ________ of the oxygen in the blood.

    a. 2%
    b. 50%
    c. 75%
    d. 98%

59. The superior portion of the heart is located in the upper chest at level of the second rib and is called the:

    a. apex
    b. base
    c. precordium
    d. apical region

60. The inferior portion of the heart is located in the left lower chest at level of 5th or 6th rib at mid-clavicular line and is called the:

    a. apex
    b. base
    c. precordium
    d. apical region

61. The left circulation is the ________ circulation.

    a. pulmonary
    b. systemic
    c. arterial
    d. venous

62. The right circulation is the ________ circulation.

    a. pulmonary
    b. systemic
    c. arterial
    d. venous

63. The valves that control flow from the atria to the ventricles are the _______ valves.

    a. semilunar
    b. atrioventricular
    c. atrial
    d. ventricular

64. The valves that control flow from the ventricles to the pulmonary arteries and aorta are the _______ valves.

    a. semilunar
    b. atrioventricular
    c. atrial
    d. ventricular

65. The amount of blood ejected from the ventricle with each contraction is called the:

a. stroke volume
b. cardiac output
c. pulmonary flow
d. tidal volume

66. Cardiac output is the stroke volume multiplied by the average ___________ per minute.

a. tidal volume
b. heart rate
c. respiratory rate
d. vital capacity

67. The first arteries to branch off the aorta and supply blood to the heart are called the _________ arteries.

a. systemic
b. brachial
c. coronary
d. pulmonary

68. Gas exchange occurs in which of the following vessels?

a. arteries
b. veins
c. capillaries
d. venules

69. Movement of particles from an area of higher concentration to an area of lower concentration best describes:

a. diffusion
b. osmosis
c. oncotic pressure
d. Starling's Law

70. The movement of water from an area of lower concentration of particles to an area of higher concentration of particles best describes:

a. diffusion
b. osmosis
c. oncotic pressure
d. Starling's law

Chapter 5

CARDIOVASCULAR EMERGENCIES

Materials and Equipment for Lesson

1. Slides, overheads, drawings or flipcharts
2. Assorted bandages and dressing
3. Adult PASG
4. Handouts
    - Bleeding control and shock
    - Arteriosclerotic heart disease
    - Pump failure and complications
    - Cardiac trauma
    - Performance sheets for bleeding control and MAST
5. Slide projector, overhead, flipchart and/or blackboard
6. Risk factor literature from American Heart Association

Section 1

Bleeding and Shock

Objectives
(Slide 5-1)

At the conclusion of the chapter the students will be able to:
1. Define shock and explain its effect upon the body cells.
2. List 3 signs of adrenaline release.
3. List 4 types of shock and explain the mechanisms.
4. Given a percentage of blood loss, indicate the likely associated signs and symptoms.
5. List 4 methods for controlling bleeding and describe the technique for each.
6. List 3 uses for Pneumatic Anti-Shock Garment (PASG).
7. List the contraindications for Pneumatic Anti-Shock Garment (PASG) and 3 reasons for not inflating the abdominal section of the garment.
8. Describe the application process for Pneumatic Anti-Shock Garment (PASG).

Instructor Preparation

Reading preparation for the lesson:

EMT Prehospital Care, Chapter 5 pages 187-209
Local cardiovascular protocols
Performance sheets for cardiovascular skills

Optional reading:

Prehospital Trauma Life Support Committee of The National Association of EMTs: Pre-Hospital Trauma Life Support, 2nd Ed, Emergency Training. Akron, Ohio, 1990

Roberts, J.R., Hedges, J.R.: Clinical Procedures in Emergency Medicine. W.B. Saunders, Philadelphia, PA 1985

Zuidema, G.D., et al (eds), The Management of Trauma, 4th Ed. W.B. Saunders, Philadelphia, PA 1985.

Suggested Learning Activities

Using a lecture format with the aid of slides, overhead transparencies or charts, provide an overview of bleeding and shock.

Demonstrate the basic techniques of bleeding control.

Demonstrate the basic technique for applying the MAST.

Content

I. Important concepts
  A. Overview **(Slide 5-2)**
    1. Definition: Shock is the failure of the respiratory and circulatory system to adequately perfuse and oxygenate tissues
    2. Shock may be present in varying degrees: slight, moderate, transient or severe
    3. Early recognition and management is essential in saving lives and recognition is dependent on knowledge of compensatory mechanisms
  B. Physiology of normal tissue perfusion **(Slide 5-3)**
    1. Normally blood flow to tissues matches their needs
    2. Arterioles regulate blood flow and open and close according to these needs
    3. Cardiac output (C.O.) can be increased when a large amount of body tissues increase their oxygen needs at a given time
    4. Cardiac output can increase several-fold according to this need
    5. Changes occur sequentially **(Slide 5-4)**
      a) Tissues need more oxygen
      b) Arteriole opens to supply more blood
      c) Increased venous return
      d) Increased cardiac output
      e) Blood flow matches tissue needs
      f) Tissue needs decrease, arterioles close
  C. Effects of epinephrine **(Slide 5-5)**
    1. "Fight or Flight" response prepares body for crisis
    2. Can be precipitated by fear or reaction to hazard
    3. Major effects of epinephrine include
      a) Increased cardiac output
      b) Increased blood flow to the brain
      c) Dilation of the pupils
      d) Increased blood flow to skeletal muscle
      e) Shunting of blood from the skin and digestive organs to the core and muscle
      f) Increased respirations
    4. Epinephrine controls blood flow via vasoconstriction and vasodilation
    5. Signs of epinephrine release are helpful to identify shock states
  D. Failure of the circulatory system to meet the body's needs **(Slide 5-6)**
    1. During blood loss venous return drops and cardiac output decreases
    2. When the existing cardiac output fails to meet body's needs, tissues become oxygen deprived and organs may dysfunction
    3. Redistribution of blood from the skin, digestive tract and muscle to vital organs occurs to assure adequate perfusion of heart, lungs and brain
    4. Poorly perfused skeletal muscle results in weakness
  E. Forces affecting venous return **(Slide 5-7)**
    1. Venous space and blood volume
      a) The size of the venous space determines the vascular resistance and can alter the pressure and venous return to the heart
      b) Changes in blood volume will increase and decrease the pressure and alter venous return

Content

2. Gravity affects venous pressure relative to the position of veins
    a) Leg veins normally have a high venous pressure
    b) Neck veins normally have a low venous pressure
    c) Change the position of your hands above and below the heart and observe changes in venous distension
3. Skeletal muscle contributes pumping force to veins in the extremities to increase venous return during exercise
4. Valves in veins prevent backward flow
5. Changes in intrathoracic pressure facilitate venous return

F. Nervous regulation of blood flow **(Slide 5-8)**
1. During shock state a "pecking order" is established in order to redistribute blood to where it is most needed
2. Less vital organs are "sacrificed" to feed more vital organs
3. The autonomic nervous system regulates redistribution and the heart and brain are the last to be deprived
4. Patients may be alert to the very end of shock states

II. Classifications of shock

A. Overview of shock **(Slide 5-9)**
1. Shock may occur due to failure of the pump, vessels, blood volume
2. Pump failure, i.e., heart attack results in decreased cardiac output due to loss of effective pumping action of the heart
3. Loss of blood volume decreases venous return and therefore decreases cardiac output
4. Dilation or loss of vascular resistance decreases system pressure and flow of blood
5. Treatment of shock may differ slightly depending on the cause
    a) Treatment of shock due to loss of blood volume is primarily directed at augmenting venous return
        (1) This treatment may be harmful for patients with pump failure
    b) Pump failure is treated by reducing venous return in order to decrease the workload of the heart

B. Cardiogenic shock (pump failure) **(Slide 5-10)**
1. Cardiogenic shock occurs when the pump is damaged or when abnormal rhythms decrease cardiac output
2. C.O. decreases due to decreases in stroke volume or heart rate
3. The most common cause of cardiogenic shock is myocardial infarction (heart attack)
4. Effects of pump failure
    a) Arterial circulation is decreased on the affected side (decreased C.O.)
        (1) Signs of decreased perfusion, i.e., hypotension, pale skin, weakness, etc.
    b) Venous circulation is affected by "backlog" of blood due to poor cardiac output
        (1) Pressure is transmitted to pulmonary or systemic capillaries, depending on the affected side

(2) In pulmonary circuit plasma is driven into alveoli and the interstitial tissues of the lung (pulmonary edema)
(3) In the systemic circuit plasma is driven into tissues (systemic edema, i.e., ankle edema)
(4) Signs of pump failure may include: **(Slide 5-11)**
(a) Dyspnea
(b) Accessory muscle use
(c) Rales (crackling breath sounds)
(d) Hemoptysis (bloody sputum)
(e) Systemic edema in the ankles, hips, abdomen
(f) Neck vein distension

C. Hypovolemic shock (low volume shock) **(Slide 5-12)**
1. Shock due to loss of body fluids from blood loss, burns, vomiting, diarrhea, etc.
2. Most common cause is acute blood loss (hemorrhage)
3. Any water loss from body spaces may lead to hypovolemic shock
4. Plasma may be decreased due to less intake or more output
a) Intake occurs through drinking and eating and reabsorption throughout the bowel
b) Output normally occurs through urination, sweat, feces and respiration
5. Signs of dehydration may include: thirst, dry skin, dry tongue and mucous membranes, skin tenting

D. Vasodilatory shock (loss of vascular tone) **(Slide 5-13)**
1. Vasodilatory shock occurs when vessels lose their ability to change diameter and widespread vasodilation occurs
2. Both arterial and venous pressure may fall, venous return will fall and cardiac output will decrease
3. Anaphylaxis or spinal injury may cause vasodilatory shock
a) Anaphylaxis causes a release of chemicals that cause vasodilation
b) Spinal cord injury may result in loss of sympathetic tone and result in widespread vasodilation
c) Direct injury to the brain and certain drugs may also cause vasodilation
4. Psychogenic shock or fainting
a) Severe emotional reactions may lead to vasodilation and slowing of the heart rate due to increase in parasympathetic tone
b) These patients may self correct or may correct after being laid supine to increase brain circulation

E. Obstructive shock **(Slide 5-14)**
1. Obstructive shock occurs when there is a blockage to blood flow in the central circulation
2. This may occur secondary to a pulmonary embolus or from traumatic conditions; tension pneumothorax and pericardial tamponade

Content

3. Tension pneumothorax
    a) The venae cavae are low pressure vessels and can collapse when the intrathoracic pressure increases
    b) In tension pneumothorax air trapped in the pleural space exerts pressure and collapses the venae cavae
    c) Pressure must be decreased with release of an airtight dressing or through needle decompression to reinstate flow
4. Pericardial tamponade
    a) Pericardial tamponade can occur as a result of penetrating wound to the heart or when wall ruptures following a massive MI
    b) Pericardial tamponade leads to obstruction when fluid or air in the pericardial space places pressure on the chambers of the heart and the venae cavae
    c) Refilling is impaired and blood flow is obstructed
5. Signs of obstructive shock **(Slide 5-15)**
    a) Venous obstruction results in distension of the neck veins due to the increase in venous pressure
    b) Signs of decreased cardiac output, i.e., pale skin, weakness, alterations of mental state, etc. may also be present

F. Septic shock (vasodilatory and hypovolemic) **(Slide 5-16)**
1. Septic shock results from widespread infection that may arise from any part of the body
2. Intestinal and urinary infections are often caused by the bacteria that lead to septic shock
3. The bacteria cause dilation of the veins which is the primary component of septic shock
4. Leakage of fluid at the site of the infection complicates the shock by a hypovolemic effect

G. Respiratory shock **(Slide 5-17)**
1. When the respiratory system fails to provide a sufficient amount of oxygen to the blood respiratory shock occurs
2. Respiratory shock can result from respiratory arrest, airway obstruction, chest trauma, etc.
3. The circulatory system may increase cardiac output but the hemoglobin is deoxygenated
4. Ultimately the heart will become hypoxic if the situation is uncorrected
5. The treatment of respiratory shock is to treat the underlying cause

H. Time constraints **(Slide 5-18)**
1. Shock must be treated promptly or tissue death will occur
2. Often surgical intervention is needed to correct the causes of shock, i.e., internal bleeding
3. Rapid access to definitive surgical care is an essential part of management

Content

III. Hypovolemic shock secondary to hemorrhage
- A. Effect of blood loss **(Slide 5-19)**
  - 1. Blood is important for its oxygen carrying capacity, its volume needed to maintain pressure and its other essential components
  - 2. Patients who suffer loss of half of their blood volume will have a circulatory arrest
  - 3. Loss of blood cells
    - a) Normally we have 3-4 times the needed red blood cells to sustain life
    - b) Patients with liver disease may live with half of their red blood cells
    - c) Patients with a reduced number of red blood cells and hemoglobin are said to be anemic
      - (1) They may be weak and have a decreased ability to perform strenuous tasks
      - (2) When anemia develops slowly the body can make adjustments to maintain an adequate blood volume
      - (3) Signs and symptoms of anemia
        - (a) Pale skin and mucous membranes
        - (b) Weakness and drowsiness
        - (c) Slight tachycardia
  - 4. Loss of blood volume **(Slide 5-20)**
    - a) Hemorrhage results in a loss of cells and volume
    - b) There may be enough cells to maintain life but the depleted volume may lead to circulatory arrest
    - c) Patients with cardiac arrest victims secondary to hemorrhage cannot be resuscitated until the volume is replaced
    - d) Some EMS systems provide volume in the field with IV solutions such as saline or plasma but whole blood is ultimately needed to restore the necessary red blood cells
  - 5. Loss of clotting factors
    - a) After severe hemorrhage the patient may need restoration of cells, volume and the clotting components (platelets) to be effectively resuscitated
- B. External bleeding
  - 1. Recognition of external bleeding **(Slide 5-21)**
    - a) Rate of flow
      - (1) Arteries result in the fastest rate of bleeding, which is pulsatile due to the direct influence of the ventricle
      - (2) Veins will result in a steady slow flow of blood, due to their low pressure
      - (3) Capillaries will ooze forth blood due to the size and low pressure

Content

b) Color of the blood
(1) Arterial bleeding is bright red in color due to the oxygenated hemoglobin
(2) Venous bleeding is dark red or maroon in color due to the deoxygenated blood
(3) Capillary bleeding is somewhere in between
c) Type of the vessel
(1) The larger the vessel the greater the rate of flow
(2) When arteries are completely cut they may retract and slow the rate of bleeding
(3) A large artery may not contract due to its large muscular wall
d) Location of the wound
(1) Veins tend to more superficial than arteries
(2) Arteries run deep, along bone and may be torn secondary to fractures

2. Clotting
a) Clotting takes place soon after bleeding (4-6 minutes)
b) It is faster for smaller vessels due to low pressure
c) Clotting may be difficult in large vessels due to high pressure

3. Bleeding control **(Slide 5-22)**
a) There are four methods of external bleeding control: direct pressure, elevation, pressure points and tourniquet
b) They are sometimes used in combination to allow clotting to take place
c) Direct pressure - primary method of bleeding control **(Slide 5-23)**
(1) Should be applied with a sterile dressing when possible
(2) Should utilize just enough pressure to control bleeding
(3) A bandage can be applied while maintaining direct pressure
(4) Pressure bandage **(Slide 5-24)**
(a) A 3-4 inch bandage should be placed over the dressing
(b) Be careful not to obstruct distal flow of blood
(c) The ideal is enough to control but not enough to obstruct
(d) If distal pulse is covered with bandage capillary refill can determine flow
(e) Do not remove dressing once it is applied or clot will be removed
(5) Care should be taken with head wound to avoid injury to brain
(6) Pressure devices - air splints and PASG **(Slide 5-25)**
d) Elevation can be utilized in extremity or head wounds to decrease pressure in the bleeding area

Content

e) Splinting can decrease the rate of flow by decreasing muscular activity and aggravation of fractures

f) Pressure points are used when the above measures fail to control bleeding

(1) Pressure over a major artery proximal to the wound can be a useful method for temporarily stopping arterial hemorrhage

(2) The brachial artery is used in the upper extremity and the femoral in the lower **(Slide 5-26)**

(3) Pressure is applied over the site and bleeding should stop immediately

(4) A pressure bandage can be applied while pressure is maintained

(5) Other sites for pressure points include

(a) The temporal for scalp bleeding

(b) The facial for bleeding in the face

(c) The carotid for uncontrolled bleeding in the neck (this should only be used as a last resort since it interrupts brain circulation)

g) A tourniquet is a method of last resort, after all other methods have failed **(Slide 5-27)**

(1) It totally obstructs blood flow and therefore can potentially result in death of the extremity

(2) The risk benefit consideration

(a) It should only be used when all other methods fail

(b) The concept of accepting total disability to save a life

(3) Method of application

(a) A 3-4 inch piece of material is applied just proximal to the wound **(Slide 5-28)**

(b) A piece of cloth should be 6-8 layers thick

(c) A dowel stick is tied to the material and tightened until bleeding stops **(Slide 5-29)**

(d) Dowel stick is secured in place **(Slide 5-30)**

(e) Clearly note the time in order to attract the attention of emergency department personnel

(f) Once applied, never remove

4. Complications of open wounds **(Slide 5-31)**

a) Infection can occur by introduction of bacteria into open wounds

(1) Use of sterile technique can reduce the chance of infection

(2) When bleeding must be controlled, concern for infection is secondary to bleeding

b) Air embolism may occur with large vein lacerations in the neck and upper chest region

(1) Air can be sucked in when intrathoracic pressure decreases during inspiration

Content

(2) The air bubble can become lodged in a pulmonary vessel causing obstruction to distal flow
(3) An airtight dressing and placing the patient in the Trendelenburg position can prevent air embolism **(Slide 5-32)**

C. Internal bleeding **(Slide 5-33)**
1. Internal bleeding may be obvious when a patient is vomiting blood or when he is bleeding actively from the mouth, nose or rectum
2. Following injury a hematoma may indicate local internal bleeding
3. At other times the EMT must maintain a high index of suspicion based on the mechanism of injury and early signs of shock
4. Major trauma should always provoke a search for these signs
5. Injuries to the trunk, pelvic region and thigh are always of potential concern
6. Medical conditions such as ulcers, ectopic pregnancy and abdominal aneurysms are also a potential cause of internal bleeding
7. Compensatory mechanisms following blood loss **(Slide 5-34)**
a) A number of compensatory mechanisms are used by the body to assure adequate perfusion
b) These mechanisms can be used as predictors of potential blood loss
c) At 10-15% blood loss the veins constrict to maintain the pressure
(1) Veins contain approximately 50% of the blood volume
(2) Constricted veins reduce the size of the vascular space and increase the peripheral resistance
(3) A person who donates blood is an excellent example of someone with this percentage of blood loss
(4) Individuals with blood loss less than 15% are likely not to exhibit signs of shock
(5) A high index of suspicion is needed to assure rapid access to definitive care
d) At 15-30% of blood loss redistribution of blood is initiated through the sympathetic nervous system and epinephrine release **(Slide 5-35)**
(1) The heart rate is increased and the ventricle pumps more forcibly to increase the stroke volume
(2) The arterial system constricts in areas of less importance to redistribute blood to vital organs
(3) Signs and symptoms reflect these compensatory mechanisms
(a) The patient will have a rapid and thready pulse, due to a narrowed pulse pressure
(b) Skin may be pale, cool and sweaty due to epinephrine release
(c) Breathing may be rapid and shallow
(d) The patient may complain of weakness due to decreased flow to skeletal muscle

Content

(e) Orthostatic changes in blood pressure (20 mm/Hg) and pulse (20 beats/min) are possible
(f) Capillary refill will be delayed (greater than 2 sec) due to redistribution
(g) Superficial veins will be flat due to decreased venous pressure
(h) The patient may complain of thirst
(i) The blood pressure and mental state will be maintained by these mechanisms

e) At approximately 30-45% blood loss the patient will begin to decompensate **(Slide 5-36)**
(1) The blood pressure will begin to fall significantly
(2) Hypotension is a late finding in hypovolemic shock
(3) The mental state will begin to deteriorate due to poor brain perfusion
(4) The brain is preserved to the very last
(5) Alteration of mental state is a late sign of shock
(6) The heart will begin to be underperfused and the pulse rate may fall

f) At greater than 45% blood loss the patient is likely to suffer a cardiac arrest **(Slide 5-37)**
(1) The poorly perfused arteries will dilate causing collapse of cardiovascular system
(2) The heart will fail to contract adequately due to hypoxia

8. Early recognition of shock is critical since prehospital cardiac arrest from hypovolemia is almost always irreversible
9. Early surgical intervention can prevent cardiac arrest

D. Treatment of hypovolemic shock **(Slide 5-38)**

1. Airway, breathing and circulation remain the priority treatment method
2. Pneumatic Anti-Shock Garment (PASG) **(Slide 5-39)**

a) Also called Military Anti-Shock Trousers (MAST)
b) The PASG have become a standard field treatment for EMTs
c) Originally used in the military, were used for the field treatment of battlefield casualties
d) The PASG is an air filled garment which surrounds the abdomen and legs and can be inflated up to 100 mm/Hg
e) They collapse the peripheral arteries and increase the peripheral vascular resistance
f) They may shunt small amounts of blood from the abdomen and legs to the central circulation
g) They tamponade bleeding in the legs and abdomen to reduce further bleeding
h) They can be used to splint fractures in the lower extremities
i) Application of the PASG
(1) Remove the clothing on the abdomen and lower extremities **(Slide 5-40)**
(2) Slide the garment beneath the patient or transfer the patient onto the garment **(Slide 5-41)**

Content

(3) Fasten the Velcro on the legs rather than on the abdomen **(Slide 5-42)**
(4) Connect the foot pump and open the valves **(Slide 5-43)**
(5) Inflate the legs then the abdomen **(Slide 5-44)**
(6) Revaluate the patient's vital signs **(Slide 5-45)**
(7) Never deflate the PASG in the field without physician order
(8) Consult local protocols for variations in the application process

j) Indications for PASG **(Slide 5-46)**
(1) PASG are used for hypovolemic and distributive shock, but are contraindicated for cardiogenic shock
(2) They are also used to control bleeding and splint fractures
(3) Consult local protocols for specific criteria, i.e., blood pressure, signs of shock

k) Contraindications **(Slide 5-47)**
(1) The absolute contraindication for PASG is pulmonary edema and uncontrolled intrathoracic bleeding
(2) The abdominal section is contraindicated in advanced stages of pregnancy when there is a probability of a viable fetus, evisceration injury, impaled objects
(3) Consult local protocols for other criteria
(4) The use of PASG has become controversial. In some areas PASG are not used in prehospital care. Consult local protocols

3. Oxygen is administered via high concentration **(Slide 5-48)**
4. Prevent further heat loss but don't overheat the patient
5. Position the patient in the supine position unless other injuries dictate placing the patient on his/her side
6. Transport rapidly to the appropriate facility
7. Again, time to definitive care is an essential aspect of treatment

Section 2

Arteriosclerotic Heart Disease

Objectives
(Slide 5-49)

At the conclusion of the chapter the student will be able to:
1. Define arteriosclerosis and atherosclerosis.
2. List the 3 major controllable risk factors of coronary heart disease.
3. Define the following terms: **Angina** **Myocardial infarction** **Ischemic chest pain**
4. List signs and symptoms of angina and the steps of management.
5. Explain 2 ways that nitroglycerin works to relieve chest pain.
6. List signs and symptoms of myocardial infarction and the steps of management.

Instructor Preparation

Reading preparation for the lesson:

EMT Prehospital Care, Chapter 5, pages 209-216
Local cardiovascular protocols
Performance sheets for cardiovascular skills

Optional reading:

American Heart Association: Advanced Cardiac Life Support Manual. Dallas, Texas, 1985

Bates, B.: A Guide to Physical Examination and History Taking, 5th Ed. J.B. Lippincott Co. Philadelphia, PA, 1991

Content

IV. Significance
A. Statistics **(Slide 5-50)**
1. Leading cause of death in United States
2. 1,500,000 heart attacks occur each year in U.S.
3. 504,000 die of myocardial infarction (M.I.), more than half in prehospital phase of care
4. Most deaths occur two hours following symptoms
B. Myocardial oxygen supply and demand **(Slide 5-51)**
1. Ordinarily coronary blood flow matches needs of myocardium
2. Mismatch occurs when the amount of oxygen needed cannot be met by vessels
a) Increased workload
b) Obstructed flow through vessel does not meet needs
C. Myocardial Ischemia **(Slide 5-52)**
1. Insufficient blood supply to meet oxygen demands
2. May be temporary (angina) or permanent (M.I.)
3. Permanently in M.I. due to sustained oxygen deprivation
D. Ischemic Chest Pain **(Slide 5-53)**
1. Pain which results from ischemia
2. Most common chief complaint for coronary artery disease
3. Review "Herberden" definition of ischemic chest pain
4. Distinction between angina vs. M.I. is primarily on the basis of time and severity
5. Always a priority call due to potential for sudden death

V. Myocardial infarction
A. Overview **(Slide 5-54)**
1. Blockage of a coronary artery resulting in death of heart tissue
2. Commonly referred to as "heart attack"
3. Greatest risk of death is in first hours of symptoms
4. EMS system required to prevent cardiac arrest
B. Pathophysiology **(Slide 5-55)**
1. Caused by arteriosclerosis, thrombus, embolus or spasm
2. Flow distal to plaque or thrombus is blocked resulting in ischemic death of heart tissue
3. Extent of damage determined by location of obstruction
C. Patient assessment
1. Chief complaint - chest pain **(Slide 5-56)**
a) Intense, continuous pain
b) Crushing, pressing, squeezing, tight, vise-like or heavy
c) May place clenched fist against chest to describe location (retrosternum)
d) May describe sense of impending doom
e) May radiate to neck, jaw and arms
f) Pain lasts more than several minutes
g) Not relieved by rest, nitroglycerin or antacids
h) In small percentage of cases patient may not have pain

Content

2. History of the present illness **(Slide 5-57)**
    a) Symptoms can present at rest or during exercise, or even during sleep
    b) Associated symptoms may include:
        (1) Nausea/vomiting
        (2) Weakness
        (3) Shortness of breath
        (4) Palpitations
        (5) Lightheadedness, dizziness
        (6) Fainting
    c) May have similar past experiences with angina or M.I.
3. Past medical history **(Slide 5-58)**
    a) Risk factors of heart disease
        (1) High cholesterol
        (2) High blood pressure
        (3) Smoking
        (4) Diabetes
        (5) Stress
        (6) Obesity
        (7) Heredity
    b) Heart disease, hypertension, diabetes and C.O.P.D.
    c) Medications may reveal a significant past medical history
    d) Previous hospitalizations
4. Physical assessment **(Slide 5-59)**
    a) May be apprehensive, anxious, or have sense of impending doom
    b) Altered mental status may indicate poor perfusion, secondary to heart failure
    c) Vital signs will vary
        (1) May be normal
        (2) May have existing hypertension
        (3) Arrythmias or pump failure may alter vital signs
    d) Head to-toe survey
        (1) Skin usually cool, pale and diaphoretic due to epinephrine release
        (2) Neck veins may be distended if heart failure exists
        (3) Accessory muscles may be active if dyspnea is present
        (4) Rales or wheezing may be present with heart failure
        (5) Check extremities for cyanosis or ankle edema
        (6) Early edema usually points to preexisting heart failure

D. Diagnosis of M.I. **(Slide 5-60)**
1. Relies on history
2. Ischemic chest pain should be considered M.I. until proven otherwise
3. In the absence of pain, other signs and symptoms should be considered
    a) Nausea and vomiting
    b) Dizziness
    c) Pale, sweaty skin
    d) Weakness
    e) Dyspnea

Content

4. Denial is possible symptom of M.I.
    a) EMT must negotiate with patient to go to hospital if M.I. is suspected
    b) Secure assistance from family and friends

E. Treatment - supply and demand **(Slide 5-61)**
1. Demand side is decreased by several factors
    a) Reducing anxiety decreases oxygen consumption
    b) Decreased activity will decrease oxygen consumption
    c) Transport quietly without siren to reduce anxiety
2. Increase the supply side
    a) Administering oxygen
        (1) Medium concentration
        (2) With hypoxia use high concentration
    b) Positioning the patient to facilitate oxygen delivery
3. Monitor patient en route
4. Prepare for cardiac arrest

VI. Angina **(Slide 5-62)**

A. Progressive development phase of arteriosclerotic heart disease

B. Ischemic chest pain caused by exertion or stress

C. Temporary mismatch in supply and demand

D. Usually lasts for 1-5 minutes

E. Relieved by rest or administration of nitroglycerin

F. Nitroglycerin **(Slide 5-63)**
1. Drug taken for angina
2. Shortens or sometimes prevents attacks
3. Reduces the workload of heart by dilating arteries
    a) Decreases peripheral resistance
    b) Dilates veins to decrease venous return
    c) Dilates coronary arteries to increase flow
4. Routes of administration
    a) Under the tongue (sublingual)
    b) Mouth (long acting)
    c) Paste to skin (long acting)
5. Dizziness, fainting and headaches may follow administration due to vasodilation

G. Presentation - chief complaint **(Slide 5-64)**
1. Chest pain for 1-5 minutes
    a) Relieved by rest
    b) Caused by exertion or stress
    c) Described as crushing or pressing

d) Usually not as severe as M.I.

e) Question about changes in the pattern
        (1) Less exertion needed to cause the pain
        (2) More nitroglycerin needed to relieve the pain
        (3) Changes in pattern should be treated as an M.I.

H. History of the present illness **(Slide 5-65)**
1. Similar previous experience is very common

Content

2. Associated signs and symptoms
    a) Nausea
    b) Dizziness
    c) Fainting
    d) Caused by angina or nitroglycerin

I. Past medical history **(Slide 5-66)**
1. May be on several cardiac drugs
2. May have risk factors such as high blood pressure, diabetes or other form of heart disease

J. Physical assessment **(Slide 5-67)**
1. Mental status - may be anxious or lightheaded due to nitroglycerin effects
2. Vital signs are usually normal; preexisting factors may alter findings
    a) Hypertension
    b) Heart failure
    c) Nitroglycerin
3. Head-to-toe survey is usually normal (signs of epinephrine release may suggest M.I.)

K. Diagnosis **(Slide 5-68)**
1. Many angina patients may refuse hospital transport
2. If pattern of disease is worse than usual, they should be treated as an M.I. Factors include:
    (1) More frequent attacks
    (2) Longer pain duration
    (3) Pain precipitated by less exertion or stress
    (4) More nitroglycerin needed to relieve pain (3 or more tablets)
3. If pattern is the same, patient may decline transport

L. Treatment **(Slide 5-69)**
1. Allow patient to take nitroglycerin if patient has prescription
2. If lightheadedness persists transport patient

Chapter 5

Section 3

Pump Failure, Trauma and Intravenous Therapy

Objectives
(Slide 5-70)

At the conclusion of the chapter the student will be able to:	
1.	**Define cardiogenic shock, chronic congestive heart failure and pulmonary edema.**
2.	**List signs and symptoms of pulmonary edema and the steps of management.**
3.	**List the signs and symptoms and steps of management for:** **Dissecting aneurysms** **Abdominal aortic aneurysms**
4.	**List the signs and symptoms and treatment for the following types of trauma to the heart:** **Cardiac contusion** **Pericardial tamponade**
5.	**Describe the technique for starting an intravenous line.**
6.	**List the indications and complications of starting an intravenous line.**

Instructor Preparation

Reading preparation for the lesson:

EMT Prehospital Care, Chapter 5, pages 216-237
Local cardiovascular protocols
Performance sheets for cardiovascular skills

Optional reading:

Bates, B.: A Guide to Physical Examination and History Taking. 5th Ed. J.B. Lippincott Co. Philadelphia, PA, 1991

Content

VII. Pump Failure **(Slide 5-71)**
- A. Causes
  - 1. Acute M.I
    - a) Massive destruction of ventricle due to infarction
    - b) Scarring of ventricular walls over more than one M.I.
  - 2. Gradual and progressive weakening of heart
    - a) Caused by overstretch of ventricle
    - b) Following prolonged hypertension or valvular disease
    - c) Past point where Starling's Law is effective
  - 3. Other causes
    - a) Overdose of cardiac toxic drugs
    - b) Metabolic problems affecting contraction
- B. Pathophysiology **(Slide 5-72)**
  - 1. Backup in veins
    - a) Ventricle cannot expel the blood
    - b) Atrium and venous system backs up
  - 2. Right side
    - a) Backup in the right atrium
    - b) Inferior and superior vena cavae
    - c) Increased pressure to systemic capillaries
    - d) Tissue edema
  - 3. Left side
    - a) Backup through the left atrium
    - b) Pulmonary veins
    - c) Increased pressure to pulmonary capillaries
    - d) Pulmonary edema
  - 4. Poor cardiac output **(Slide 5-73)**
    - a) Weak heart will not eject normal stroke volume
    - b) Cardiac output will fall
    - c) Sympathetic nervous system will increase rate and force of contraction
    - d) Peripheral vasoconstriction
    - e) Physical exam findings
      - (1) Tachycardia
      - (2) Pale, cool and clammy skin
      - (3) Severe cases of hypotension
    - f) Digoxin
      - (1) Taken for chronic heart failure
      - (2) Increases power of contraction
      - (3) Can also affect the conduction system
- C. Right and left heart failure **(Slide 5-74)**
  - 1. Left Heart Failure
    - a) Decreased cardiac output - arterial side signs
      - (1) Altered mental status or weakness
      - (2) Rapid and thready pulse
      - (3) Pallor and cool, clammy skin
      - (4) Dyspnea on exertion

Content

b) Venous backup
(1) Fluid forced into capillaries
(2) Dyspnea
(3) Sitting upright, using accessory muscles
(4) Cyanosis
(5) Coughing up foamy, pink tinged sputum
2. Right heart failure **(Slide 5-75)**
a) Causes
(1) Left heart failure
(2) C.O.P.D.
b) Signs and symptoms
(1) Tissue edema (peripheral edema) **(Slide 5-76)**
(2) Effect of gravity
(a) Dependent portions of the body first
(b) Feet, then ankles with upright patient
(c) Sacrum for supine patient
(d) Legs, sacrum and ascites as disease progresses
(e) In severe cases total body edema (anasarca)
(3) Neck vein distension **(Slide 5-77)**
(a) Increased back-pressure distends veins
(b) Veins in neck visible
(c) Patient is placed at a 45 degree angle to provide baseline
3. Paroxysmal nocturnal dyspnea (PND) **(Slide 5-78)**
a) Sudden dyspnea awaking patient during night
b) During sleep edema in ankle and legs may reenter circulation
c) Increased venous return
d) Left heart failure and pulmonary edema
e) Patient awakes with dyspnea (PND)
f) Dyspnea dissipates when erect due to fluid shifts
4. Orthopnea
a) Patient compensates for PND by sleeping more upright
b) Adds pillows or sleeps in chair
c) Degree of orthopnea characterized by number of pillows (or chair)
D. History and physical findings with heart failure
1. History **(Slide 5-79)**
a) Chief complaint
(1) Most common is dyspnea
(2) Chest pain may be present in some patients
(3) Other complaints
(a) Weakness
(b) Dizziness
(c) Altered mental state
(d) Fainting

Content

b) History of present illness **(Slide 5-80)**
   (1) Paroxysmal nocturnal dyspnea
   (2) Dyspnea on exertion
   (3) Orthopnea
   (4) Pink tinged sputum or cough
   (5) Progressive fatigue
   (6) Systemic edema
   (7) Associated with chest pain or palpitations

c) Past medical history **(Slide 5-81)**
   (1) Heart failure
   (2) Angina
   (3) Myocardial infarction
   (4) Hypertension
   (5) C.O.P.D.

d) Medications **(Slide 5-82)**
   (1) Digoxin
   (2) Lasix
   (3) Other cardiac medications

e) Physical examination **(Slide 5-83)**
   (1) Mental status
      (a) Early - agitated, anxious or restless
      (b) Late - hypoxic, lethargic, unresponsive
   (2) Vital signs
      (a) May vary depending on condition and past history
      (b) Tachycardia is common early but hypoxia may result in arrhythmias, i.e., bradycardia
      (c) Rapid, deep breathing in early phase
      (d) Slow or shallow breathing as hypoxia becomes worse
      (e) Blood pressure
         i) May be hypertensive due to preexisting condition
         ii) Hypotension is ominous sign related to cardiogenic shock
   (3) Head-to-toe survey
      (a) Skin may be pale, cool, diaphoretic or cyanotic
      (b) Accessory muscle use and distended neck veins
      (c) Breath sounds may reveal rales, rhonchi or wheezes
         i) Early - rales at bases
         ii) Late - rales higher up
         iii) Position may affect location of rales
         iv) Describing rales
            i) Basilar
            ii) According to level
            iii) Atelectasis may produce false rales
      (d) Pink tinged sputum
      (e) Edema
         i) Ankle
         ii) Ascites
         iii) Anasarca

Content

2. Treatment **(Slide 5-84)**
    a) Increase oxygen delivery
        (1) High - concentration oxygen via nonrebreather
        (2) Adjusted for C.O.P.D. patients as needed
        (3) Positive pressure ventilation if needed
            (a) Mental state - depressed
            (b) Signs of severe hypoxia
    b) Position
        (1) Sitting position if responsive
        (2) Supine if positive pressure is required
    c) Decreasing oxygen demand
        (1) Calming patient reduces oxygen consumption
        (2) Siren and lights may increase oxygen demand

VIII. Aneurysms of the aorta **(Slide 5-85)**
- A. Outpouching of the wall of the aorta
- B. Dissection (the thoracic aorta) or rupture (the abdominal aorta)
- C. Caused by arteriosclerosis
- D. May have a history of aneurysm
- E. Survival requires rapid surgical intervention
- F. Thoracic dissecting aneurysm **(Slide 5-86)**
- G. Abdominal aortic aneurysm **(Slide 5-87)**
    1. Occurs primarily in older patients
    2. If the aorta ruptures, severe and often fatal hemorrhage results
    3. Signs and symptoms
        a) Abdominal tenderness, rigidity and guarding
        b) Pulsatile mass in midabdomen
        c) Pulsations may be felt normally, particularly in thin people
        d) Signs of hypovolemic shock
            (1) Delayed capillary refill
            (2) Tachycardia
            (3) Cool, pale and sweaty skin
            (4) Hypotension
            (5) Altered mental state
    4. Treatment **(Slide 5-88)**
        a) Surgical intervention is a major factor in outcome
        b) PASG may be useful to elevate blood pressure and tamponade bleeding

IX. Pulmonary embolus **(Slide 5-89)**
- A. Causes
    1. Embolism can become lodged in the pulmonary artery
    2. Venous thrombosis is the source for most emboli (thrombophlebitis)
    3. Prolonged bed rest following surgery
    4. Birth control pills
    5. Fat emboli from long bone fractures
    6. Large emboli may obstruct a major pulmonary artery causing right heart failure
- B. Signs and symptoms **(Slide 5-90)**
    1. Sudden onset of chest pain or dyspnea
        a) Usually sharp, pleuritic pain
        b) May be unilateral chest pain

Content

2. Cough and possibly bloody expectorations (hemoptysis)
3. History **(Slide 5-91)**
    a) Phlebitis
    b) Unilateral leg swelling
    c) Calf tenderness
    d) Prolonged bedrest or travel (car trip)
    e) Recent surgery
    f) Use of birth control pills
4. Pertinent Physical Findings **(Slide 5-92)**
    a) Tachypnea is almost always present
    b) Pleural friction rub or normal breath sounds
    c) Tachycardia and hypotension in severe cases
    d) Significant obstruction to flow out of the right ventricle (rare)
        (1) Neck vein distension
        (2) Systemic edema
        (3) Cyanosis
        (4) Altered mental status may be present

C. Treatment **(Slide 5-93)**
1. High concentration oxygen
2. Signs of severe hypoxia or hypotension or distension of neck veins = rapid transport

X. Dysrhythmias **(Slide 5-94)**

A. Most common cause of sudden death in patients suffering from heart disease and myocardial infarction

B. May result in heart failure and pulmonary edema and cardiogenic shock

C. Treatment
1. Administration of drugs
2. Electric shock
3. Pacemaker therapy
4. Treatment of the underlying cause
5. EMT has limited ability to recognize and treat
6. Must rely on supportive therapy, i.e., oxygen which may abolish some dysrhymtias

D. EMT must rely on physical findings, especially pulse rate, quality and rhythm to suspect dysrhythmias

E. Slow rates: bradycardia **(Slide 5-95)**
1. Can reduce cardiac output
    a) Cardiac output = pulse rate x stroke volume
    b) Decreased rate can decrease C.O.
2. Examples
    a) Normal - (HR) 70 x (SV) 70 = (C.O.) 4900 ml per minute
    b) Bradycardia - (HR) 40 x (SV) 70 = (C.O.) 2800 ml per minute
        (1) Reduced cardiac output
        (2) Hypotension and shock may occur

F. Too fast: tachycardia **(Slide 5-96)**
1. Increased heart rate will generally increase cardiac output
    a) Response to exercise or fever
    b) Compensatory response to hypovolemia
    c) Mediated by autonomic nervous system

Content

2. If the heart rate exceeds 180, the cardiac output will usually begin to fall
   a) Decreased ventricular filling time
   b) 70% occurs during diastole
   c) 30% via atrial contraction
3. Heart rate and myocardial oxygen needs
   a) Rest period of the heart is during diastole
   b) Heart rate of 75/min = 40 seconds of rest
   c) Heart rate of 200/min 28 seconds of rest.
   d) Faster rates = increased oxygen use and increased need
   e) Coronaries fill during diastole
   f) Some areas of the ventricles perfused during diastole
4. Examples **(Slide 5-97)**
   a) Normal - (HR) 70 x (SV) 70 = (CO) 4900 ml per minute
   b) Fast - (HR) 130 x (SV) 70 = (CO) 9100 ml per minute
5. Palpitations **(Slide 5-98)**
   a) Patients with rapid heart rhythms or extra beats may describe sensation of palpitations
   b) If the patient shows signs of shock, treat as you would a patient with cardiogenic shock
   c) Other secondary effects
      (1) Heart failure
      (2) Myocardial infarction
      (3) Syncope
      (4) Dyspnea
      (5) Dizziness

G. Irregular rhythms **(Slide 5-99)**
1. An EMT may note an irregularity when checking the pulse
2. Some irregular rhythms may cause a fall in cardiac output
3. May be quite stable
4. May be precursors of fatal events
5. Field diagnosis and treatment impossible without ECG
6. Prepare for cardiac arrest in setting of MI

H. Syncope **(Slide 5-100)**
1. Syncope or a sudden loss of consciousness may be by dysrhythmias
2. Prolonged pause between beats
3. Very rapid rhythms
4. May be caused by a number of other conditions

I. Pacemakers **(Slide 5-101)**
1. Implanted to control certain dysrhythmias, and to provide a backup if the pacemaker fails
2. Pacemakers also can fail if:
   a) Patients return to their own rhythm
   b) Own rhythm is too slow for adequate cardiac output
3. Does not alter assessment and treatment of a patient except location during defibrillation

Content

XI. Traumatic cardiac emergencies **(Slide 5-102)**

A. Cardiac contusion **(Slide 5-103)**

1. Significance
   - a) Blunt trauma to the chest can bruise the heart
   - b) May range from a minor bruise to disruption of myocardium with pericardial tamponade
   - c) Most do not result in severe complications
   - d) Main complication is dysrhythmias
2. Causes
   - a) Any blunt chest trauma
   - b) Steering wheel injury most common
3. Signs and symptoms **(Slide 5-104)**
   - a) Suspected from the mechanism of injury
   - b) Signs of trauma over the anterior chest
   - c) Cannot be diagnosed definitively in the field
   - d) Irregular pulse or a slow pulse should increase your index of suspicion
4. Treatment **(Slide 5-105)**
   - a) No definite treatment for this condition in the field
   - b) Be aware of the possibility of tamponade
   - c) High - concentration oxygen
   - d) Treat for shock

B. Cardiac tamponade or pericardial tamponade **(Slide 5-106)**

1. Heart may bleed into the pericardium due to penetrating wounds or rupture of ventricle
2. Signs can develop at different rates depending on the size of the wound and affected chamber
3. Gunshot wounds usually cause rapid and fatal hemorrhage if the ventricles are penetrated
4. Signs and symptoms **(Slide 5-107)**
   - a) Site of chest injury
   - b) Signs of shock
   - c) Neck vein distension
   - d) Capillary refill test may be normal
   - e) Decrease pulse pressure
5. Treatment **(Slide 5-108)**
   - a) Rapid transport to the hospital
   - b) PASG may be useful; check local protocols
   - c) High concentration oxygen
   - d) Patient's require decompression of sac with a needle in hospital

XII. Intravenous therapy **(Slide 5-109)**

A. Purposes of an IV in prehospital care

1. Administer fluid
2. Administer medications
3. Sample of blood

B. Risk benefit considerations

1. Fluid administration is a temporary resuscitation method
2. Often bleeding exceeds potential for fluid replacement
3. Time needed to start an IV may negatively impact patient care
4. Ideally IV should be started en route to hospital

Content

C. Types of fluid **(Slide 5-110)**
1. Crystalloids
a) Fluids containing water electrolytes and glucose
b) Used to establish medication administration route or fluid replacement
c) Types and most common use
(1) Normal saline - fluid replacement
(2) Ringers lactate - fluid replacement
(3) Dextrose 5% and water - keep vein open for medication administration
(4) 50% dextrose to treat hypoglycemia
2. Colloids
a) Contain large molecules, i.e., proteins which cannot diffuse out of vascular space
b) Are used to create "pulling" (osmotic) force to hold fluid within vascular space
c) Examples
(1) Plasmanate
(2) Albumin
(3) Dextran
d) Important in the treatment of hypovolemia
e) Not often used in prehospital care due to shelf life and expense

D. Intravenous equipment **(Slide 5-111)**
1. IV administration sets
a) Tubing connected to solutions to administer fluid or medication
b) Inserts in IV bag at one end and IV catheter at other end
c) Varies according to volume and rate of administration
d) Macrodrip
(1) Used to administer high volume quickly
(2) 10 gtts = 1 ml
(3) Used commonly with normal saline and ringer's
e) Microdrip
(1) Used to keep vein open and administer medications
(2) 60 gtts = 1 ml
(3) Prevents fluid overload
f) Volutrols or Burotrols
(1) Used to limit the volume of fluid during medication administration
(2) Contain no more than 100 ml
(3) Chamber is filled from a larger IV bag and clamped between bag and chamber of Volutrol or Burotrol
g) Extension sets are used to lengthen the tubing, making it easier to change solutions

Content

2. Catheters **(Slide 5-112)**
    a) Most common is over-the-needle catheter
        (1) Needle is inserted in vein and removed after insertion
        (2) Needle must be disposed of properly
        (3) Several sizes ranging from 12 gauge to 25 gauge are available
            (a) Larger gauges (12-16) are used to administer high volume or viscous solutions
            (b) Medium gauges (18-20) are used for medication administration and KVO lines
            (c) Smaller gauges (21-25) are used for difficult venipunctures or children and infants
    b) Over-the-catheter needle is used for central IV insertion
    c) Butterfly needles
        (1) Used for difficult venipunctures and children and infants
        (2) Not commonly used in prehospital care
        (3) More likely to "infiltrate" into

E. Starting an IV
1. Checks for necessary equipment **(Slide 5-113)**
    a) IV solution (D_5W, Ringer's lactate)
    b) IV tubing
    c) IV catheter
    d) Venous constricting band
    e) Band-Aid
    f) Betadine swab
    g) Tape
    h) Gloves
    i) Goggles
2. Properly examines IV bag for leaks **(Slide 5-114)**
    a) Type of solution
    b) Contamination
    c) Expiration date
3. Connects IV tubing and solution aseptically **(Slide 5-115)**
4. Correctly prepares IV solution and administration set **(Slide 5-116)**
    a) Drip chamber 1/2 full
    b) IV solution in tubing without air
5. Prepares patient psychologically
6. Applies venous constricting band, and checks for radial pulse **(Slide 5-117)**
7. Palpates vein for resilience
8. Cleanses puncture site area with Betadine in increasing concentric circles which spiral outward **(Slide 5-118)**
9. Stabilizes vein aseptically with thumb and fingers **(Slide 5-119)**
10. Enter skin aseptically at a 45 degree angle with the over-the-needle catheter bevel-up **(Slide 5-120)**
11. Punctures vein, observes for flashback, and advances the over-the-needle catheter 1 mm more into vein **(Slide 5-121)**
12. Stabilizes the needle, and advances the catheter aseptically **(Slide 5-122)**

Content

13. Withdraws needle with digital pressure proximal to venipuncture site to inhibit bleeding **(Slide 5-123)**
14. Connects IV tubing to IV catheter **(Slide 5-124)**
15. Removes venous constricting band **(Slide 5-125)**
16. Opens drip chamber clamp to assure free flow and adjusts to appropriate drip rate **(Slide 5-126)**
17. Applies Band-Aid over puncture site, and anchors IV catheter with chevron **(Slide 5-127)**
18. Secures tubing with tape, leaving the tubing/catheter communication area exposed **(Slide 5-128)**
19. Rechecks drip rate
20. Labels IV puncture area with the IV catheter gauge size, date, time, and candidate's initials

F. Complications **(Slide 5-129)**
1. Infection
    a) Poor sterile technique can lead to infections
    b) When sterile technique has been compromised the emergency department should be notified
    c) With seriously ill patients the IV line may have to remain until hospital arrival
2. Pyrogenic reaction
    a) Allergic reaction to IV solution
    b) Signs and symptoms
        (1) Fever
        (2) Chills
        (3) Vomiting
        (4) Back pain
        (5) Cardiovascular collapse
    c) Stop IV and change solution and advise hospital personnel
3. Infiltration
    a) Fluid leaks into subcutaneous tissues
    b) Due to misplaced catheter or rupture of vein
    c) Rupture of vein may be due to fluid administration with tourniquet in place
4. Thrombophlebitis (inflammation of vein) may occur due to poor sterile technique or prolonged IV therapy
5. Circulatory overload **(Slide 5-130)**
    a) Due to runaway IV solution
    b) Minimized by use of microdrip, careful observation and small IV bags
    c) May cause heart failure with MI and other heart patients
    d) careful monitoring is essential
6. Air embolism
    a) Caused by introducing air from injection or IV line
    b) Be careful to clear syringe and IV line prior to administration
    c) Large boluses of air may cause heart or lung embolus

Content

7. Catheter shear
    a) Caused by tearing of catheter during insertion
    b) May cause pulmonary embolism
    c) Never reinsert needle into catheter after removing
    d) Avoid twisting catheter around needle
    e) If occurs, report to hospital staff
8. Arterial puncture
    a) Artery may be cannulated accidentally during insertion
    b) Evidenced by bright red blood running up IV line
    c) Remove immediately and start new IV line
    d) Hold pressure over site for at least 5 minutes
    e) Avoid venipuncture over sites of arteries

G. EMT safety **(Slide 5-131)**
1. Wear protective gear whenever dealing with body fluids
2. Gloves, goggles and sometimes masks
3. Report needle sticks to self
4. Carry sharps container to scene

Chapter 5

CARDIOVASCULAR EMERGENCIES

Examination

1. Inadequate tissue perfusion and oxygenation is referred to as:

    a. clinical death
    b. heart failure
    c. shock
    d. respiratory failure

2. Each tissue and organ has the ability to control its own blood flow through the __________ in direct response to oxygen needs.

    a. arterioles
    b. veins
    c. lungs
    d. capillaries

3. The _______________ if a large number of tissues in the body require more oxygen at the same time.

    a. cardiac output will increase
    b. peripheral vascular resistance will increase
    c. cardiac output will decrease
    d. venous return will decrease

4. The "fight or flight" response is mediated by the hormone:

    a. histamine
    b. epinephrine
    c. atropine
    d. dopamine

5. Which of the following are effects of adrenaline release?

    a. decrease in cardiac output, increased blood flow to the brain, pupils dilate
    b. decrease in cardiac output, increased blood flow to the brain, pupils constrict
    c. increase in cardiac output, increased blood flow to the brain, pupils dilate
    d. increase in cardiac output, increase in blood flow to the brain, pupils constrict

6. During shock, there is a redistribution of blood away from some organs to assure perfusion of more vital organs. Of the following organs, which one would be the first to be deprived of blood in shock?

   a. heart
   b. kidneys
   c. lungs
   d. brain

7. Receptors located in the __________ monitor blood pressure as well as the oxygen and carbon dioxide content of blood:

   a. lungs and heart
   b. lungs and aorta
   c. pulmonary artery and carotid artery
   d. carotid artery and aorta

8. Shock that occurs secondary to blood loss is called:

   a. cardiogenic shock
   b. distributive shock
   c. obstructive shock
   d. hypovolemic shock

9. Another term for vasodilatory shock is:

   a. neurogenic shock
   b. hypovolemic shock
   c. cardiogenic shock
   d. septic shock

10. Which of the following may cause vasodilatory shock?

    a. bilateral fractured femurs
    b. spinal cord injury
    c. blood clot in the brain
    d. dehydration

11. The collapse of a lung on the side of an injury associated with a shift of the mediastinum to the opposite side of the chest and the collapse of the lung is called:

    a. cardiac tamponade
    b. hemothorax
    c. tension pneumothorax
    d. subcutaneous emphysema

12. Signs of cardiac tamponade include:

    a. distended neck veins and absent breath sounds on the left side
    b. flat neck veins and absent breath sounds on the left side
    c. distended neck veins and normal breath sounds
    d. flat neck veins and normal breath sounds

13. Severe anemia is characterized by:

    a. hypotension
    b. a decrease in the amount of hemoglobin
    c. an increase in the amount of hemoglobin
    d. hypovolemia

14. Bleeding characterized by a steady flow dark red color is termed:

    a. peripheral
    b. venous
    c. systemic
    d. arterial

15. Which of the following is a characteristic of arterial bleeding?

    a. pulsatile flow
    b. dark red color
    c. occurs in abrasion type injuries
    d. always requires pressure point to control

16. The proper order to be used to control bleeding is:

    a. pressure point, elevation, direct pressure, tourniquet
    b. elevation, direct pressure, tourniquet, pressure point
    c. elevation, direct pressure, pressure point, tourniquet
    d. direct pressure, elevation, pressure point, tourniquet

17. The pressure point for the lower extremity is located over the:

    a. femoral artery
    b. radial artery
    c. ulnar artery
    d. brachial artery

18. The pressure point for the scalp is located over the:

    a. carotid artery
    b. facial artery
    c. temporal artery
    d. brachial artery

19. An appropriate device to be used for a tourniquet is:

    a. a wire
    b. a rope
    c. a hanger
    d. a folded triangular bandage

20. Orthostatic changes are first appreciated by a pulse rate _________ beats per minute when a patient is placed upright.

    a. increase of 5
    b. increase of 20
    c. decrease of 5
    d. decrease of 20

21. Which of the following signs is the first to occur following acute blood loss?

    a. pale skin
    b. tachycardia
    c. delayed capillary refill
    d. hypotension

22. Pulse rate increase, delayed capillary refill and orthostatic hypotension usually first appear when blood loss exceeds ____________ of total volume.

    a. 5%
    b. 10%
    c. 15%
    d. 30%

23. Which of the following best describes the sequence of the signs of hypovolemic shock?

    a. rapid pulse, delayed capillary refill, hypotension, coma
    b. hypotension, rapid pulse, delayed capillary refill, coma
    c. coma, rapid pulse, hypotension, delayed capillary refill
    d. rapid pulse, coma, hypotension, delayed capillary refill

24. Use of the Pneumatic Anti-Shock Garment (PASG) is contraindicated in the presence of:

    a. pulmonary edema
    b. hypovolemic shock
    c. septic shock
    d. anaphylactic shock

25. The PASG may be useful in the prehospital treatment of all of the following forms of shock except:

a. cardiogenic shock
b. distributive shock
c. obstructive shock
d. hypovolemic shock

26. When removing the PASG in the hospital, the blood pressure should be maintained by:

a. deflating legs first
b. deflating slowly while administering IV fluids
c. increasing the heart rate
d. leg elevation

27. Any patient in shock who also requires the PASG must also:

a. have their cervical spine immobilized
b. be given oxygen
c. have two large bore IV's started prior to transport
d. have their blood pressure stabilized prior to transport

28. The upper margin of the abdominal section of the PASG should be placed no higher than the:

a. umbilicus
b. iliac crest of the pelvis
c. lower margin of the rib cage
d. suprapubic region

29. Unavoidable risk factors of coronary artery disease include:

a. age, race, and high blood pressure
b. cigarette smoking, diet, and high blood pressure
c. age, sex, and race
d. sex, race, and high blood pressure

30. The leading cause of death in the United States is ________________ and its resulting complications.

a. cancer
b. accidental death
c. arteriosclerotic heart disease
d. AIDS

31. Angina pectoris:

a. usually results from exertion or stress
b. is also known as a myocardial infarction
c. causes permanent damage to the heart
d. is usually not relieved by rest

32. The term infarction refers to:

    a. a state of decreased blood flow to an organ or tissue
    b. an obstruction of blood flow resulting in death of heart cells
    c. a reversible condition that affects the myocardium
    d. the pain felt by a patient experiencing a myocardial infarction

33. All of the following are major **avoidable** risk factors of coronary artery disease, except:

    a. smoking
    b. diet
    c. hypertension
    d. heredity

34. All of the following are methods through which patients take nitroglycerin:

    a. swallow tablets, apply paste to skin, inject into muscle
    b. inject into muscles, swallow tablet, place under tongue
    c. apply paste to skin, swallow tablet, place under tongue
    d. place under tongue, inject into muscle, apply paste to skin

35. An insufficient supply of blood through a vessel that results in oxygen deprivation to tissue best describes:

    a. ischemia
    b. hypoxia
    c. anoxia
    d. anemia

36. Sudden cardiac death is characterized by:

    a. pressure-like chest pain
    b. pleuritic chest pain
    c. cardiac arrest
    d. nausea and vomiting

37. Nausea, vomiting, weakness, shortness of breath, palpitations, light-headedness, sweating, dizziness and loss of consciousness are all possible associated signs of:

    a. cardiac arrest
    b. angina pectoris
    c. myocardial infarction
    d. oxygen toxicity

38. Chest pain which can be increased by breathing best describes:

a. pleuritic chest pain
b. angina pectoris
c. myocardial infarction
d. cardiogenic shock

39. The duration of the pain and whether the pain was caused and relieved in its typical pattern is part of the:

a. chief complaint
b. history of present illness
c. medications and allergies
d. past medical history

40. Most people who die from myocardial infarctions die

a. within 30 minutes of the onset of symptoms
b. after bypass surgery
c. within 1 hour of the onset of symptoms
d. before the patient reaches a hospital

41. Nitroglycerin acts to relieve chest pain by which of the following mechanisms?

a. increases heart rate
b. increases the force of contraction
c. vasodilation
d. increases blood pressure

42. Which of the following terms best describes the classic pain of coronary artery diseases, such as angina or myocardial infarction?

a. sharp
b. squeezing
c. pleuritic
d. stabbing

43. A common side effect of taking nitroglycerin is:

a. hives
b. arrhythmias
c. headache
d. edema

44. The two most important factors in the treatment of cardiac arrest are defibrillation and:

a. CPR
b. drug therapy
c. intubation
d. catheterization

Match the type of heart failure in column B with the signs and symptoms in column A:

Column A	Column B
45. rales	a. right heart failure
46. ankle edema	b. left heart failure
47. frothy sputum	
48. distended neck veins	
49. ascites	

50. Paroxsymal nocturnal dyspnea is characterized by:

    a. waking up in the middle of the night with difficulty breathing
    b. sleeping on two or more pillows
    c. cessation of breathing during sleep
    d. sudden onset of chest pain while sleeping

51. A patient tells you that he must sleep on three pillows or he experiences difficulty breathing. This condition is called:

    a. eupnea
    b. tachypnea
    c. orthopnea
    d. dyspnea

52. An acute myocardial infarction is a common cause of:

    a. hypovolemic shock
    b. angina pectoris
    c. cor pulmonale
    d. cardiogenic shock

53. When the left ventricle cannot pump out an adequate amount of blood and blood backs up through the atria and pulmonary system, this best describes:

    a. hypovolemia
    b. obstructive shock
    c. acute pulmonary edema
    d. distributive shock

54. The most common cause of right heart failure is

    a. C.O.P.D.
    b. pericarditis
    c. angina
    d. pneumonia

55. It is best to auscultate lungs with the patient in the:

    a. supine position
    b. prone position
    c. sitting position
    d. Trendelenburg position

56 A patient with acute pulmonary edema who is becoming sleepy, is cyanotic and has barely perceptible chest wall movement should be treated with:

    a. supplemental oxygen via Venturi mask
    b. supplemental oxygen via bag valve mask
    c. supplemental oxygen via nasal cannula
    d. supplemental oxygen via simple face mask

57. Pink frothy sputum which may be present in a patient with pulmonary edema is caused by:

    a. leakage of red blood cells through the pulmonary capillaries
    b. a rupture of the arterioles in the lungs
    c. trauma to the pulmonary system
    d. usage of the PASG

58. The term used to describe a fast heart rate (greater than 100) is:

    a. bradycardia
    b. tachycardia
    c. hypocardia
    d. hypercardia

59. Very rapid heart rates may cause decreased cardiac output due to a shortened:

    a. contraction
    b. relaxation period (diastole)
    c. atrial contraction
    d. depolarization

60. Palpitations can best be described as:

    a. a spasm of the myocardium
    b. an extra beat, skipping, or jumping in the chest
    c. sharp chest pain radiating to the left arm
    d. chest discomfort relieved with nitroglycerin

61. Your first action to control arterial bleeding from the arm is:

    a. apply a tourniquet between the wound and heart
    b. apply a pressure point over the brachial artery
    c. clamp the vessel with a hemostat
    d. apply direct pressure to the wound and elevate the arm

62. If the above action is not successful, then you should:

    a. apply a tourniquet between the wound and heart
    b. apply a pressure point over the popliteal artery
    c. clamp the vessel with a hemostat
    d. apply a pressure point over the brachial artery

63. If this is not successful, then you should:

    a. apply a tourniquet between the wound and heart
    b. apply a pressure point over the popliteal artery
    c. clamp the vessel with a hemostat
    d. apply a pressure point over the brachial artery

64. A patient complaining of a tearing type of pain in his abdomen radiating to his back appears to be cool, pale and diaphoretic. His neck veins are flat and you note a pulsatile mass in his abdomen. His blood pressure is 72/40, pulse is 132, and respiratory rate is 26. Based on the above you suspect the patient has:

    a. an acute myocardial infarction
    b. severe heart failure
    c. a bleeding ulcer
    d. an abdominal aortic aneurysm

65. Your initial treatment of the above patient includes:

    a. administering oxygen via nasal cannula, application of the PASG, and rapid transport
    b. administering oxygen via non-rebreather mask, application of the PASG, and rapid transport
    c. placing the patient in Fowler's position, administering oxygen via non-rebreather mask, and application of the PASG
    d. placing the patient in Fowler's position, rapid transport, and application of the PASG

66. This patient is in __________ shock:

    a. septic
    b. neurogenic
    c. hypovolemic
    d. cardiogenic

67. You respond to a call and find a 30 year old female who "fainted" while being the bridesmaid at a wedding. The patient is now alert and oriented and has perfectly normal physical exam. This patient most likely suffered a transient form of ___________ shock.

a. obstructive
b. vasodilatory
c. hypovolemic
d. cardiogenic

68. What action should her friend have taken to facilitate her recovery?

a. sit the patient up.
b. administer ammonia capsules
c. elevate her legs while supine
d. administer glucose by mouth

69. A patient who has "squeezing" substernal chest pain that was relieved by nitroglycerin after 3 minutes has most likely suffered from:

a. heart failure
b. cardiac syncope
c. cardiogenic shock
d. angina pectoris

70. What is the most common cause of death related to patients with an MI?

a. shock
b. ventricular fibrillation
c. pulmonary edema
d. respiratory failure

Chapter 6

CARDIOPULMONARY RESUSCITATION AND EMT-DEFIBRILLATION

Materials and Equipment for Lesson

1. Slides, overhead transparencies, drawings or flipcharts
2. Adult and pediatric CPR training manikins and infection control supplies
3. Mechanical CPR device (optional)
4. Stretcher with CPR board
5. Ventilation devices (BVM, pocket mask, etc.) and airways
6. Manual, automatic or semi-automatic defibrillator
7. Training electrode pads and arrhythmia simulator
8. Handouts
    - CPR critical performance sheets
    - CPR handout
    - EMT-D critical performance sheets
    - EMT-D handout
9. Slide projector, overhead projector, flipchart and/or blackboard

Section 1

Cardiopulmonary Resuscitation

Objectives
(Slide 6-1)

At the conclusion of the chapter the students will be able to:

1. **Describe the correct steps of performance for:**
    - **One rescuer CPR**
    - **Two rescuer CPR**
    - **Child CPR**
    - **Infant CPR**

2. **List 3 complications of CPR.**

3. **List 5 instances when CPR can be stopped by an EMT.**

4. **Provide 1 special consideration for each of the following cardiac arrest victims:**
    - **Drowning**
    - **Accident**
    - **Electrocution**
    - **Patients with a stoma**

5. **Describe the appropriate actions for performing CPR under the following conditions:**
    - **Down a stairway**
    - **Ground level**
    - **In a moving ambulance**

Instructor Preparation

Reading preparation for the lesson:

EMT Prehospital Care, Chapter 6, pages 238-260
Local protocols for cardiac arrest
Performance sheets for CPR

Optional reading:

Safer P., Bircher N.: Cardiopulmonary Cerebral Resuscitation. 3rd Edition, W.B. Saunders. Philadelphia, PA, 1988

Suggested Learning Activities
Using a lecture format with the aid of slides, overhead transparencies or charts, provide an overview of cardiopulmonary resuscitation. **Demonstrate the adult and pediatric skills.** **Provide a scenario demonstration of a typical cardiac arrest with integration between lay rescuers and EMTs.** **Demonstrate CPR while moving along ground level, down stairs and if possible in the ambulance.**

Content

I. Overview **(Slide 6-2)**

- A. Airway obstruction, respiratory and circulatory arrest are primary concerns of the EMT
- B. CPR is major component of the primary survey and resuscitation process
- C. It incorporates management of several problems
  - 1. Airway obstruction i.e. by the tongue
  - 2. Respiratory failure or arrest
  - 3. Cardiac arrest
- D. CPR is usually a temporary measure prior to defibrillation or other ALS interventions
- E. Must be performed with careful attention to performance to assure oxygenation and perfusion of the brain

II. Performance of one rescuer CPR

- A. Establishing unresponsiveness and positioning the patient **(Slide 6-3)**
  - 1. Gently shake the patient and shout "Are you okay?"
  - 2. Suspected spinal injury - apply a painful stimulus such as a pinch
- B. Call for help
  - 1. Most arrest victims are discovered by lay rescuers
  - 2. Alerts others within the sound of his/her voice to
    - a) Activate EMS system
    - b) Assist in the care of the patient
- C. Position the patient **(Slide 6-4)**
  - 1. Position supine
  - 2. Log roll if spinal injury is suspected
  - 3. Support head and spine during the procedure
- D. Airway **(Slide 6-5)**
  - 1. The tongue is the most common cause of obstruction
  - 2. Tilting the head and lifting the jaw opens the airway
  - 3. Two basic procedures for opening the airway
    - a) Head tilt-chin lift **(Slide 6-6)**
      - (1) Fingers of one hand along margin of jaw
      - (2) Lift jaw anteriorly without closing mouth
      - (3) Perform a head tilt with the other hand
    - b) Jaw thrust (without head tilt) **(Slide 6-7)**
      - (1) Used with suspected cervical spine injury
      - (2) Index and middle fingers at angle of the jaw
      - (3) Thumbs on the cheekbones
      - (4) Displace the jaw without tilting the head
- E. Breathing
  - 1. Assessment **(Slide 6-8)**
    - a) Look for chest rise
    - b) Listen for the movement of air
    - c) Feel for the movement of air
    - d) Breathing patient, maintain airway patency
    - e) Not breathing, positive pressure ventilations

Content

2. Positive pressure ventilation
    a) Methods (advantages - disadvantages)
        (1) Mouth to mouth **(Slide 6-9)**
            (a) Reliable tidal volumes
            (b) Low concentration of oxygen
            (c) Infection control issues
        (2) Pocket mask **(Slide 6-10)**
            (a) Reliable tidal volumes
            (b) Moderate oxygen concentrations
        (3) Bag-valve-mask **(Slide 6-11)**
            (a) Low tidal volumes
            (b) High concentration of oxygen
            (c) Two handed technique recommended
        (4) Manually triggered demand valve resuscitator **(Slide 6-12)**
            (a) Reliable tidal volumes
            (b) 100% oxygen
            (c) May lead to gastric distension
    b) Technique **(Slide 6-13)**
        (1) Administer two smooth breaths (1-1.5 seconds per breath) while observing for chest rise
        (2) Chest excursion is the best indicator of an effective ventilation
        (3) Average adult requires tidal volume of approximately 800-1200 ml of air
        (4) After each breath, remove your mouth from the victim's mouth and inhale
        (5) If you encounter resistance, reopen the airway and attempt to ventilate again
        (6) If still unsuccessful, then the obstructed airway procedure should be followed

F. Circulation
    1. Pulse check **(Slide 6-14)**
        a) The absence of a pulse is the primary indicator of cardiac arrest
        b) Slide your index and middle finger in the groove between the larynx and sternocleidomastoid muscle
        c) Palpate gently for 5-10 seconds
        d) If you feel a pulse, continue to maintain the airway and provide positive pressure ventilations
        e) If no pulse is felt, the need for cardiac compressions has been established
    2. Activation of EMS system
        a) Lay rescuers would activate the EMS system at this point
    3. External cardiac compressions **(Slide 6-15)**
        a) Provide blood flow in two ways
            (1) Changes in the intrathoracic pressure
            (2) Squeezing the heart between the sternum and the spine
            (3) Provides blood flow of approximately 1/3 normal
            (4) Usually not sufficient to support consciousness

Content

b) Technique **(Slide 6-16)**
(1) Place patient on hard surface
(a) Floor
(b) Cardiac compression board
(c) Spine board
(2) Hand and rescuer body position **(Slide 6-17)**
(a) Position yourself to the side of the patient with your knees close to the patient
(b) Slightly separate knees
(c) Find the lower margin of ribcage and slide your fingers upward to the xiphoid
(d) Place the heel of your other hand next to the index finger on the sternum
(e) Only the heel of the hand should be in contact with the breastbone
(f) Place the heel of your other hand directly on top of the hand on the sternum
(g) Keep fingers up and off the chest wall
(h) Position your shoulders directly over the lower half of the sternum and lock your elbows
(i) Straight line from the shoulders to the heel of your hand
(3) Compression technique
(a) Compress straight down, bending slightly at the hips during the downward thrust
(b) Compress the sternum approximately 1 1/2" to 2" in the adult patient
(c) Smooth and rhythmic, with approximately 50% compression and 50% release

4. Rate and ratio of compression and ventilation **(Slide 6-18)**
a) 15 compressions and 2 ventilations are performed after the initial two breaths
b) Compressions rate of approximately 80-100 per minute
c) Commonly used mnemonic that can achieve this approximate rate is: "1 and 2 and 3 and 4...and 15"

5. Pulse check
a) Check pulse after four complete cycles (one minute)
b) If no pulse, give two breaths and continue CPR

III. Performance of two rescuer CPR **(Slide 6-19)**
A. Advantages
1. Less fatiguing
2. Increases the frequency of ventilations per minute (12 instead of 8)
3. Permits the employment of mechanical aids and supplemental oxygen

B. Transition of one rescuer to two rescuer CPR **(Slide 6-20)**
1. Second rescuer advises first rescuer that he/she will assist
2. Second rescuer positions himself on the opposite side from the first rescuer

Content

3. First rescuer completes compression cycle and gives two breaths and checks the pulse
4. First rescuer gives one breath and signals you to begin compressions
5. Rate and ratio
    a) Ratio of compressions to ventilation is 5:1
    b) Compression rate is also 80-100 compressions per minute
    c) After 5 compressions, the compressor pauses to allow the ventilator to give one breath
6. Switch and pulse check
    a) CPR is a physically fatiguing process
    b) Switch is initiated at direction of compressor
    c) Ventilator administers one breath after fifth compression
    d) Both rescuers switch places
    e) New ventilator checks pulse, administers one breath and tells compressor to resume CPR
    f) Performed every few minutes or when the compressor becomes fatigued

C. Two rescuers starting together
1. One assumes role of ventilator and other the role of compressor
2. All initial evaluation procedures are performed by the ventilator
3. Upon documenting breathlessness the ventilator administers two breaths and checks the pulse
4. If there is no pulse, the ventilator signals the beginning of compressions and proceeds as described above

IV. Infant and child CPR **(Slide 6-21)**

A. Most cardiac arrests in children are a result of accidents or respiratory problems
1. Leading causes of death below the age of one
    a) Congenital malformations
    b) Infections
    c) Sudden Infant Death Syndrome (SIDS)
2. Leading causes of death over the age of 1 year
    a) Accidental and violent injuries (#1 cause)
    b) Airway obstruction
    c) Drowning
    d) Infections
3. Definition of infant vs. child for CPR performance
    a) Infant is someone less than one year of age
    b) Child is someone between one and eight
    c) Ages are guidelines and the size of infant may dictate selection of the procedure

B. Performance of infant CPR
1. Establishing unresponsiveness **(Slide 6-22)**
    a) Gently shake the infant and shout "Are you okay?"
    b) Briskly tap the bottom of the feet or apply a painful stimulus such as a pinch
2. Positioning the victim **(Slide 6-23)**
    a) Place the infant on a hard surface in the supine position
    b) Turn the patient carefully to avoid spinal injury

Content

3. Airway and breathing assessment
    a) Opening the airway
        (1) Hyperextension of the neck should be avoided. Head should be placed in the neutral or sniffing position
        (2) Head tilt-chin lift **(Slide 6-24)**
            (a) Place one finger at the base of the chin
            (b) Rotate the head slightly backward, being careful not to overextend
            (c) Lift the chin toward the front of the body being careful not to close the mouth
        (3) Jaw thrust-without head tilt **(Slide 6-25)**
            (a) Place your thumbs on the cheek bones of the victim
            (b) Place your index and middle fingers beneath the angle of the jaw
            (c) Displace the jaw upward while maintaining counter-pressure with your thumbs
            (d) Do not tilt the head
    b) Breathing assessment **(Slide 6-26)**
        (1) Look for chest rise
        (2) Listen for air escaping during exhalation
        (3) Feel the victim's breath on your cheek
        (4) If the patient is breathing spontaneously, continue to ensure a clear airway
        (5) If the patient is not breathing, begin positive pressure ventilation
    c) Breathing **(Slide 6-27)**
        (1) Administer two slow breaths
        (2) Mouth to mouth and nose
        (3) Chest rise is the indication to stop an individual breath to avoid gastric distension. Each breath should take approximately 1-1.5 seconds to deliver
4. Circulation
    a) Pulse check **(Slide 6-28)**
        (1) Pulse of an infant is felt over the brachial artery
            (a) Located on the inner side of the upper arm between the elbow and the axilla
            (b) Gently palpate with your index and middle fingers for 5-10 seconds
        (2) If you feel a pulse, continue to maintain the airway and provide positive pressure ventilation
            (a) 1 breath every 3 seconds
            (b) Reevaluate the pulse periodically
        (3) If no pulse is felt begin cardiac compressions
    b) External cardiac compressions **(Slide 6-29)**
        (1) Place your index, middle and ring fingers on the sternum starting at nipple line
        (2) Lift the finger closest to nipple line

Content

(3) Use the tips of these two fingers and compress down 1/2-1 inch
(4) Rate of 100 compressions per minute
(5) Ratio of compressions to ventilations is 5:1. Pause briefly after five compressions and breathe while observing for chest rise
(6) Reevaluate the pulse after 1 minute (approximately 10 cycles)

C. Performance of CPR in a child **(Slide 6-30)**
1. The initial sequence remains the same
a) Check for unresponsiveness
b) Call for help
c) Position the victim
d) Head tilt-chin lift or jaw thrust-without head tilt to open the airway **(Slide 6-31)**
e) Establish breathlessness **(Slide 6-32)**
2. Breathing
a) Mouth to mouth breathing is utilized rather than mouth to mouth and nose **(Slide 6-33)**
b) Pinch the nose with the fingers of the hand on the forehead
c) Seal your mouth around the child's mouth and administer two slow breaths
d) Observe chest rise
3. Pulse check **(Slide 6-34)**
a) Carotid artery in the neck
b) Check the pulse for 5-10 seconds
4. Cardiac compressions **(Slide 6-35)**
a) The heel of one hand is placed over the lower half of the sternum
b) Follow the margin of the ribs to the base of the breastbone
c) Place the heel of the same hand on the breastbone just above the location of the fingers
d) The head tilt is maintained during this procedure
e) Position your shoulder directly over your hand on the lower half of the sternum and lock your elbow
f) There should be a straight line from the shoulder to the heel of your hand, perpendicular to the sternum
g) Compress downward approximately 1-1 1/2 inches
h) Rate of 80-100 compressions per minute
i) 5:1 ratio of compressions to ventilations
j) At the end of 5 compressions, 1 breath is administered
k) Check the pulse after one minute

V. Special considerations **(Slide 6-36)**
A. When to start CPR **(Slide 6-37)**
1. In general CPR should be started unless there is definitive evidence of death

Content

2. Many factors may delay brain death time
    a) Children
    b) Drowning
    c) Hypothermia
3. Give the patient the benefit of the doubt

B. Evaluating the effectiveness **(Slide 6-38)**
1. Most patients require defibrillation to be resuscitated
2. Certain signs might be helpful to judge the effectiveness of CPR performance
    a) Chest rise to monitor correct breathing technique
    b) Improvement in skin color
    c) Pupillary narrowing and reactivity to light
    d) Spontaneous breathing
    e) Patient movement and responsiveness
    f) Pulse return
3. Resuscitated experience return of normal function gradually
    a) Return of a pulse
    b) Then spontaneous respiratory efforts which may be inadequate to support life
    c) Airway and the breathing must be monitored and positive pressure ventilations are provided as necessary

C. When to stop **(Slide 6-39)**
1. Relieved by another rescuer
2. A physician assumes responsibility for the patient
3. The rescuer is exhausted and unable to continue
4. Patient is delivered to the emergency department
5. Patient develops spontaneous breathing and a pulse.

D. Complications of CPR **(Slide 6-40)**
1. Some complications are the result of improper performance
2. Other complications may occur even with proper technique
3. Specific complications
    a) Broken ribs
    b) Fracture of the sternum
    c) Cardiac contusions
    d) Lung lacerations
    e) Liver lacerations

VI. Mechanical CPR devices **(Slide 6-41)**

A. Range from simple hand operated units through sophisticated oxygen powered machines which compress and ventilate

B. When utilized properly are capable of providing excellent CPR

C. If applied improperly or if left unattended, may be ineffective or may cause severe injuries

D. Advantages of mechanical CPR **(Slide 6-42)**
1. Avoid rescuer fatigue
2. Potential to perform optimal compressions as long as there is an adequate supply of oxygen
3. Useful in prolonged resuscitation, i.e., hypothermia
4. Valuable during transport

Content

E. Technique of operation
1. Vary from unit to unit
2. Never delay application of CPR while preparing device
2. Manual CPR should always be started while a second rescuer readies the device **(Slide 6-43)**
3. Do not interrupt CPR for more than 30 seconds
4. Place the patient on the CPR board and continue manual CPR **(Slide 6-44)**
5. The piston arm is then attached to the CPR board **(Slide 6-43)**
6. Compression piston should be positioned in the same location as manual cardiac compressions **(Slide 6-44)**
7. Compression piston is engaged according to the manufacturer's criteria **(Slide 6-45)**
8. The unit should be constantly monitored to avoid accidental displacement of the compression piston
9. Ventilation device can be attached to the mask or endotracheal tube to administer positive pressure **(Slide 6-46)**
10. Oxygen source must be monitored closely

F. Disadvantages of mechanical CPR **(Slide 6-47)**
1. Injury resulting from operator error or inattentiveness
2. Size and weight
3. Storage space in ambulance

VII. Special resuscitation situations

A. Mouth to stoma ventilation **(Slide 6-48)**
1. EMTs may encounter "neck breathers" (persons who breathe through a surgical opening in the neck)
2. Ventilation must be provided through stoma
3. Opening may or may not communicate with the mouth and nose
4. Check for air escape through mouth and cover mouth and nose as needed

B. Drowning **(Slide 6-49)**
1. EMTs first concern is his own safety
2. When possible, a floatable rescue device should be tossed to the drowning person
3. Where the distance prevents such actions, a boat or raft should be utilized
4. If the EMT must swim, he or she should be aware of own abilities and limitations
5. Breathing should begin as soon as possible (in shallow water or on a floatable object)
6. If neck injury is suspected spinal precautions should be taken, i.e., backboard
7. Length of submersion should not affect the decision to resuscitate
8. Water in the mouth can be removed by turning the patient
9. Water in the stomach should be left alone unless excessive gastric distension interferes with ventilation

Content

C. Electric shock **(Slide 6-50)**

1. May cause either respiratory or cardiac arrest
2. There may also be burns or trauma resulting from falls
3. Approach the patient with concern for the cervical spine
4. If the victim is still in contact with the source of electricity
   a) Electrical source should be unplugged or turned off
   b) Wire should be cleared away from the patient with a non-conductive object
   c) Where the electric current is fixed or cannot be moved, then the patient can be separated from the source with a non-conductive object

D. CPR during movement **(Slide 6-51)**

1. Time to defibrillation is most important variable
2. Whenever possible coordinate patient movement in relation to access to defibrillation
   a) If EMT-P, EMT-P, or EMT-D is less response time than time to hospital, wait on scene
   b) If hospital is closer than EMT-D or EMT-P response time, transport to hospital
   c) If patient movement is essential, apply the following principles:
   d) Stairway **(Slide 6-52)**
      (1) Secure the patient to the device selected for transport
      (2) Removal should be done with no less than four people
      (3) CPR should be done on each landing
      (4) Patient should be moved to the next landing quickly and CPR resumed
      (5) If possible, CPR should not be interrupted for more than 30 seconds
   e) Ground level and into the ambulance **(Slide 6-53)**
      (1) Rolling cot should be placed in half way upright position, CPR should continue
      (2) Ventilator is at top of stretcher
      (3) Compressor at side
      (4) Helpers should position themselves at the top and bottom ends of stretcher
      (5) Stretcher should be advanced feet first toward the ambulance
      (6) Care should be taken to traverse obstacles, i.e., curbs
      (7) At ambulance, helpers should lower the cot to its lowest position while CPR continues
      (8) To lift the patient in the ambulance, CPR should be stopped briefly
      (9) Compressor and one helper lift from the side position
      (10) Ventilator can resume CPR as soon as the stretcher is locked in place
      (11) Patient should be hyperventilated after any period when CPR was interrupted

Content

f) CPR during transport **(Slide 6-54)**

(1) Ideally, four people should be involved to provide both good CPR and safety

(2) Person should be positioned at the head administering positive pressure ventilation

(3) Second EMT should be administering cardiac compressions

(4) Third helper supports the compressor from behind

(5) Driver should exercise great care in departure and when stopping to avoid abrupt movements

(6) At hospital, the driver and helper can receive the stretcher while CPR stops for a very short period of time

(7) Movement into the emergency department should proceed as described previously

Section 2

EMT - Defibrillation (EMT-D)

Objectives
(Slide 6-55)

At the conclusion of the chapter the students will be able to:

1. **Describe the history of prehospital defibrillation.**
2. **Explain why EMTs are an ideal population to provide prehospital defibrillation.**
3. **Explain the following concepts related to the function of the heart:**
   - **Automaticity**
   - **Depolarization**
   - **Conductivity**
   - **Repolarization**
   - **The Rest Period**
4. **Define the following terms:**
   - **Electrodes**
   - **Leads**
   - **Standardization**
5. **Describe the operation of the monitor.**
6. **Explain how to calculate rate using the following methods:**
   - **Six second strip**
   - **Large box method**
   - **Small box method**
7. **Correctly label an ECG complex and explain its relationship to mechanical events within the heart.**
8. **List your actions when presented with the following ECG rhythms with conventional and semiautomatic defibrillators:**
   - **Asystole**
   - **An organized rhythm without a pulse (EMD)**
   - **Ventricular tachycardia without a pulse**
   - **Ventricular fibrillation**
9. **Describe the operation of a manual, automatic or semiautomatic defibrillator.**
10. **State the AHA recommended energy levels for defibrillation.**
11. **Describe the care of the patient following successful defibrillation.**

Instructor Preparation

Reading preparation for the lesson:

EMT Prehospital Care, Chapter 6, pages 260-287
Local EMT-D protocols
Performance sheets for EMT-D

Optional reading:

American Heart Association: Advanced Cardiac Life Support Manual. Dallas Texas, 1985

Suggested Learning Activities
Using a lecture format with the aid of slides, overhead transparencies or charts, provide an overview of EMT-defibrillation. **Provide a scenario demonstration of the following scenarios:** **Ventricular fibrillation converting to NSR** **Asystole arrest** **Unconscious patient with NSR** **Ventricular fibrillation converting to asystole** **Discuss access to ALS when EMT-D does not resuscitate patient.**

Content

VIII. EMT-defibrillation overview **(Slide 6-56)**

A. The most common and treatable cause of sudden death is ventricular fibrillation

1. A chaotic quivering of the heart that results in cardiac arrest
2. Up to 70% of cardiac arrest victims have been found in this rhythm
3. Require early application and delivery of an external electrical shock
4. Early CPR and defibrillation can result in conversion to a functional rhythm

B. Evolution of the concept **(Slide 6-57)**

1. Prior to the 1960's, patients who suffered sudden death outside the hospital rarely survived
2. In 1960 CPR was developed and improved the chances for survival
3. In the late 1960s portable defibrillation and biotelemetry allowed prehospital advanced life support
4. The combination of CPR and ALS (especially defibrillation) significantly improves survival
5. Prehospital care and defibrillation
   - a) Pantridge in Belfast, Northern Ireland developed first mobile ICU
   - b) Grace in New York City introduced the concept of mobile intensive care units in US
   - c) Early paramedic programs in Miami, Pittsburgh, Seattle first used paramedics
   - d) In 1973 federal Emergency Medical Services Systems legislation stimulated advanced life support
   - e) Studies documented the effectiveness of prehospital ALS systems
     - (1) Survival rates of 43% were reported when victims of ventricular fibrillation received
       - (a) CPR less than 4 minutes
       - (b) ALS less than 8 minutes
     - (2) These skills were in the hands of a small number of prehospital providers
   - f) In the 1970's, Eisenberg, Copass and others from Seattle studied EMT-D
   - g) Many other programs have demonstrated the effectiveness of the EMT-D concept

C. Conceptual framework **(Slide 6-58)**

1. Knowledge to administer defibrillation is minimal
   - a) Recognition of cardiac arrest
   - b) CPR
   - c) Basic ECG recognition (not needed with automated defibrillators)
2. Medical control
   - a) Medical director needed to supervise training and monitor effectiveness
   - b) Done through initial training, refresher and monitoring of field care

Content

3. Knowledge needed varies with type of defibrillator
    a) Automated defibrillator minimal knowledge is needed
        (1) CPR
        (2) Cardiac arrest assessment
        (3) Operation of the machine
    b) Manual defibrillator
        (1) Same as above
        (2) Plus minimal ECG knowledge
            (a) Cardiac arrest rhythms
            (b) Basic appearance of organized rhythms
            (c) Potentially confusing rhythms

IX. EMT-D with manual defibrillator **(Slide 6-59)**
  A. The electrocardiogram
    1. Electrical activity of the heart is detected, amplified, and displayed as an electrocardiogram or ECG
    2. ECG machine is connected to the body's surface by electrodes and cables
        a) Electrodes pick up the heart's signal
        b) Cables transmit the signal to the ECG machine
        c) Signal is amplified and displayed on an oscilloscope or paper readout
    3. Electrodes and ECG leads **(Slide 6-60)**
        a) Can be placed at various locations
        b) Placement creates a `lead`
        c) Positive and negative electrode and a ground
            (1) Electrical event received by the electrodes
            (2) Depolarization toward positive electrode = upward wave
            (3) Depolarization toward negative electrode = downward wave
            (4) Depolarization at right angle to electrode = upward/downward wave
        d) Electrodes form a triangle around the heart **(Slide 6-61)**
            (1) Attached to the extremities or to the torso
            (2) Most common leads are called I, II, and III
            (3) Lead II is best for monitoring since wave is most positive
    4. ECG monitor
        a) Screen or CRT **(Slide 6-62)**
            (1) Cathode ray tube or CRT
            (2) Similar to a television or computer screen
            (3) Blue/green background with bright line waves
            (4) Some allow "freeze" for closer observation
        b) Paper readout
            (1) Monitors may have paper readout
            (2) Hot stylus records ECG waves on paper
            (3) Can be adjusted to darken or lighten
            (4) Rolled at predetermined speed
            (5) Lines permit calculation of rate and size and duration of the wave forms
            (6) Provides permanent record

Content

c) Amplification and standardization **(Slide 6-63)**
   (1) Size of wave can be adjusted
   (2) Standard marker allows measure against a "standard"
      (a) 10 small boxes = 1 millivolt
      (b) Push standard button each time you use the monitor
      (c) If amplification is turned down, all recordings may appear as a flat line

d) Operation of the monitor **(Slide 6-64)**
   (1) Remove sweat from skin surface
   (2) Attach the electrodes to the patient **(Slide 6-65)**
   (3) Attach the cables to the electrodes **(Slide 6-66)**
   (4) Instruct patient to lay still/not touch metal
   (5) Select lead II for routine monitoring **(Slide 6-67)**
   (6) Turn on recorder and press standard button
   (7) Adjust the amplitude as needed
   (8) Adjust audible "beep" as needed

e) Paddle monitoring **(Slide 6-68)**
   (1) Some monitors permit paddle monitoring
   (2) Permits rapid assessment and defibrillation
   (3) Paddles act as electrodes
   (4) Lead switch must be turned to PADDLE MODE
   (5) May be poor quality tracing

5. ECG recognition
   a) Waves and intervals **(Slide 6-69)**
      (1) P wave = depolarization of the atria
      (2) QRS complex = depolarization of ventricles
         (a) Q = first downward deflection occurring before first positive deflection-R wave
         (b) Negative deflection following the R wave is called the S wave
         (c) QRS takes various forms
      (3) T wave represents ventricular repolarization
      (4) U wave may follow the T wave
      (5) PR interval = beginning of P wave to QRS
         (a) Normal PR interval - .12 to .20 seconds
         (b) Longer intervals reflect delay or blocked conduction through the AV node
      (6) QRS wave is normally less than 0.12 seconds
   b) Analyzing rate
      (1) 6 second strip **(Slide 6-70)**
         (a) 3 second marks on the top of the paper
         (b) Number of QRS within 2 top markings x 10 = rate
      (2) Large box method **(Slide 6-71)**
         (a) Dark vertical markings correspond to 0.2 seconds
         (b) 5 dark lines = one second
         (c) 300 dark lines = one minute
         (d) Number of dark lines between 2 complexes divided into 300 = rate

Content

(e) The dividends for successive large boxes are
i) 1 = 300
ii) 2 = 150
iii) 3 = 100
iv) 4 = 75
v) 5 = 60
vi) 6 = 50

(3) Small box method **(Slide 6-72)**
(a) Each large box contains 5 smaller boxes. Each small box represents 0.04 seconds
(b) 1500 small boxes = one minute
(c) Number of small boxes between 2 complexes divided into 1500 = rate

c) Rhythm
(1) Regular **(Slide 6-73)**
(a) Rhythms with P waves/QRS complexes occurring at regular intervals
(b) Example - normal sinus rhythm
(2) Irregularly irregular **(Slide 6-74)**
(a) No predictable pattern
(b) Random with no fixed order
(c) Example - atrial fibrillation
(3) Regularly irregular **(Slide 6-75)**
(a) Irregular but distinct pattern
(b) Extra beat occurs at regular intervals
(c) Example - premature ventricular contractions (bigeminy)

d) Relationships between the P and QRS **(Slide 6-76)**
(1) Normally P wave and QRS wave are coupled together
(2) PR interval is relatively constant
(3) Rates of P wave and QRS are same
(4) Beats which originate in ventricle have no P wave
(5) With blocks P and QRS may not be related

6. Rhythm recognition and decision to defibrillate **(Slide 6-77)**
a) EMT needs to know basic patterns of a few rhythms
b) Extensive ECG knowledge not needed for EMT-D
c) Basic concept
(1) Normally heart cells are driven by pacemaker
(2) Ventricular fibrillation is chaotic discharge of ventricles cells
(3) Defibrillation causes simultaneous depolarization of all cells
(4) The pacemaker, first to recharge, may regain control of the rhythm (usually SA node)
(4) Forced discharge is called defibrillation
d) Decision to defibrillate **(Slide 6-78)**
(1) Based upon pulselessness and the recognition of ventricular fibrillation on an ECG

Content

(2) Distinguishing v-fib from organized rhythms is not difficult
(a) Ventricular fibrillation has a disorganized appearance
(b) Organized rhythms have ventricular complexes
(3) Pulselessness and ventricular fibrillation must be present to defibrillate
(a) Some rhythms may appear as v-fib
(b) Some cardiac arrest rhythms have organized complexes
e) Important Rhythms for EMT-D **(Slide 6-79)**
(1) Rhythm with organized ventricular complexes
(a) Normal sinus rhythm **(Slide 6-80)**
i) Rhythm with P, QRS, T
ii) Rate of 60-100 times a minute
iii) Most common rhythm
(b) Sinus tachycardia **(Slide 6-81)**
i) Same as NSR
ii) Rate greater than 100/minute
(c) Sinus bradycardia **(Slide 6-82)**
i) Same as NSR
ii) Rate less than 60/minute
(2) Cardiac arrest rhythms
(a) Ventricular fibrillation **(Slide 6-83)**
i) Wide, multiformed complexes
ii) Vary in size and regularity
iii) Jagged, disorganized, chaotic appearance
iv) No organization or synchronized electrical or mechanical event
v) May be fine or course
vi) No cardiac output = no pulse
(b) Ventricular tachycardia **(Slide 6-84)**
i) Rapid dysrhythmia (rate 100-220)
ii) Originates within ventricles
iii) May or may not produce a pulse
iv) Wide complexes without P or T waves
v) Occasionally P waves may be noted
vi) Not treated, evolves to V-fib
vii) Defibrillated when no pulse is present
viii) Check local protocols
(c) Asystole/agonal rhythm **(Slide 6-85)**
i) Simply means without contraction
ii) No electrical/mechanical activity
iii) Other terms - cardiac standstill and flat line
iv) Initial arrest rhythm or evolves from other rhythms
v) May be accompanied by wide occasional complexes (agonal)
vi) Check other leads (could be v-fib)

(d) Electrical mechanical dissociation (EMD) **(Slide 6-86)**
- i) Organized electrical complexes without a pulse
- ii) May have the P, QRS and T components
- iii) Other times only ventricular complexes
- iv) May suggest hypovolemia, tension pneumothorax, cardiac tamponade

(3) Potentially confusing rhythms

(a) Artifact **(Slide 6-87)**
- i) Disturbance in ECG tracing caused by
  - i) Electrical interference (60 cycle)
  - ii) Patient or cable movement
  - iii) Dislodging of the cables
  - iv) Muscle tremors and seizures
  - v) Poor attachment of electrodes
  - vi) Sweaty patients
  - vii) Defective pads or cables
  - viii) Touching other person

(b) Atrial flutter **(Slide 6-88)**
- i) Atria discharging 220 to 350 times a minute
- ii) Abnormal electrical mechanism pacemaker
- iii) "Sawtooth" pattern may appear as v-fib
  - i) Look for QRS complexes
  - ii) Check for pulse

(c) Atrial fibrillation **(Slide 6-89)**
- i) Discharge of atria exceeds 350/minute
- ii) May be mistaken for ventricular fibrillation
- iii) Irregularly - irregular pattern
- iv) Waves vary from course to fine
  - i) Look for QRS
  - ii) Check for pulse

(d) Pacemaker spikes with ventricular fibrillation **(Slide 6-90)**
- i) Artificial pacemakers may produce spikes with ventricular fibrillation
- ii) Should be defibrillated
- iii) Defibrillator paddles 5" from pacemaker generator

f) Decision to defibrillate **(Slide 6-91)**

(1) Pulse absent

(a) CPR

(b) ECG tracing
- i) Ventricular fibrillation or
- ii) Ventricular tachycardia
  - i) Defibrillate
  - ii) CPR
- iii) Asystole or
- iv) Organized rhythm
  - i) CPR
  - ii) Transport

Content

B. Defibrillation
  1. Conceptual **(Slide 6-92)**
    a) Application of electric shock across the heart
    b) Depolarizes heart's cells simultaneously
    c) Cells enter a rest period
    d) Pacemaker recharges fastest
    e) Pacemaker (hopefully) gains control
  2. Devices
    a) Three types of monitor - defibrillators for EMT-D
      (1) Manual (conventional) **(Slide 6-93)**
        (a) Require ECG recognition
        (b) Manual energy selection
        (c) Manual charging
        (d) Manual discharge
        (e) No directions
      (2) Semi-automatic **(Slide 6-94)**
        (a) No ECG recognition needed
        (b) Screen may be available
        (c) Automatic or manual energy selection
        (d) Automatic or manual charging
        (e) Voice or screen directions
        (f) Discharge by operator
      (3) Automatic
        (a) No ECG recognition needed
        (b) No screen
        (c) Automatic energy selection
        (d) Automatic charging
        (e) Voice directions
        (f) Discharge by machine
      (4) Common features **(Slide 6-95)**
        (a) Rhythm evaluation
        (b) Defibrillation
        (c) Recording of rhythm and voice on tape cassette
        (d) Battery power source
        (e) Capacitors to store direct current
        (f) Energy select switches (not on some automatics)
        (g) Charge switches (not on some automatics)
        (h) Discharge switches (not on automatics)
  3. Technique using conventional defibrillators
    a) Confirm pulselessness and start CPR **(Slide 6-96)**
      (1) One rescuer if only two EMTs are available
      (2) Two rescuer if more than two EMTs are available
      (3) If only one EMT is available he or she should attach monitor and defibrillate if needed
    b) Monitor operation **(Slide 6-97)**
      (1) Patient cables and electrodes are attached
      (2) Main power switch is turned on
      (3) ECG will appear on the screen
      (4) Adjust size as needed

(5) Paper recording switch is turned on and the standardization is pressed
(6) Check to see that medical control device is on
(7) Lead selection to lead II (unless paddle monitoring)
(8) Verbally describe events as you proceed
(a) Pulselessness
(b) Rhythm interpretation
(c) Energy selection
(d) Discharge
(e) Post defibrillation rhythm and pulse
(9) The ECG pattern is evaluated and the pulse is rechecked
(10) Change lead selection if a flat line appears

c) Defibrillation operation **(Slide 6-98)**
(1) Energy selection and charging
(a) Expressed in joules or watt-seconds
(b) AHA recommendation are 200, 200-300 and 360 joules for the first three defibrillations
(c) If ventricular fibrillation persists 360 joules is used thereafter
(d) Energy selection **(Slide 6-99)**
i) Controls may be located on the paddles or machine
ii) Select energy
iii) Push "charge" button
i) An audible or visual device will indicate when charging is complete
ii) Discharge occurs by depressing both buttons simultaneously
(e) If the patient is not defibrillated immediately paddles may lose their charge
(f) Recharging may be necessary
(2) Disarming the defibrillator **(Slide 6-100)**
(a) If the patient is not defibrillated you may have to "dump" the charge
(b) Common ways to dump charge
i) Turning power off
ii) Changing energy selection
iii) Placing paddles into cradle
(3) Paddle Placement **(Slide 6-101)**
(a) Paddle placement will direct energy flow
(b) A "critical mass" of the heart cells must be defibrillated
(c) If paddles are placed too close together, a smaller number of cells will be depolarized

(d) Paddles are placed in two locations on the anterior chest wall **(Slide 6-102)**

i) Just below the right clavicle on the right sternal border

ii) Just to the left of the left nipple on the mid-axillary line

(e) Anterior - posterior placement of paddle electrodes **(Slide 6-103)**

i) Less commonly used

ii) Anterior pad is placed on the precordium to the left of the sternal border

iii) Posterior pad behind the heart beneath the scapula and lateral to the spine

(4) Conductive mediums **(Slide 6-104)**

(a) The chest surface provides resistance to energy flow

(b) Conductive mediums reduce resistance

i) Gels or creams

ii) Saline - soaked gauze pads

iii) Pre-gelled defibrillator pads

(c) Care should be taken to prevent bridging and burns to the patient

(d) Bridging - transfer of energy from one paddle to another over surface of body

i) Via gel, cream, saline, sweat or other moisture

ii) Results from excessive conductive gel or other material on chest's surface

(5) Paddle Pressure **(Slide 6-105)**

(a) Chest wall is irregular due to ribs and other bony prominences

(b) Pressure is needed to ensure firm contact between the paddle and surface of the skin

i) Approximately 25 pounds of muscular pressure

ii) Use arm pressure instead of body weight to avoid slipping

(6) Paddle size **(Slide 6-106)**

(a) Paddle size can influence the energy delivery

(b) EMT-D equipment is designed for adult patients

i) Smaller paddles would be indicated for children (8 cm diameter)

ii) Infants (4.5 cm diameter)

iii) Ventricular fibrillation is a very rare event in children and infants

iv) Energy setting for children should be 2 joules per kilogram of body weight

Content

(7) Energy delivery **(Slide 6-107)**
(a) Clear rescuers and bystanders prior to defibrillation
(b) Say "all clear" and view all sides of patient and stretcher
(c) Push defibrillation buttons simultaneously
(d) Observe for muscular contraction of patient

d) Procedure for defibrillation
(1) Time to defibrillation is the most important variable for successful resuscitation
(2) You should practice for fastest possible time
(3) Protocol **(Slide 6-108)**
(a) Confirm cardiac arrest
(b) Initiate CPR
(c) Attach leads
(d) Turn on recorder and medical control recording device
(e) Assess rhythm
(f) If ventricular fibrillation or pulseless ventricular tachycardia, defibrillate
(g) Apply conductive gel, etc.
(h) Apply paddles and charge to 200 joules
(i) Apply 25 pound of muscular pressure
(j) Announces "all clear"
(k) Make sure no one is in contact with patient, stretcher or equipment
(l) Press the discharge buttons on the paddles to defibrillate
(m) Reevaluate pulse and rhythm
(n) If pulseless and still in ventricular fibrillation, defibrillate 200-300 joules
(o) If pulseless and still in ventricular fibrillation, defibrillate with 360 joules
(p) If rhythm changes, always evaluate for need for CPR

e) Defibrillation and the ECG **(Slide 6-109)**
(1) After defibrillation an isoelectric (flat) line may appear on the ECG
(a) Reflects forced rest period of the myocardial cells
(b) Gives a chance for the normal pacemaker to assume control of the heart's rhythm
(2) Flatline may last for several seconds before organized rhythm appears

f) Post defibrillation care
(1) Three possible results can be encountered **(Slide 6-110)**
(a) Ventricular fibrillation or tachycardia can persist
(b) Asystole or EMD
(c) Patient will have a pulse and a rhythm with organized ventricular complexes

Content

(2) Patients remaining in ventricular fibrillation or tachycardia **(Slide 6-111)**
(a) After three defibrillations, the patient will probably require advanced life support
(b) Some protocols suggest three additional defibrillations after a short period of CPR
(c) Decision after these shocks should be determined by time to ALS
i) Paramedic unit close, wait for arrival
ii) Hospital closer, transport
(3) Patients converting to asystole or EMD **(Slide 6-112)**
(a) Try a second lead when asystole first appears (may be v-fib)
(b) Drug therapy is needed to treat these rhythms
(c) Continue CPR and access ALS
(d) Consider hypovolemia, tension pneumothorax or other conditions
(4) Patients with return of pulse **(Slide 6-113)**
(a) Varying clinical and ECG responses are possible
(b) Monitor ventilations and administer positive pressure ventilations as needed
i) Usually a lapse from conversion to normal breathing and consciousness
ii) Often related to time in arrest
iii) When in doubt ventilate
(c) Types of rhythms
i) Normal rhythms may refibrillate
ii) Oxygenation is critical for preventing return of v-fib
iii) Refibrillation
i) If patient refibrillates use same energies used when conversion occurred
g) Recorder devices **(Slide 6-114)**
(1) Documentation of rhythm before and after defibrillation is essential
(2) Manual defibrillators have a built-in recorder which documents ECG, defibrillation and voice
(3) EMTs should record their actions verbally during all phases of assessment and treatment
(4) Used as part of the medical control record and is essential for quality assurance

X. Automatic and semiautomatic defibrillators **(Slide 6-115)**
A. Automatic
1. Defibrillators are fully automatic
a) Interpret rhythm
b) Spontaneously initiate a defibrillation
c) Remove the necessity of ECG recognition
d) Eliminate concerns about operator error

Content

B. Use rate and shape of ECG waves to differentiate ventricular fibrillation from organized rhythms
   1. Very reliable for not shocking organized rhythms
   2. May direct operator to not shock ventricular tachycardia (depends on rate)

C. Operation
   1. Cardiac arrest is confirmed **(Slide 6-116)**
   2. Attach to the patient and turn on **(Slide 6-117)**
   3. EMTs stand clear of the patient **(Slide 6-118)**
   4. Audible signal notifies the rescuers of the impending defibrillation
   5. Following defibrillation the rescuers check the pulse and recharge the machine if pulselessness still exists.
   6. Extreme caution should be exercised to clear rescuers or bystanders

D. Semiautomatic **(Slide 6-118)**
   1. Same as automatic defibrillators but allow operator to defibrillate
   2. May or may not have video screen
   3. May have voice or screen messages to guide operation
   4. Protocol
      a) Confirm cardiac arrest with pulse check **(Slide 6-119)**
      b) Begin CPR **(Slide 6-120)**
      c) Attach the electrodes and turn on the device **(Slide 6-121)**
      d) Press button to analyze the rhythm (do not touch patient) **(Slide 6-122)**
      e) If ventricular fibrillation is present the machine will charge to 200 joules **(Slide 6-121)**
      f) Machine advises the EMT to press the defibrillation button **(Slide 6-122)**
      g) Make sure that everyone is clear from the patient and deliver the shock **(Slide 6-123)**
      h) Push the analyze button (do not touch patient) **(Slide 6-124)**
      i) If shock advised, repeat at 200-300 joules
      j) If shock advised, repeat at 360 joules
      k) If ventricular fibrillation persists reevaluate pulse and perform CPR for 1 minute
      l) Perform a second set of 3 "stacked shocks"
      m) If the patient is still in v-fib consider transport to ALS
      n) If distance is great consider continued defibrillation
      o) Check local protocols

E. Medical control **(Slide 6-125)**
   1. Essential part of EMT-D program
   2. Physicians must assume responsibility for:
      a) Initial training
      b) Refresher training
      c) Protocol development
      d) Continuing education
      e) Case review
      f) Outcome evaluation
   3. Standing orders are used to initiate defibrillation

Content
Content

F. Defibrillator maintenance **(Slide 6-126)**
1. Must be carefully maintained to assure readiness and prevent operational failure
2. According to manufactures instructions
    a) Adhere to a regular schedule of maintenance
    b) Visual checks
    c) Regular testing of delivered energy
    d) Rotation of batteries
    e) Log of maintenance

G. Medical control unit **(Slide 6-127)**
1. May consist of a card, cassette or module
2. May include voice, ECG and call summary of events
3. Reviewed by medical control after each call
4. Unit can be erased and reused
5. Printed record can be attached to record for documentation

Chapter 6

CPR AND EMT DEFIBRILLATION

Examination

1. When assessing a patient you should check the pulse for:

   a. 2-5 seconds
   b. 5-10 seconds
   c. 10-15 seconds
   d. 15-20 seconds

2. When assessing a patient to determine if the patient is breathing you should check for:

   a. 3-5 seconds
   b. 5-10 seconds
   c. 10-15 seconds
   d. 15-20 seconds

3. When we look, listen and feel we are checking for:

   a. adequate circulation
   b. adequate respiration
   c. obvious external bleeding
   d. medic alert tags and medications

4. The appropriate location to check for a pulse in an unconscious adult patient is the:

   a. radial artery
   b. brachial artery
   c. femoral artery
   d. carotid artery

5. The appropriate location to check for a pulse in an unconscious infant is the:

   a. radial artery
   b. brachial artery
   c. femoral artery
   d. carotid artery

6. Infant CPR is performed on patients:

   a. less than 6 months of age
   b. less than 1 year of age
   c. less than 2 years of age
   d. less than 5 years of age

7. Child CPR is performed on patients __________ to __________ years of age.

   a. newborn to 1
   b. 1 to 5
   c. 1 to 8
   d. 1 to 10

8. During infant CPR the rate of compressions is:

   a. 60 per minute
   b. 80 per minute
   c. 80-100 per minute
   d. at least 100 per minute

9. During child CPR the rate of compressions is:

   a. 60 per minute
   b. 80 per minute
   c. 80-100 per minute
   d. at least 100 per minute

10. During adult CPR the rate of compressions is:

    a. 60 per minute
    b. 80 per minute
    c. 80-100 per minute
    d. at least 100 per minute

11. During infant CPR the sternum is depressed:

    a. 1/4 to 1/2 inch
    b. 1/2 to 1 inch
    c. 1 to 1 1/2 inches
    d. 1 1/2 to 2 inches

12. During child CPR the sternum is depressed:

    a. 1/4 to 1/2 inch
    b. 1/2 to 1 inch
    c. 1 to 1 1/2 inches
    d. 1 1/2 to 2 inches

13. During adult CPR the sternum is depressed:

    a. 1/4 to 1/2 inch
    b. 1/2 to 1 inch
    c. 1 to 1 1/2 inches
    d. 1 1/2 to 2 inches

14. The ratio of compressions to ventilations during one person CPR for an infant is:

    a. 5:1
    b. 5:2
    c. 15:1
    d. 15:2

15. The ratio of compressions to ventilations during one person CPR for a child is:

    a. 5:1
    b. 5:2
    c. 15:1
    d. 15:2

16. The ratio of compressions to ventilations during one person CPR for an adult is:

    a. 5:1
    b. 5:2
    c. 15:1
    d. 15:2

17. The ratio of compressions to ventilations during two person CPR for an adult is:

    a. 5:1
    b. 5:2
    c. 15:1
    d. 15:2

18. The likelihood of success of CPR is <u>primarily</u> determined by the:

    a. sex of the patient
    b. time to initiation of CPR and ALS
    c. previous medical condition of the patient
    d. distance to the hospital

19. The most common cause of airway obstruction in an unconscious adult patient is:

    a. trauma
    b. foreign body
    c. the tongue
    d. loose dentures

20. The currently recommended procedure for opening the airway of an unconscious patient is the:

    a. head tilt-chin lift
    b. tongue pull
    c. chin pull
    d. triple airway maneuver

21. The airway maneuver of choice when dealing with a suspected cervical spine injury patient is:

    a. jaw thrust-without head tilt
    b. chin pull maneuver
    c. head tilt-neck lift
    d. head tilt-chin lift

22. During mouth to mouth resuscitation each breath should take approximately __________ to __________ seconds to deliver:

    a. .5 to 1
    b. 1 to 1.5
    c. 1.5 to 2
    d. 2 to 2.5

23. The best indicator of an effective ventilation is:

    a. chest excursion
    b. pupillary response
    c. pinking of the skin
    d. patient skin temperature

24. The end point of each breath should be based upon:

    a. delivering the maximum amount of air possible
    b. chest rise
    c. delivering only a small puff when ventilating an infant
    d. when the patient begins to exhale passively

25. Overinflation of the lungs:

    a. is not a primary concern in the unconscious patient
    b. will cause a pneumothorax in most patients
    c. results in gastric distension
    d. can be treated with the Heimlich maneuver

26. The volume of air required to effectively ventilate a nonbreathing adult is approximately ____________ ml.

    a. 250-500
    b. 500-700
    c. 800-1200
    d. 2000-3000

27. Ventilations for an infant respiratory arrest victim should be provided at a rate of 1 breath every ____ seconds.

    a. 3
    b. 4
    c. 5
    d. 10

28. Ventilations for a child respiratory arrest victim should be provided at a rate of 1 breath every ____ seconds.

    a. 3
    b. 4
    c. 5
    d. 10

29. Ventilations for an adult respiratory arrest victim should be provided at a rate of 1 breath every ____ seconds.

    a. 3
    b. 4
    c. 5
    d. 10

30. If you encounter resistance to your initial ventilation you should:

    a. reopen the airway and attempt to ventilate again.
    b. ventilate more forcefully
    c. provide an abdominal thrust immediately
    d. check for a pulse

31. To ensure maximum blood flow during compressions, the compression-relaxation ratio should be:

    a. 20 % compression to 80% relaxation
    b. 30 % compression to 70% relaxation
    c. 40 % compression to 60% relaxation
    d. 50 % compression to 50% relaxation

32. During the performance of compressions, you hear a rib break. Your action should be:

    a. compress more forcefully
    b. reassess your compression technique and continue
    c. discontinue compressions
    d. have someone else perform compressions

33. The point at which pulse and breathing stop is referred to as:

    a. biological death
    b. irreversible death
    c. temporary death
    d. clinical death

34. To locate the correct position for compressions you should initially locate the ______________ with the fingers of the hand closest to the patient's feet.

    a. lower margin of the rib cage
    b. suprasternal notch
    c. manubrium of the sternum
    d. left sternal border

35. Most cardiac arrests in children over 1 year old are a result of:

    a. accidents or respiratory problems
    b. coronary artery disease
    c. genetic defects
    d. arrhythmias

36. The appropriate location to check for a pulse in an unconscious child is the:

    a. radial artery
    b. brachial artery
    c. femoral artery
    d. carotid artery

37. An adult patient is standing up and clutching his throat. You are concerned that he may have an obstructed airway. Your first response is to:

    a. perform the Heimlich maneuver
    b. deliver 4 back blows
    c. have the patient open his mouth and look for any obstruction
    d. ask the patient if he is choking

38. An adult patient is choking on a piece of meat. He is coughing forcefully. You should:

    a. perform the Heimlich maneuver
    b. deliver 4 back blows
    c. observe the patient but do not interfere
    d. attempt to remove the obstruction with your fingers

39. You are administering the Heimlich maneuver to an adult patient when she becomes unconscious. You first response is to:

    a. check for breathing
    b. perform a finger sweep
    c. deliver the abdominal thrust
    d. attempt to ventilate the patient

40. When you perform the Heimlich maneuver on a conscious child, you should repeat the maneuver:

    a. 2-4 times
    b. 6-10 times
    c. until the airway is cleared or the patient becomes unconscious
    d. 2-4 times and then deliver 4 back blows

41. The proper position for the rescuer to place his hands in to perform the Heimlich maneuver on a conscious patient is:

    a. 1 inch below the navel
    b. between the navel and the xiphoid process
    c. on the xiphoid process
    d. on the rib cage

42. You should deliver the abdominal thrust to an unconscious patient with an airway obstruction:

    a. 2-4 times
    b. 6-10 times
    c. 12 times
    d. until the airway is cleared

43. After delivering abdominal thrusts to an unconscious adult patient with an airway obstruction your next step is to:

    a. perform a blind finger sweep
    b. attempt to ventilate
    c. deliver 4 back blows
    d. reposition the head

44. When opening the airway of an infant you should:

    a. slightly extend the neck
    b. hyperextend the neck
    c. flex the neck
    d. flex the neck to 90 degrees

45. Ventilation for the infant is provided via:

    a. mouth to mouth
    b. mouth to nose
    c. mouth to mouth and nose
    d. mouth to stoma

46. Chest compressions for the infant are initiated with the tips of 2 fingers at which of the following locations?

    a. lower half of the sternum
    b. 1 finger breadth below nipple line
    c. just below the suprasternal notch
    d. just above the xiphoid process

47. When performing compressions on a child you should use one hand:

    a. on the lower half of the sternum
    b. on the upper half of the sternum
    c. on nipple line
    d. just above nipple line

48. While performing compressions on a child you should ____________ with the hand closest to the child's head.

    a. check a pulse
    b. maintain an open airway
    c. provide pressure on the cricoid
    d. monitor your compression position

49. In which of the following circumstances can CPR be discontinued?

    a. when the rescuer is too exhausted to continue
    b. when a physician assumes responsibility for the patient
    c. when the patient becomes pink
    d. when a rescuer breaks a patient's rib during compressions

50. The physiologic response that conserves oxygen utilization by the body's cells (along with hypothermia) in a drowning victim is called the:

    a. cell preservation response
    b. dormant response
    c. mammalian diving reflex
    d. hibernation reflex

51. Water in the stomach following a near drowning should be:

    a. suctioned out with a long catheter
    b. left alone unless it interferes with ventilation efforts
    c. removed by a "breaking" maneuver
    d. removed by applying a chest thrust

52. The chaotic electrical rhythm that most cardiac arrest patients develop is called:

    a. ventricular asystole
    b. ventricular fibrillation
    c. ventricular tachycardia
    d. ventricular standstill

53. The origin of prehospital defibrillation dates back to the:

    a: 1940's
    b. 1950's
    c. 1960's
    d. 1970's

Match the electrical and mechanical events in column B to the wave in column A.

Column A	Column B
54. P wave	a. ventricles repolarize, no mechanical event
55. QRS	b. atria depolarize and contract
56. T wave	c. ventricles depolarize and contract

57. The rate of discharge of the SA node or pacemaker is approximately ______ beats per minute.

    a. 20-40
    b. 60-80
    c. 100-120
    d. 140- 160

Match the definition in column B with the correct term in column A.

Column A	Column B
58. automaticity	a. change in electric potential across a cell membrane that leads to contraction
59. depolarization	b. ability of a cell to generate an electrical impulse
60. conductivity	c. ability of the heart cell to receive a stimulus from a neighboring cell and pass it on
61. repolarization	d. recharging of the cell membrane to its original "polarized" state

62. Immediately following contraction, the heart's cells enter a _______ period during which they cannot be depolarized.

    a. excitation
    b. refractory
    c. interlude
    d. stimulation

63. The first part of the conduction system to recharge or repolarize the fastest is the ____________.

    a. SA node (pacemaker)
    b. AV node
    c. Bundle of his
    d. Purkinje fibers

64. If the SA node or pacemaker fails, the AV node can fire at a rate of ____________ beats per minute.

    a. 20-40
    b. 40-60
    c. 60-80
    d. 80-100

65. If the SA node and AV node fail, the ventricles can fire at a rate of ______ beats per minute.

  a. 20-40
  b. 40-60
  c. 60-80
  d. 80-100

66. The electrical activity of the heart is commonly measured by an instrument which detects and amplifies the electrical signals called the:

  a. defibrillator
  b. electrocardiogram
  c. electroencephalogram
  d. electrograph

67. An ECG machine is connected to the body's surface by __________ and cables.

  a. electrodes
  b. interfacers
  c. connection modules
  d. resistance inhibitors

68. The dark vertical markings on the ECG paper correspond to ____ seconds in time.

  a. .1
  b. .2
  c. .3
  d. .5

Match the time in seconds in column B with the related number of dark vertical lines on an ECG tracing in column A.

Column A	Column B
69. 5 lines	a. .6 seconds
70. 3 lines	b. 1.0 seconds
71. 10 lines	c. 4.0 seconds
72. 20 lines	d. 2.0 seconds

73. The periodic marks that measure time marks on the top of the paper appear every _____ seconds of time.

    a. 1
    b. 2
    c. 3
    d. 5

74. By counting the number of ventricular complexes within 2 top periodic markings on ECG paper and multiplying times _____, you can estimate the ECG rate.

    a. 2
    b. 3
    c. 5
    d. 10

75. Standardization is usually calibrated so that a ____ mm deflection (10 small boxes on the ECG paper) corresponds to 1 millivolt.

    a. 1
    b. 3
    c. 5
    d. 10

76. The type of defibrillator that will identify the rhythm, charge and discharge automatically without any further direction from the operator is called:

    a. automatic
    b. semi-automatic
    c. manual
    d. controllable

77. Energy settings currently recommended by the American Heart Association are ____ joules for the first defibrillation.

    a. 100
    b. 200
    c. 300
    d. 400

78. If ventricular fibrillation persists, the AHA recommends _______ joules for the second defibrillation.

    a. 100-200
    b. 200-300
    c. 300-400
    d. 400-500

79. After the initial pulse check with automatic and semi-automatic defibrillators, the AHA recommends that _____ successive shocks be performed for the patient in ventricular fibrillation without intervening pulse checks.

a. 2
b. 3
c. 4
d. 5

80. During the initial successive shocks for a patient in v-fib, the AHA recommends that:

a. CPR be performed for 30 seconds
b. CPR be performed for 60 seconds
c. each shock should be delivered as soon as possible with no pause between them
d. the patient should be ventilated and CPR continued for 60 seconds

81. The recommended placement of paddles on the anterior chest wall includes one placed just left of the left nipple, midaxillary line, and the other:

a. below the right clavicle on the sternum
b. below the left clavicle on the sternum
c. below the right clavicle on the right sternal border
d. below the right clavicle on the left sternal border

82. Which of the following is not considered an adequate approach to improving conduction across the skin?

a. gels
b. creams
c. alcohol
d. saline pads

83. The transfer of electricity directly across the chest wall from one paddle to another via the conductive medium, sweat or other forms of moisture is called:.

a. depolarization
b. bridging
c. resistance
d. repolarization

84. There should be sufficient pressure to ensure firm contact between the paddle and the surface of the skin. Approximately ____ pounds of muscular pressure is recommended.

a. 5
b. 10
c. 15
d. 25

Skill Performance Sheet

Adult One Rescuer CPR

Student's Name ____________________________ Date _________

Performance Standard	**Performed**	**Failed**
Check for unresponsiveness		
Open airway with appropriate maneuver (head tilt-chin lift or jaw thrust)		
Assess breathing (look, listen and feel)		
Seal mouth around the patient's mouth and pinch nose		
Give two smooth breaths while observing chest rise (1-1.5 seconds per breath)		
Take mouth away between breaths		
Check carotid pulse (pulse is present)		
If no pulse, locate correct hand position		
Maintain vertical position and provide 15 compressions (80-100/min)		
Provide two ventilations		
After four cycles of 15:2, give two ventilations and check a pulse		
If no pulse, continue 15:2 cycle		

Comments____

____

____

Instructor __________________ Circle One: Pass Fail

Skill Performance Sheet

Adult Two Rescuer CPR

Student's Name ______________________ Date ________

Performance Standard	**Performed**	**Failed**
RESCUER #1		
Check for unresponsiveness		
Open airway with appropriate maneuver (head tilt-chin lift or jaw thrust)		
Assess breathing (look, listen and feel)		
Seal mouth around the patient's mouth and pinch nose		
Give two smooth breaths while observing chest rise (1-1.5 seconds per breath)		
Take mouth away between breaths		
Check carotid pulse (pulse is present)		
RESCUER #2		
If no pulse, locate correct hand position		
Maintain vertical position and provide five compressions (80-100/min)		
Rescuer #1 provide one ventilation		
After four cycles of 5:1, check a pulse		
If no pulse, continue 5:1 cycle		

Comments ____

____

Instructor ________________ Circle One: Pass Fail

Skill Performance Sheet

Child One Rescuer CPR

Student's Name ______________________________ Date __________

Performance Standard	**Performed**	**Failed**
Check for unresponsiveness		
Open airway with appropriate maneuver (head tilt-chin lift or jaw thrust)		
Assess breathing (look, listen and feel)		
Seal mouth around the patient's mouth and pinch nose		
Give two smooth breaths while observing chest rise (1-1.5 seconds per breath)		
Take mouth away between breaths		
Check carotid pulse (pulse is present)		
If no pulse, locate correct hand position		
Maintain vertical position and provide five compressions (80-100/min) while continuing to maintain head tilt		
Provide two ventilations		
After ten cycles of 5:1, give two ventilations and check a pulse		
If no pulse, continue 5:1 cycle		

Comments ____

____

Instructor ____________________ Circle One: Pass Fail

Skill Performance Sheet

Infant One Rescuer CPR

Student's Name ____________________ Date ________

Performance Standard	**Performed**	**Failed**
Check for unresponsiveness		
Open airway with appropriate maneuver (head tilt-chin lift or jaw thrust)		
Assess breathing (look, listen and feel)		
Seal mouth around the patient's mouth and nose		
Give two smooth breaths while observing chest rise (1-1.5 seconds per breath)		
Take mouth away between breaths		
Check brachial pulse (pulse is present)		
Locate correct finger position (one finger below nipple line)		
Maintain head tilt		
Provide compressions at a rate of 100/min (1/2 to 1 inch)		
After ten cycles of 5:1, give two ventilations and check a pulse		
If no pulse, continue CPR		

Comments ____

____

Instructor ______________ Circle One: Pass Fail

Skill Performance Sheet

Defibrillation - Manual Defibrillator

Student's Name ____________________________ Date _________

Performance Standard	**Performed**	**Failed**
Check pulselessness		
If witnessed arrest, perform precordial thump		
If pulseless, EMT #1 performs CPR		
EMT #2 attaches electrodes and leads		
Turn on recorder and medical control device		
Assess rhythm		
If ventricular fibrillation or ventricular tachycardia, defibrillate:		
Apply gel or other conductive medium to paddles		
Charge paddles to 200 joules		
Properly place paddles and apply 25 pounds of muscular pressure		
Announce "all clear" and confirm that no person is in contact with the patient		
Press the discharge buttons		
Reevaluate pulse and rhythm		
If still in ventricular fibrillation or ventricular tachycardia, repeat defibrillation process at 200-300 joules.		

CONTINUED ON NEXT PAGE

Skill Performance Sheet

Defibrillation - Manual Defibrillator (continued)

Performance Standard	**Performed**	**Failed**
Reevaluate pulse and rhythm		
If still in ventricular fibrillation or ventricular tachycardia, repeat defibrillation process at 360 joules		
Continue process according to local protocol		

Comments____

____

____

____

Instructor __________________ Circle One: Pass Fail

Skill Performance Sheet

Defibrillation - Semiautomatic Defibrillator

Student's Name ____________________________ Date _________

Performance Standard	Performed	Failed
Check pulselessness		
If witnessed arrest, perform precordial thump		
If pulseless, EMT #1 performs CPR		
EMT #2 attaches electrodes and leads		
Turn on device		
Push analyze and stand clear of patient		
If ventricular fibrillation or ventricular tachycardia, the machine will advise defibrillation		
Machine will either charge or advise operator to charge (200 joules)		
Announce "all clear" and confirm that no person is in contact with the patient		
Press the discharge buttons		
Push analyze and stand clear of patient		
If ventricular fibrillation or ventricular tachycardia, the machine will advise defibrillation		
Machine will either charge or advise operator to charge (300 joules)		

CONTINUED ON NEXT PAGE

Skill Performance Sheet

Defibrillation - Semiautomatic Defibrillator (continued)

Performance Standard	Performed	Failed
Announce "all clear" and confirm that no person is in contact with the patient		
Press the discharge buttons		
Push analyze and stand clear of patient		
If ventricular fibrillation or ventricular tachycardia, the machine will advise defibrillation		
Machine will either charge or advise operator to charge (360 joules)		
Announce "all clear" and confirm that no person is in contact with the patient		
Press the discharge buttons		
Reevaluate pulse and rhythm		
If pulseless, perform CPR for 1 minute		
If still in ventricular fibrillation or ventricular tachycardia, repeat process of three stacked shocks at 360 joules.		
Continue process according to local protocol		

Comments____

____

____

Instructor ________________ Circle One: Pass Fail

Chapter 7

CENTRAL NERVOUS SYSTEM EMERGENCIES

Materials and Equipment for Lesson

1. Anatomy slides, overhead transparencies or flipcharts
2. Handouts
   - Anatomy and physiology
   - Head trauma
   - Spinal trauma
   - Performance sheets for CNS skills
3. Model of the central nervous system
4. Slide projector, overhead projector, flipchart and/or blackboard

Section 1

Anatomy and Physiology

Objectives
(Slide 7-1)

At the conclusion of the chapter the students will be able to:

1. **List the bones of the skull and spinal column.**
2. **Describe how brain is protected from injury.**
3. **List the parts and functions of the central and peripheral nervous system.**
4. **List the divisions and functions of the autonomic nervous system.**

Instructor Preparation

Reading preparation for the lesson:

EMT Prehospital Care, Chapter 7, pages 289-304

Optional reading:

Guyton, AC: Textbook of Medical Physiology, 8th Ed. W.B. Saunders, Philadelphia, PA 1991

Solomon, EP, Phillips, GA: Understanding Human Anatomy and Physiology. W.B. Saunders, Philadelphia, PA 1987

Suggested Learning Activities

Using a lecture format with the aid of slides, overhead transparencies or charts, provide an overview of CNS anatomy and physiology.

Pass a CNS model throughout the class and have the students observe key structures.

When possible, have students palpate anatomical structures on self or classmates and monitor activities.

Content

I. Overview **(Slide 7-2)**
- A. Major goal of prehospital care is to ensure brain viability
  - 1. Large number of deaths result from brain trauma
  - 2. Death may result from vital systems failure due to central nervous system control
- B. The central nervous system is the controlling system of the body
  - 1. It is our consciousness and intellectual/emotional/behavioral center
  - 2. It receives and interprets information from environment
  - 3. It directs and regulates organs and tissues
  - 4. Some activity is conscious, while some is unconscious

II. Divisions of the nervous system **(Slide 7-3)**
- A. Central and peripheral nervous systems are two divisions
  - 1. Central nervous system is the computer and consists of brain, brain stem, and spinal cord
    - a) It receives information about environment and internal functions
    - b) All voluntary functions require willful or conscious actions
  - 2. Peripheral nervous system connects the central nervous system to the target organs
    - a) Sensory nerves transmit information to the brain via the spinal cord
    - b) Motor nerves carry information from the brain to skeletal muscle via the spinal cord
    - c) Cranial nerves communicate directly from brain to organs
- B. Voluntary vs. autonomic nervous system **(Slide 7-4)**
  - 1. Voluntary nervous system controls conscious functions
    - a) Connects sensory nerves from sense organs and skin to the brain
    - b) Directs activities via motor nerves to skeletal muscle
  - 2. The autonomic division controls involuntary body functions
    - a) Controls vital functions, such as heart rate, vessel dilation and constriction, digestion, etc.
    - b) Sensory nerves detect changes, such as oxygen, blood pressure, etc.
    - c) Motor nerves direct changes, i.e., increase in heart rate
    - d) The autonomic nervous system has two divisions: the parasympathetic and sympathetic
    - e) The parasympathetic slows the heart rate while the sympathetic speeds it up
    - f) The parasympathetic constricts the pupil while the sympathetic dilates it **(Slide 7-5)**
    - g) These divisions allow the autonomic nervous system to counterbalance and regulate vital functions

Content

III. Regeneration of nerve cells, and oxygen and glucose requirement **(Slide 7-6)**
A. When peripheral cells are injured, regeneration is possible
1. Amputated body part can be reattached in some instances
2. Function can be partially restored when peripheral nerves are cuts
B. Central nervous System structures cannot regenerate
1. When brain tissue or spinal cord are destroyed, they cannot regenerate
2. Other parts of the brain can take over some functions but disability is usually present
C. Nerve cells are very dependent on oxygen
1. When oxygen delivery ceases, the brain will die in 4 - 6 minutes
2. This explains irreversible brain death after prolonged cardiac arrest
3. CPR must be applied quickly to affect survival
4. Hypoxia is often manifested by altered mental state or brain dysfunction
5. Altered mental state may include agitation, combativeness, confusion, and unresponsiveness
6. The check for unresponsiveness is part of the primary survey
D. The brain is also dependent on glucose for proper function
1. Low glucose may cause the same alteration in mental state
2. Patients with altered mental states who are able to swallow are often given sugar solutions
3. Prolonged glucose deprivation can result in brain damage
4. Many EMS systems have glucose protocols to address this problem
E. Nerve cells and pressure **(Slide 7-7)**
1. Nerve cells are very sensitive to pressure
2. When pressure is exerted on nerve cells, dysfunction is possible
3. The degree of dysfunction depends on the amount of pressure and the length of time it is applied
4. Strong forces over short time or lesser forces over longer time may result in similar damage
5. Provide examples of intracranial bleeding and Saturday night palsy

IV. Protection of brain and spinal cord **(Slide 7-8)**
A. The brain and spinal cord are well protected by bone and membranous coverings
1. The bone consists of the skull and vertebral column
2. The membrane consists of three layers and fluid between two layers
B. The skull consists of several bones comprising the cranium and face
1. Knowledge of these bones allow the EMT to effectively communicate the location of injuries
2. Bones of the skull at birth are flat/irregular
a) Separate at birth
b) Fused during childhood
3. Bones of the skull include: **(Slide 7-9)**
a) Frontal (1) (forehead)
b) Occipital (1) (posterior region)
c) Parietal (2) (superior lateral)
d) Temporal (2) (anterolateral)
4. Fontanelles at birth are located on top of skull in anterior-posterior areas **(Slide 7-10)**

Content

5. The base of the skull consists of several bones fused together
    a) The foramen magnum is an opening for the spinal cord
    b) The brain rests at the base
6. The skull has approximately a 1 liter capacity and is filled by brain
7. There is no room for expansion; bleeding can cause pressure and herniation through the foramen magnum
8. Pressure and herniation is a potentially lethal problem that must be addressed quickly

C. The facial bones consist of the orbits, nasal bone, maxilla, mandible and zygoma **(Slide 7-11)**
1. The zygomatic bone connects the temporal bone to the maxilla
2. The mandible is connected to the skull at the temporomandibular joints

D. The spinal column consists of 33 vertebrae that surround the spinal cord and nerves **(Slide 7-12)**
1. They extend from the base of the skull to the tail bone (coccyx)
2. They are held together by ligaments and separated by discs
3. The structure permits rotation and bending, and proper alignment is essential
4. The vertebrae are named for their location:
    a) Cervical (7) are located in the neck
    b) Thoracic (12) are connected to each rib in the chest
    c) Lumbar (5) form the lower back
    d) Sacrum (5 fused) form the posterior aspect of the pelvic girdle
    e) Coccyx (4 fused) form the tail bone
5. Each vertebrae have similar characteristics **(Slide 7-13)**
    a) Anterior body separated by discs with ligament attachments
    b) Posterior spinous processes with ligament attachments
    c) Arcs connect anterior and posterior components to form canal for cord
    d) Nerves exit and enter at each level
6. The spinal cord ends at the first lumbar vertebrae
7. Nerves continue to lumbar and sacral region

E. Membranous coverings surround the brain and spinal cord **(Slide 7-14)**
1. The meninges consists of three layers of membranes
2. The outer layer is a tough leathery layer called the dura
    a) Arteries are located between bone and dura
    b) Bleeding from these arteries causes epidural hemorrhage
3. The middle layer is called the arachnoid
    a) Veins and venous sinuses are located between the dura and arachnoid
    b) Bleeding from these veins cause subdural hemorrhage
4. The inner layer is called the pia mater and is adhered to the brain
    a) The space between the arachnoid and pia mater contains spinal fluid
    b) This fluid lubricates the brain and provides a cushion
    c) The fluid circulates to all aspects of the brain and cord
    d) The cerebral spinal fluid contains nutrients
    e) It is continually produced and absorbed from blood plexes

Content

V. The central nervous system **(Slide 7-15)**
   A. The central nervous system consists of the brain, brain stem and spinal cord
   B. It acts as the central computer for body functions
      1. It receives and interprets all sensory input
      2. It receives input on vital functions and regulates vital organs
      3. All information is processed at incredible speed
   C. The cerebrum is the largest and most superior component
      1. It is divided into left and right halves at the middle called hemispheres
         a) The right side controls the left body, and the left side controls the right body
         b) The hemispheres communicate through the corpus callosum
      2. Each hemisphere is divided into lobes which have specific functions
         a) Frontal lobes control intellect and motor functions
         b) The parietal lobe controls sensory functions
         c) The occipital lobe controls vision
         d) The temporal lobe controls smelling and hearing
      3. Loss of or damage to a given area will result in specific function loss
      4. The homunculus is a representative map of brain function
      5. Review areas of the homunculus **(Slide 7-16)**
      6. The inner cerebrum is composed of dense nerve tracts that journey to the brain stem and cord
      7. Nerve tracts cross over to opposite sides in brain stem
      8. The outer cell bodies on the brain appear gray (gray matter) while the nerve tracts appear white (white matter)
      9. Basic knowledge of anatomy allows understanding of regional injuries
      10. Provide examples of injury
   D. The brain stem is the controlling center for vital autonomic functions **(Slide 7-17)**
      1. It is located at the base of the cerebrum
      2. It consists of its own nerve cells and nerve tracts traveling down from the cerebrum
      3. Vital centers in the brain stem communicate to organs via cranial nerves
      4. Vital centers control respiration and circulatory functions
         a) Respiratory arrest can result from damage
         b) Structures such as pupils are also controlled from these centers
         c) For this reason, pupils are important to evaluate brain stem function
         d) Abnormal respiratory patterns are also signs of brain stem function
      5. Gathering baseline information about brain stem function is an essential role of the EMT's assessment
      6. The cerebellum is the outpocketing behind the brain stem and is responsible for balance and coordination
   E. The spinal cord is a continuation of the brain
      1. It contains nerve tracts and also has its own cell bodies
      2. Reflex activity of the spinal cord
         a) Immediate reactions to stimulus, i.e., removal of hand from hot stove

Content

b) This type of action occurs through the reflex arc

F. Actions mediated by the central nervous system **(Slide 7-18)**

1. Automatic action includes heart rate, bleed pressure, temperature regulation, etc., and occurs through the autonomic nervous system
2. Reflex action refers to actions mediated through the spinal cord via a reflex arc (pain withdrawal, reflex) **(Slide 7-19)**
3. Conscious action requires sensory input and motor response through the appropriate parts of the cerebrum
4. Voluntary muscle control occurs in skeletal muscle through conscious controls
5. Involuntary muscle control occurs in smooth muscle lining vessels, G.I. tract, etc., and occurs automatically

G. Blood supply to the brain **(Slide 7-20)**

1. 80% of blood supply occurs through carotids
    a) Carotid pulse should be felt gently to avoid blockage
    b) Embolus can be released if plaques are dislodged
2. Remainder of blood supply occurs through vertebral arteries
3. Vertebral arteries merge to form basilar artery
4. Basilar arteries join carotids to form network to feed entire brain
5. Damage or blockage of specific arteries will result in damage to respective area of brain

H. Overview of pathophysiology of central nervous system **(Slide 7-21)**

1. Structural injuries occur when specific sections of the brain are injured. These include:
    a) Disruption of focal brain tissue, i.e., penetrating wounds
    b) Blockage of blood supply due to clot or vessel rupture to that part of the brain
    c) Blunt trauma to a specific area
    d) Any other medical condition or trauma that affects specific region
    e) Structural injuries result in localized findings (unequal pupils, paralysis, one-sided sensory loss)
2. Metabolic injuries occur when the entire central nervous system is affected equally
    a) Poisoning, hypoxia, low blood sugar are examples of metabolic injury
    b) Metabolic injuries result in symmetry of findings
    c) Provide examples of metabolic versus structural injuries
3. Secondary complications of brain injury include hypoxia, hypotension, hypoglycemia, infections, increased intracranial pressure **(Slide 7-22)**
    a) Secondary conditions can occur with direct brain injury and complicate brain function
    b) Hypoxia can occur as a result of airway blockage, respiratory arrest or other respiratory or cardiovascular problems
    c) Hypotension can result from shock states
    d) Hypoglycemia may have caused a fall or accident
    e) Increased intracranial pressure can result from brain edema or bleeding within the skull
    f) Infection can occur following open wounds to the brain

Chapter 7

Section 2

HEAD INJURIES

Objectives
(Slide 7-23)

At the conclusion of the chapter the student will be able to:

1. **Provide 1 condition that may result from each of the following mechanisms of injury to the head and spine:**
   Deceleration
   Compression
   Penetrating; knife vs. missile

2. **Describe the correct steps of assessment for a patient with suspected head and spinal injury**

3. **Given a scenario, recognize and provide the appropriate treatment for the following types of head trauma:**
   Skull fracture
   Subdural and epidural hematoma

4. **List 4 types of brain injury and how they occur.**

5. **List 5 types of "secondary" brain injury.**

Instructor Preparation

Reading preparation for the lesson:

EMT Prehospital Care, Chapter 7, pages 304-319

Optional reading:

Prehospital Trauma Life Support Committee of The National Association of EMTs: Pre-Hospital Trauma Life Support, 2nd Ed., Emergency Training, Akron, Ohio, 1990

Safer P., Bircher N.: Cardiopulmonary Cerebral Resuscitation, 3rd Ed., W.B. Saunders, Philadelphia, PA 1988

Suggested Learning Activities

Using lecture format with handouts, provide a presentation on the assessment and management of head trauma.

Provide case history examples of various problems.

Content

VI. Overview **(Slide 7-24)**
- A. More than half of all head trauma is a result of motor vehicle accidents
- B. Falls, sports accidents, penetrating wounds are other causes
- C. Blunt trauma results from:
  - 1. Static forces (i.e., car, falls on head)
  - 2. Dynamic (movement of brain following initial blow)
  - 3. Most instances involve both static and dynamic
  - 4. Contrecoup results from dynamic forces when skull is struck **(Slide 7-25)**
    - a) After impact, brain continues to move forward within skull
    - b) Brain may strike opposite side of skull during movement
    - c) Patient may exhibit occipital neurological signs with frontal impact
- D. Penetrating trauma results from: **(Slide 7-26)**
  - 1. Missiles, knives, etc
  - 2. Brain tissue is damaged in path of object
  - 3. Bleeding may occur in cranium
  - 4. Shock waves may injure adjacent tissue
- E. Cervical spine injuries may result from head trauma
  - 1. Movement of head following trauma may cause cervical spine injury
  - 2. Cervical spine injury can result in paralysis or death
  - 3. A high index of suspicion is essential in managing these patients

VII. Specific head injuries
- A. Scalp wounds may occur from blunt or penetrating trauma **(Slide 7-27)**
  - 1. May or may not be associated with brain injury.
  - 2. Direct pressure must be gentle and over a broad area to avoid compression of bone fragments into brain
  - 3. Scalp is highly vascular and hypovolemia may develop through extensive blood loss
  - 4. Don't irrigate or explore wound due to potential for brain infection
- B. Skull fractures may occur from blunt or penetrating wounds **(Slide 7-28)**
  - 1. Skull fractures not always associated with brain injury
  - 2. Significant injury may result from forces or bone fragments in the brain
  - 3. Fractures of bone may lead to bleeding due to location of arteries
  - 4. Open fractures
    - a) Cause communication of with the brain
    - b) Infection is more possible
  - 5. Closed fractures exist without the skin being broken
  - 6. There are specific types of skull fractures
    - a) Linear fractures are lines of fractures without displacement
    - b) Comminuted fractures are fragments of bone usually caused by a severe force
    - c) Depressed fractures are segments of bone pushed downward toward brain

Content

d) Basilar skull fractures are fractures in the base of the skull
(1) External palpation/inspection not possible
(2) Other signs are needed to identify
(a) Blood/fluid leaks from ears or nose
(b) Raccoon sign (bilateral black eyes) **(Slide 7-29)**
(c) Battle's sign (ecchymosis behind ears) **(Slide 7-30)**

C. Specific brain injuries **(Slide 7-31)**
1. Concussion is transient loss of consciousness or neurological deficit due to injury
a) Reversible injury that usually has no permanent damage
b) Caused by shock waves to the "waking" brain centers
c) Least severe is a brief disturbance of consciousness with full recall of accident
d) More severe concussion patients may have amnesia of events before and after accident
e) Most severe may have sustained unconsciousness and have risk of other injuries
2. Cerebral contusions may occur following blunt trauma **(Slide 7-32)**
a) Localized brain injury results with focal findings
b) May involve either motor or sensory malfunction, consistent with area injured
3. Intracerebral hematoma is bleeding within the brain **(Slide 7-33)**
a) It can occur when arteries tear within the brain tissue
b) Bleeding can affect the local brain tissue
c) Bleeding can also lead to increased intracranial pressure causing more diffuse signs
4. Signs of increased intracranial pressure **(Slide 7-34)**
a) Headaches, nausea, and vomiting (sometimes projectile)
b) Alterations in consciousness may occur
c) Alterations immediately following injury may be related to the blow
d) Later episodes may be related to continued bleeding, edema and increased pressure
e) Other secondary brain injury must also be considered (hypoxia, hypertension, etc.)
f) Eye and motor findings may be unilateral during herniation of brain and may then extend to both sides
(1) Eyes - unequal pupils, bilateral pinpointing or dilated are possible during expansion
(2) Motor - unilateral paralysis or sensory loss are possible
(3) Posture - classic postures, decorticate (flexion), decerebrate (extension) and flaccid extremities are possible
g) Vital signs can be affected by increased pressure
(1) Respirations can vary according to level of injury
(a) Cheyne-Stokes
(b) Central neurogenic hyperventilation
(c) Apneustic
(d) Ataxic
(e) Biot's

Content

(2) Cushing reflex involves slowing of pulse and increase in blood pressure

5. Epidural hematoma is bleeding above dura mater **(Slide 7-35)**
   a) Bleeding is arterial and pressure may rise quickly.
   b) Definitive treatment is evacuation of blood at hospital operating room
   c) Classic history is loss of consciousness, lucid interval, loss of consciousness
   d) Patients may never regain consciousness
   e) May not immediately lose consciousness but become unconscious later
   f) Lateralizing motor signs may be present
   g) Respiratory and cardiovascular signs (i.e., Cushing reflex)
   h) Provide a few scenario examples of variations
6. Subdural hematoma is bleeding between dura **(Slide 7-36)**
   a) Bleeding is venous
   b) Subdurals carry highest mortality rate due to expanding bleeding
   c) Signs of increased pressure may present in days to months
   d) The same signs as epidural are present in subdural.
   e) Access to surgical intervention is essential

VIII. Assessment of head injury patients **(Slide 7-37)**

A. History
1. The mechanism of injury is critical since signs may develop late
2. Key questions about injury include:
   a) Facts about motor vehicle accident, i.e., speed, location of patient, seat belt use, and type of impact
   b) Loss of consciousness and lucid intervals followed by deterioration of mental status?
   c) Was injury direct blow (i.e., windshield) or not, deceleration?
   d) Was there apnea or cyanosis at the scene to indicate hypoxia?
   e) Was there evidence of blood loss to suggest hypovolemia?
   f) Are there known diseases that may have contributed to the accident?

B. Physical exam **(Slide 7-38)**
1. Should be rapid so as to not delay time to definitive care
2. ABC's should be done with consideration for possible cervical spine injury
   a) Modified jaw thrust
   b) Immobilized routinely when mechanism of injury suggests possible spinal injury
3. Mental status is assessed by use of the Glasgow Coma Scale **(Slide 7-39)**
   a) Stimulus is applied sequentially from verbal to painful to identify highest possible score
   b) Painful stimuli are applied with
      (1) Pressure on nailbed
      (2) Pinching arm
      (3) Pain should be applied bilaterally (in case of one-sided sensory loss)

Content

c) Eyes are evaluated according to:
   (1) 4 - open spontaneously (no stimuli)
   (2) 3 - open to verbal stimuli
   (3) 2 - open to painful stimuli
   (4) 1 - do not open

d) Verbal is evaluated according to:
   (1) 5 - alert and oriented
   (2) 4 - confused (attention can be maintained)
   (3) 3 - inappropriate (attention cannot be maintained)
   (4) 2 - incomprehensible sounds
   (5) 1 - nod response

e) Motor is evaluated according to:
   (1) 6 - obeys verbal commands
   (2) 5 - localized to pain (reaches to source of pain)
   (3) 4 - withdraws (rolls or moves from pain)
   (4) 3 - flexion (flexes arms to pain) or decorticate **(Slide 7-40)**
   (5) 2 - extension (extends arms to pain) or decerebrate **(Slide 7-41)**
   (6) 1 - no response to pain

f) Communicated Glasgow test results to emergency department with description of individual findings and total score

g) Provide example of communication of score

h) Glasgow Coma Scale may be used
   (1) To initiate treatments (i.e., hyperventilation of head trauma)
   (2) For facility selection in conjunction with trauma score

i) Injuries may prevent developing total score
   (1) Quadriplegia, closed contused eyes, intubated patient
   (2) Communicate measurable components and indicate limitations of testing

4. Vital signs may include several variations
   a) Respiration assessment should include rate, depth, and especially patterns **(Slide 7-42)**
   b) Temperature may be altered in central nervous system injuries
      (1) Damage of control center hypothalamus
      (2) Note variations
      (3) Pulse and blood pressure should be evaluated
         (a) To identify hypovolemia or other shock states
         (b) To identify classic Cushing reflex (increased blood pressure, slow pulse)

5. Head and scalp are examined gently and carefully for evidence of skull fractures **(Slide 7-43)**
   a) Look for Battle's, raccoon and signs of CSF from ears or nose
   b) Crepitus, swelling or wounds should be searched for throughout the scalp region

Content

6. Pupils are evaluated for size, equality, reactivity **(Slide 7-44)**
    a) Size is described as constrictive, midposition, or dilated (mm system can also be used)
    b) Pupils may vary for many reasons, review variations
    c) Equality is evaluated to identify unilateral signs (5% normally have unequal pupils). Differences are usually greater than 2 mm
    d) Reactivity is evaluated by light exposure to eyes
    e) Note relative response (i.e., bilateral or unilateral failure to react should be noted)
    f) Traumatic iritis (injury to the iris) may hamper reactivity and vary size
7. Neck and spine are evaluated by observation and gentle palpitation **(Slide 7-45)**
    a) Absence of physical signs does not rule out cervical spine injury
    b) When unsure, you should immobilize
    c) Combative or disoriented patients may have to be manually immobilized
8. Motor and sensory function is evaluated in upper and lower extremities, trunk and bilaterally **(Slide 7-46)**
    a) Conscious patients should be asked to move hands and feet and evaluate for sensory function
    b) Unconscious patients are evaluated with painful stimuli and checked for symmetry
9. Serial exams should be performed en route to the hospital to note evaluation of findings

IX. Treatment **(Slide 7-47)**
  A. Directed at assuring adequate ventilation, oxygenation and circulation
  B. Treatment of secondary head injury and immobilization
  C. The airway is established with the use of the modified jaw thrust or the chin lift without head tilt
    1. Patients who can tolerate an oropharyngeal of nasopharyngeal airway should have it inserted
    2. If gag reflex is present, it should be removed immediately to avoid vomiting and increases in intracranial pressure caused by gag reflex
    3. If protocols permit, the EGTA or endotracheal intubation can be performed. However, care should be taken not to hyperextend neck
  D. Ventilations should be evaluated
    1. In hypoventilation, positive pressure should be instituted quickly **(Slide 7-48)**
      a) CO_2 buildup can cause cerebral vasodilation which can lead to increased cerebral edema
      b) This concept can be used to decrease cerebral edema
      c) Hyperventilation causes cerebral vasoconstriction reducing blood flow to head
      d) This decreases cerebral edema. Check local protocols for treatment based on this concept

Content

2. Oxygenation is assured by free flow or positive pressure as needed **(Slide 7-49)**
    a) High-concentration oxygen should be used whenever significant head trauma exists, (in C.O.P.D. patients consult local protocols)
    b) Nonrebreather mask is the free flow device of choice
    c) Manually triggered resuscitation or bag valve mask with high oxygen reservoir, etc., when positive pressure is needed

E. Circulation should be evaluated to identify shock states and evidence of poor brain perfusion **(Slide 7-50)**
F. Increased intracranial pressure should be identified by a search of signs (i.e., mental status, nausea, vomiting, one-sided signs, Cushing reflex, etc.)
G. If protocols permit, hyperventilation should be instituted
H. Low blood sugar should be considered particularly in the face of a diabetic history
I. If protocols permit, glucose or glucagon should be administered
J. Infection should be prevented by use of sterile dressing, and never irrigate head wounds
K. Immobilize patient with cervical collar, short spine or long spine when time permits
L. If critical injuries, i.e., epidural hematoma, are present, rapid extrication should be utilized with c-spine precautions
M. If possible, patient can be placed in semi-sitting position in case of vomiting
N. Suction should be available in case of vomiting during transport, particularly if patient is supine and attached to a long spine board **(Slide 7-51)**
O. Transport and Notification **(Slide 7-52)**

1. Quiet transport to avoid aggravating injuries is essential
2. Trauma center, CNS center or hospital should be notified so that preparations (i.e., neurosurgeon on standby) can be made
3. An accurate precise history should be given including sequential neurological exam to hospital staff

Section 3

SPINAL INJURIES

Objectives
(Slide 7-53)

At the conclusion of the chapter the student will be able to:

1. **State the body locations for the following dermatomes:**
   Cervical-4 Thoracic-4-
   Thoracic-10 Lumbar-1
   Lumbar-5

2. **List the steps of assessment for a patient with spinal injury.**

3. **Describe proper spinal immobilization for the following patients:**
   Stable automobile accident victim
   Unstable automobile accident victim

4. **Describe the proper steps for removing a helmet from a suspected spinal injury victim.**

Instructor Preparation

Reading preparation for the lesson:

EMT Prehospital Care, Chapter 7, pages 319-338

Optional reading:

Prehospital Trauma Life Support Committee of The National Association of EMTs: Pre-Hospital Trauma Life Support, 2nd Ed., Emergency Training, Akron, Ohio, 1990

Safer P., Bircher N.: Cardiopulmonary Cerebral Resuscitation, 3rd Ed., W.B. Saunders, Philadelphia, PA, 1988

Suggested Learning Activities

Using lecture format with handouts, provide a presentation on the assessment and management of spinal trauma.

Provide case history examples of various problems.

Content

X. Overview **(Slide 7-54)**

A. Incidence between 3 and 5 per 100,000 population.

B. Careful prehospital management makes the difference between good recovery vs. paralysis or even death

C. Spinal injury should assumed in all suspected trauma patients

The spinal column **(Slide 7-55)**

D. Spinal cord injuries are usually associated with injuries to the bony vertebrae

E. Basic structure of spinal column and vertebrae

1. Spinal column consists of 33 vertebrae from the base of the skull to the tip of the coccyx
2. Held together by ligaments and separated by discs
3. Most vertebrae are separate bones, some are fused
4. Specific vertebrae
    - a) 7 cervical vertebrae
    - b) 12 thoracic vertebrae
    - c) 5 lumbar vertebrae
    - d) 5 sacral vertebrae (fused)
    - e) 4 coccygeal vertebrae (fused)
5. Basic components of the vertebrae
    - a) Anterior body which gives support to the column
    - b) Posterior spinous process
    - c) Transverse processes
    - d) Anterior, posterior and transverse bones form a circular vertebral foramen or spinal canal
    - e) Ligaments on the anterior, lateral and posterior surfaces
        - (1) Hold the vertebrae in position
        - (2) Allow a limited degree of movement
6. Intervertebral discs
    - a) Made of fibrocartilage
    - b) Allow the vertebrae to move upon one another
    - c) Act as shock absorbers
7. Spinal nerves and vessels exit on each side **(Slide 7-56)**
    - a) 31 pairs of spinal nerves
        - (1) 8 cervical
        - (2) 12 thoracic
        - (3) 5 lumbar
        - (4) 5 sacral
        - (5) 1 coccygeal
    - b) Spinal cord ends at first lumbar vertebra

F. Spinal nerves

1. Sensory and motor components
    - a) Exit from each side of the vertebral column
    - b) 31 pairs
    - c) Provide communication between all body structures and CNS
    - d) Sensory nerves bring information to the spinal cord and brain
    - e) Motor nerves transmit information to organs, muscles and tissues, regulating their activity
    - f) Disruption of nerves can cause loss of organ function

Content

2. Dermatones (sensory) **(Slide 7-57)**
    a) EMTs are not expected to memorize all dermatomes
    b) Some are helpful to appreciate level of injury
        (1) Cervical 4 - above collar bone
        (2) Thoracic 4 - nipple line
        (3) Thoracic 10 - umbilicus
        (4) Lumbar 1 - groin
3. Motor (innervation of muscles)
    a) Muscles of arm and shoulder - C4-T1
    b) Muscles of legs - lumbar and sacrum
4. Nerves and the muscles of respiration
    a) Respiratory nerves pass through cervical and thoracic spinal column
    b) Injuries to the cervical and thoracic spine may affect patient's ability to breath
        (1) Phrenic nerve - third, fourth and fifth cervical vertebrae
        (2) Intercostals - T2-T8
        (3) Abdominal muscles T8 - T11
    c) Possible respiratory effects of spinal injury
        (1) Low cervical (below C5) or high thoracic - diaphragmatic breathing only
        (2) High cervical - respiratory arrest

XI. Autonomic nervous system **(Slide 7-58)**
  A. Two main divisions
    1. Actions tend to counterbalance each other
    2. Parasympathetic
        a) Effects tend to be localized
        b) Effects tend to be limited to a particular organ
        c) Nerves arise of brain stem and sacrum
    3. Sympathetic
        a) Concerned with mass response
        b) Affects many parts of the body at the same time
        c) Example during crisis "fight or flight"
            (1) Increase the heart rate
            (2) Increase the blood flow to skeletal muscles
            (3) Regulate the blood pressure
            (4) Decrease circulation to the skin and digestive system
            (5) Direct blood flow to the muscles, heart and brain
        d) Nerves arise along thoracic and upper lumbar spinal cord (the sympathetic chain)
        e) If spinal cord is damaged above upper thoracic - sympathetic tone is lost
    4. Neurogenic shock **(Slide 7-59)**
        a) Shock resulting from widespread vasodilation
        b) Loss of sympathetic chain has several effects
            (1) Hypotension from vasodilatation
            (2) Pulse rate will appear normal in the range of 60-80
            (3) Cannot compensate by increasing the heart rate

Content

(4) Signs of hypovolemic shock may be masked
(5) Priapism - sustained penile erection
(6) Inability to urinate
(7) Loss of bowel function
c) Treated with oxygen, PASG and rapid transport

XII. Mechanism of injury **(Slide 7-60)**
A. Types of injuries
1. Open injuries
a) Produced by penetrating wounds
b) Primarily from gunshot wounds or knives
2. Closed injuries
a) Most common type of injury
b) Motor vehicle accidents cause greater than 50%
c) Other causes
(1) Falls
(2) Sports related accidents
(3) Diving accidents
B. Vulnerable vertebrae **(Slide 7-61)**
1. Most common where fixed vertebrae meet mobile
2. Thoracic and sacral are fixed to ribs and pelvis
3. Cervical and lumbar are mobile
4. Fractures at junctions are common (examples)
a) Cervical 7 (mobile) - thoracic 1 (fixed)
b) Thoracic 10 (fixed) - thoracic 11 (mobile)
c) Lumbar 5 (mobile) - sacral 1 (fixed)
C. Specific mechanisms
1. Compression forces **(Slide 7-62)**
a) One spinal vertebrae is driven onto another
b) Force may be come from above or below
c) Examples
(1) Diving into shallow water with head and neck in normal alignment (not flexed)
(2) Falls with the victim landing on his feet and/or buttocks
(3) Bone fragments can intrude on spinal canal
2. Flexion injuries **(Slide 7-63)**
a) Usually involve fixed and mobile vertebrae
b) Head is hyperflexed when force is applied to the back of the skull
c) Lumbar is flexed with fall while body is flexed or over a lap belt during deceleration
d) Vertebrae flex forward and fracture body
e) Vertebrae may be dislocated anteriorly
3. Extension injuries **(Slide 7-64)**
a) Occur when the head is suddenly jolted backward
(1) Forehead striking windshield
(2) Forehead striking tub
(3) Whiplash injury
b) Anterior ligaments supporting the spine can tear resulting in dislocation

Content

4. Open wounds - missile injuries **(Slide 7-65)**
    a) Gunshot wounds
    b) Directly or indirectly
5. Patients should be immobilized based on the mechanism of injury

XIII. Types of injuries **(Slide 7-66)**

A. Concussion, or a temporary loss of function
1. May disrupt nerve tracts resulting in temporary but complete paralysis
2. Cannot distinguish temporary vs. total disruption of the spinal cord at the scene
3. Always give the patient the benefit of the doubt

B. Lacerations
1. Bony fragments or penetrating injuries can lacerate the cord
2. Degree of laceration again will vary from minor wounds to complete transection of the cord
3. Open wounds run risk of infection

C. Contusions
1. Bruised against the bony spinal column
2. Various degrees of motor and sensory loss

D. Epidural vs subdural
1. Epidural and subdural bleeding in coverings of cord
2. Blood may disperse along the entire length of the spinal canal resulting in little or no pressure
3. May cause localized compression and signs

E. Complete and incomplete **(Slide 7-67)**
1. Spinal cord may be complete or incomplete
2. Complete injury, no nerve function below the level of the spinal cord is evident
3. Only structures innervated above the level of injury will function
4. No motor or sensory function below
5. Incomplete injury results in some nerve tracts damaged while others are spared
    a) Normal findings above the level of injury
    b) Variable findings below
6. Recognition of signs related to spinal cord injury help the EMT treat patients
7. The absence of signs does not suggest the absence of spinal vertebrae injury
8. Immobilization is performed based on the mechanism of injury

XIV. Patient assessment **(Slide 7-68)**

A. Goals
1. Determine if the possibility of spinal injury
2. Determine and document the level of injury
3. Prevent further injury
4. Anticipate complications requiring respiratory and circulatory support

B. Scene survey **(Slide 7-69)**
1. Determine the mechanism of injury
2. Anticipate the possible injuries
3. Assume spinal injury if the patient is unconscious

Content

4. Bruising or lacerations about the head, face and forehead should raise your suspicion
5. Signs of trauma to the shoulders or pelvis should also raise suspicion

C. The primary survey **(Slide 7-70)**
1. Check for responsiveness
   a) Provide immediate in-line immobilization of the cervical spine
   b) Do not move the patient to establish unresponsiveness
   c) Log roll the patient as a unit if prone
2. Airway
   a) Jaw thrust-without head tilt
   b) Tongue jaw lift
   c) If head flexed, return it to the neutral position and support the head
      (1) If resistance is encountered, attempt to evaluate in flexed position
      (2) Evaluate the adequacy of ventilations in the position found
      (3) Dislocation injuries can become locked in a dislocated position
3. Breathing **(Slide 7-71)**
   a) If hypoventilating or apneic, provide positive pressure ventilations
   b) Check for diaphragmatic breathing
      (1) If present use care with PASG abdominal section
      (2) Administer high-concentration oxygen
4. Circulation **(Slide 7-72)**
   a) Look for signs of neurogenic shock
      (1) Hypotension
      (2) Pale or pink skin
      (3) Normal pulse rate
   b) If patient is unstable, transport immediately
5. History **(Slides 7-73, 7-74)**
   a) Important questions
      (1) When did the injury occur?
      (2) Was he thrown by the impact (i.e., pedestrian struck)?
      (3) What does the car look like?
      (4) Position of the victim at time of injury?
      (5) Wearing a seat belt at time of injury?
      (6) Was the patient moved?
      (7) Did the patient have motor function initially?
      (8) Did the patient pass out prior to the accident?
      Was there a period of cyanosis or apnea?
      Height of the fall and surface struck on landing?
      (a) Do you suspect alcohol or drug use?
      (10) Previous medical history?
      Is it in any way related to the cause of the accident? (e.g., diabetic)

Content

6. Vital signs **(Slide 7-75)**
   a) Respirations
      (1) Rate and depth of respirations
      (2) Abdominal breathing only?
   b) Pulse and blood pressure
      (1) Evidence of neurogenic shock (hypotension with a normal or slow pulse)?
      (2) Neurogenic shock may mask hypovolemia
   c) Temperature
      (1) Loss of thermoregulatory mechanisms with some severe spinal injuries
      (2) Vasodilated patient will lose heat rapidly to the environment
7. Head-to-toe survey
   a) Special attention to the spine
      (1) Slide your hand under cervical, thoracic and lumbar spine
         (a) Tenderness or deformities
         (b) Bruises on the shoulders or pelvis
   b) Inspect neck before a cervical collar is applied
   c) Sensory exam
      (1) Check for sensation in feet, legs, abdomen, torso, hands, arms **(Slide 7-76)**
      (2) Document the findings where sensory findings change (i.e. 2 inches below the nipple)
      (3) Line of demarcation appears where the skin is moist or clammy above and dry below
   d) Motor exam **(Slide 7-77)**
      (1) Ask the patient to move his toes up and down and lift his feet 3-4 inches
      (2) Place your hands against the soles of his feet and ask him to push against your hands **(Slide 7-78)**
      (3) Muscle strength should be noted as absent, weak or present **(Slide 7-79)**
      (4) Proceed in the same way with the arms, starting at the hands **(Slide 7-80)**
      (5) If patient is unconscious, use a sharp object to stimulate the feet, then the hands **(Slide 7-81)**
         (a) Check the face for any grimacing
         (b) Observe the limbs for signs of movement.
      (6) Perform sequential exams

XV. Treatment **(Slide 7-82)**
   A. Getting to the patient
      1. Most victims are in motor vehicle accidents
      2. Many may be trapped
      3. Patients should be evaluated with due attention to the cervical spine
      4. Maintain neutral in-line immobilization

Content

B. Extrication **(Slide 7-83)**

1. If primary survey is normal
    a) Apply rigid collar
    b) Short spine board
    c) Extricate carefully
    d) Attach patient to long spine board
2. If life-threatening injuries are present
    a) Apply rigid collar
    b) Rapidly extricate
    c) Rapidly transport
3. Combative patients may require one person to support the head throughout the pre-hospital treatment
4. Consider hypoxia as the explanation for agitated or combative behavior

C. Airway, ventilation, oxygenation **(Slide 7-84)**

1. Patients with altered mental status/neurological signs should be given high-concentration oxygen
2. Care should be taken to maintain airway and secretions
    a) Have suction on standby
    b) Immobilize patient if he/she must be turned on side
3. Positive pressure ventilation if needed

D. Immobilization **(Slide 7-85)**

1. Assume spinal injury based on mechanism of injury
2. Manual immobilization first step of assessment for all suspected trauma victims
3. Immobilize the patient before moving except in the setting of a hazardous condition
4. Do not delay transport of patient in shock for the sake of comprehensive immobilization
5. Neurological deficits need not exist to suspect spinal injury
6. Cervical collar alone does not constitute spinal immobilization
7. Prepare for vomiting
    a) Be ready to log roll the patient
    b) Have suction ready
8. Specific techniques **(Slide 7-86)**
    a) Patient found lying on the ground
        (1) Log rolled or scooped onto a long spine board
        (2) Must be secured with straps which prevent movement during carry
        (3) Must be turned as a unit should vomiting occur
        (4) The log roll
            (a) Suitable movement technique for potential spinal injury victims
            (b) Used to place a patient on a spinal immobilization device
            (c) Used to move patient without disturbing the alignment of the spinal column

Content

(d) Technique
i) Team leader maintains gentle in-line immobilization to the cervical spine **(Slide 7-87)**
ii) Cervical collar is applied **(Slide 7-88)**
iii) Three other rescuers are positioned along one side **(Slide 7-89)**
iv) Spine board is placed on opposite side **(Slide 7-90)**
v) Upon command of the team leader the patient is
1) Rolled toward the three rescuers **(Slide 7-91)**
2) Position the board behind the patient **(Slide 7-92)**
3) Patient is then rolled onto the spine board **(Slide 7-92)**
vi) Patient is securely attached
1) Upper chest, pelvis, thighs and lower leg first **(Slide 7-93)**
2) Then attached at head **(Slide 7-94)**
vii) Log roll should be performed slowly and carefully
viii) Team leader must observe movement to assure good alignment

b) Patient found in sitting position **(Slide 7-95)**
(1) Adequate time to fully immobilize
(a) Apply collar
(b) Kendrick extrication device or short spine board
(c) Remove to long spine board
(2) Rapid extrication needed
(a) Apply cervical collar
(b) Maintain in-line immobilization
(c) Rotate and slide onto long board

c) Water accidents **(Slide 7-96)**
(1) Floated on the back into the shallow water
(2) Avoid hyperextension if mouth-to-mouth resuscitation is necessary
(3) Place a long spine board, or other board (surfboard), allow it to float up

d) Helmet removal **(Slide 7-97)**
(1) Following motorcycle accidents, it may be necessary to remove helmets
(2) Technique
(a) EMT #1 is positioned behind patient and grasps each side of the helmet **(Slide 7-98)**
i) Grasping angles of the mandible applies in-line immobilization **(Slide 7-99)**
ii) Other EMT cuts or loosens the chin strap **(Slide 7-100)**

Content

(b) EMT #2 after loosening the chin strap assumes the in-line immobilization **(Slide 7-101)**
- i) Supports occiput with hand closest to head with arm resting on ground **(Slide 7-102)**
- ii) Supports mandible with other hand
- iii) Must be ready to support weight of head when helmet is removed

(c) EMT #1 removes helmet
- i) Carefully stretches side of helmet laterally **(Slide 7-103)**
- ii) Removes carefully past ears
- iii) Full face helmets will have to be tilted back to clear the nose
- iv) Move the helmet, not the head, during the procedure

(d) After the helmet is removed **(Slide 7-104)**
- i) EMT #1 assumes in-line immobilization
- ii) EMT #2 applies a cervical collar and other immobilization measures **(Slide 7-105)**

E. Psychological support **(Slide 7-106)**

1. Patients with fractures of the spine and paralysis may be conscious
2. They will become aware of their problems as you proceed through assessment
   - a) Be thorough and attentive and finish your assessment
   - b) Maintain a positive attitude
   - c) Be honest but keep in mind that recovery is possible

Section 4

MEDICAL CENTRAL NERVOUS SYSTEM EMERGENCIES

Objectives
(Slide 7-107)

At the conclusion of the chapter the student will be able to:

1. **Define stroke.**
2. **List 3 types of stroke.**
3. **Describe steps of assessment and treatment of stroke patient.**
4. **List 2 types of seizure disorders and describe their effects.**
5. **List steps in the emergency care of a patient during and after a convulsion.**
6. **Describe the treatment for status epilepticus.**

Instructor Preparation

Reading preparation for the lesson:

EMT Prehospital Care, Chapter 7, pages 338-348

Optional reading:

Safer P., Bircher N.: Cardiopulmonary Cerebral Resuscitation, 3rd Ed., W.B. Saunders, Philadelphia, PA, 1988

Suggested Learning Activities

Using lecture format with handouts, provide a presentation on the assessment and management of CNS emergencies.

Provide case history examples of various problems.

Content

XVI. Overview **(Slide 7-108)**
- A. Alteration in central nervous system function is a common call for emergency care
- B. CNS problems have a wide range of possible dysfunctions including
    - 1. Loss of consciousness
    - 2. Sensory problems
    - 3. Loss of motor ability
    - 4. Loss of vital functions
        - a) Respiratory arrest
        - b) Organ failure
- C. Two general mechanisms **(Slide 7-109)**
    - 1. Disease problems originating in CNS
        - a) Stroke
        - b) Brain tumors
        - c) Intracranial bleeding
    - 2. General metabolic problems
        - a) Hypoxia
        - b) Hypercarbia
        - c) Hypoglycemia
- D. General goals of prehospital care **(Slide 7-110)**
    - 1. Assure adequate ventilations and circulation
    - 2. Rule out the possibility of trauma
    - 3. Give supplemental oxygen and perhaps glucose
    - 4. If possible, treat the underlying cause

XVII. Altered mental status **(Slide 7-111)**
- A. Often first indication of central nervous system problems
- B. Ranges from mild confusion and abnormal behavior through deep coma
- C. Assessing adequacy of ventilations is priority
    - 1. Central nervous system depressant may lead to respiratory arrest
    - 2. Most common cause of death from overdoses is failure of the respiratory system
    - 3. Respiratory problems may also occur with strokes or seizures
- D. Patient with CNS problem or unconsciousness may also block airway or aspirate
- E. Terminology **(Slide 7-112)**
    - 1. Lethargy
        - a) Sluggishness or sleepiness
        - b) Easily aroused but drifts into a sleepy state without stimulation
    - 2. Stupor
        - a) A state of lessened responsiveness
        - b) Can be aroused but more stimuli is required than for the lethargic patient
        - c) Stuporous patient does not reach a normal level of consciousness and function
        - d) Speech may be slurred or garbled
        - e) Motor ability may be sluggish and uncoordinated

Content

3. Semi-coma
   a) A condition of unconsciousness or lack of awareness of one's environment
   b) Patient may be aroused
4. Coma
   a) A lack of responsiveness to the environment
   b) Patient is unconscious and cannot be aroused by external stimuli
5. Limitations of terms
   a) These terms are commonly used but have certain disadvantages
      (1) May be used differently by other observers
      (2) EMT may have difficulty as mental state varies
   b) Glasgow Coma Scale provides a standardized method for documenting level of CNS function
6. Orientation
   a) In conscious patients there are degrees of intellectual and memory function
   b) One can determine whether a patient is oriented to their environment
   c) The patient is assessed for his orientation to person, time, and place
      (1) A confused patient may not be aware of the time of day, date, or even year
      (2) A patient may not be aware of his immediate surroundings
      (3) Less common are patients who are not aware of their own name
      (4) Patient is described as oriented x 3 if he is aware of all three variables
      (5) If he is not aware of one of the variables, he is said to be "oriented to person and place but not to time," etc.

F. Causes of altered mental status **(Slide 7-113)**
1. There are numerous causes of altered mental status
2. Structural
   a) Most common is a stroke or cerebral vascular accident (CVA)
   b) Blood supply to part of the brain is disrupted
   c) Portion of the brain fails to function from lack of oxygen
   d) Findings on the physical exam are one-sided or asymmetric
   e) History of recent head trauma
      (1) Subdural hematoma
      (2) Occurred a week or a month ago
3. Metabolic
   a) Majority of patients with altered mental status suffer from metabolic problems
   b) Originate outside the CNS
   c) Affect both sides of the brain equally
   d) Physical findings will generally be bilateral and symmetrical rather than one-sided

Content

e) Examples
(1) Poisoning and overdose
(2) Environmental conditions such as hypothermia or hyperthermia
(3) Infectious organisms
(4) Diabetic states
(5) Failure of organs of excretion [liver, kidney]
(6) Causes of hypoxia, i.e., cardiac arrest

XVIII. Cerebral vascular accidents
A. Overview **(Slide 7-114)**
1. A blockage or disruption of blood flow in an artery feeding the brain
2. Obstruction of the vessel [by a thrombus or embolus]
3. Rupture of the vessel itself
4. Brain tissue distal to the obstruction will be deprived of oxygen and nutrients
5. Damage to the section of the brain supplied by that artery
6. Functions controlled by that part of the brain will be affected
7. When a vessel in the brain ruptures
a) Not only is the distal brain affected
b) Bleeding within the brain can result in increased pressure and damage to surrounding structures
c) If bleeding is extensive, herniation and massive destruction of brain tissue can occur
8. Risk factors for stroke are same as heart disease

B. Causes **(Slide 7-115)**
1. Thrombus **(Slide 7-116)**
a) Most common cause of a CVA is from thrombus or blood clot formation within artery
b) Signs and symptoms correlate with the part of the brain being deprived of blood flow
c) Examples
(1) Occipital lobe - patient may complain of visual disturbances
(2) Frontal lobe - may experience intellectual or motor disturbances
(3) Parietal area - sensory loss may occur
(4) Major artery is blocked, the loss of function is widespread
d) Transient ischemic attacks
(1) Thrombotic stroke may be preceded by a transient ischemic attack or TIA
(2) A temporary loss of brain function secondary to diminished blood supply
(3) Neurological deficit which completely resolves within 12 hours
(4) Can only be diagnosed after signs or symptoms disappear

Content

2. Embolus **(Slide 7-117)**
    a) Less common cause of CVAs is embolism
    b) Substance which travels through the circulation and lodges in artery smaller than its own size
    c) Blood flow distal to the obstruction is then compromised
    d) Signs and symptoms come on suddenly
3. Hemorrhage
    a) Cerebral artery bursts
    b) Onset of signs and symptoms is rapid
    c) Signs may progress and the neurological exam can change with continued bleeding
    d) May be confined within the brain tissue
    e) May occur along the subarachnoid space
        (1) Subarachnoid hemorrhage
        (2) Patients may exhibit signs of neck stiffness
        (3) May resist flexion of the neck because it irritates brain coverings
    f) Hemorrhagic strokes and subarachnoid hemorrhage have the highest mortality

C. Signs and symptoms of CVAs **(Slide 7-118)**
1. Signs and symptoms of strokes are quite varied
2. They reflect the portion of the brain which is deprived of blood

Motor and sensory findings are usually asymmetric
    a) One-sided paralysis
    b) Facial droop
    c) Eyelid droop
    d) One-sided sensory loss
3. Patients will have intellectual impairment and difficulty in communicating
4. Mental status may vary from confusion to coma
5. Urinary and rectal incontinence
6. Nausea and vomiting
7. Some patients may have seizures or convulsions

D. Management considerations **(Slide 7-119)**
1. Perform Glasgow Coma Scale
2. Document neurological deficits
3. Maintain airway
4. Administer high-concentration oxygen
5. Place in semi-sitting position if conscious
6. Left lateral recumbent position if unconscious
7. Monitor vitals and ventilations
8. Document changes in condition
9. Communication requires patience and understanding

Content

XIX. Seizures **(Slide 7-120)**
- A. A temporary alteration in behavior due to abnormal electrical activity in the brain
- B. Also called convulsions or epilepsy
- C. Causes
  1. Scars on the brain or its meningeal covering
  2. Drug or alcohol withdrawal
  3. Eclampsia (toxemia of pregnancy)
  4. Trauma
  5. Hypoglycemia
  6. Unknown cause
- D. Types of seizures
  1. Grand mal **(Slide 7-121)**
     - a) Type that most people think of when they use terms such as convulsions or epilepsy
     - b) Consists of three phases; tonic, clonic, postictal
     - c) Tonic phase is a sustained contraction of all voluntary muscles
       - (1) Extension of the body and the extremities
       - (2) Lasts up to 30 seconds
       - (3) Ventilations are compromised due to sustained respiratory muscle contraction
     - d) Clonic phase characterized by intermittent contractions/relaxations of muscles **(Slide 7-122)**
       - (1) Results in rapid jerking movements
       - (2) Patient may injure himself if he strikes surrounding objects
       - (3) Lasts for seconds up to a few minutes
       - (4) Spasms of contractions and relaxations interfere with ventilation
       - (5) Patient can become cyanotic
       - (6) May be followed by a short period (up to 30 seconds) of flaccid paralysis
       - (7) Breathing is slowly re-established
       - (8) May suffer loss of urine
       - (9) May bite tongue during the tonic or clonic phase
     - e) Postictal is final phase **(Slide 7-123)**
       - (1) Patient shows a depressed level of consciousness and confusion
       - (2) Will slowly awake but may feel confused and drowsy
       - (3) May complain of headache, some muscle aching, and perhaps a sore tongue
     - f) Aura
       - (1) Some seizures originate in part of the brain with early warning signs
       - (2) Peculiar to the site of origin
       - (3) Strange smells, visual or auditory sensations, or motor events
       - (4) May herald the onset of a generalized convulsion

Content

2. Focal seizures **(Slide 7-124)**
   Some patients have focal seizures which do not generalize and involve the entire brain
   a) May affect only a portion of the body
   b) Manifest as an alteration in consciousness with bizarre behavior
3. Status epilepticus
   a) A rapid succession of epileptic attacks without an intervening period of consciousness
   b) A definite threat to life due to sustained respiratory compromise
4. Febrile convulsion
   a) Seizure in a child between 6 months and 6 years
   b) Precipitated by a high temperature in the setting of an infection
   c) Occur in up to 5% of children
5. Petite mal
   a) Brief lapses of attention and awareness lasting 10-20 seconds
   b) More common in childhood but sometimes persists into adult life
   c) Can occur many times a day
   d) Child may suddenly stare, eyes turned upward or to the side, and his eyelids flutter
   e) Episode is always brief (seconds)

E. Management considerations **(Slide 7-125)**
1. General goals of management are the same as those for any patient with altered mental status
2. Protection of patient from injuring himself during seizure
3. Airway and ventilation
   a) Airway may not be possible during tonic and clonic phase
   b) Do not force objects in mouth during seizure
   c) During the postictal phase manual and mechanical maneuvers may be necessary
   d) Suction should be available in the event of vomiting
   e) With status epilepticus, respiratory compromise becomes the major concern
   f) High-oxygen concentrations should be given and assistance with positive pressure ventilation
   g) May be difficult due to muscle contractions
   h) Rapid transport is of high priority to minimize the time with hypoxia
   i) Drugs, i.e., diazepam are needed to break seizure
4. Psychological aspects **(Slide 7-126)**
   a) Patients may be very sensitive to the perceptions of those around them
   b) May not acknowledge disease in the presence of co-workers or friends
   c) Clear crowds away from the patient and create private environment before interviewing

XX. Meningitis **(Slide 7-127)**

A. Can be life threatening and require prompt evaluation and therapy
B. Caused by bacteria or viruses
C. Can present with signs of meningeal irritation

Content

D. Usually follows an infection in another area of the body
E. Signs and symptoms **(Slide 7-128)**
   1. Can be abrupt or gradual
   2. Signs and symptoms
      a) Change in mental status
      b) Severe headache
      c) Stiff neck
      d) Photophobia
      e) Nausea, loss of appetite
      f) Fever
   3. Patient may initially be irritable but depression of the mental status can be rapid
   4. May have a rash characterized by small red spots or small sites of hemorrhage visible under the skin
   5. Signs leading to early recognition can be lost in coma
   6. Infants may have few signs other than high fever, vomiting, and irritability and/or convulsions
   7. Nuchal rigidity **(Slide 7-129)**
      a) Elicited by flexing the neck forward 45 degrees
      b) Patient will respond by flexing his legs at the hip and the knee
      c) Caused by irritation of the pain-sensitive spinal nerves
      d) Patients complaining of stiff neck may assume a fetal position
      e) Nuchal rigidity is also encountered in cases of subarachnoid hemorrhage
F. Special considerations
   1. Prophylaxis **(Slide 7-130)**
      a) EMT in rare situations may be advised to take drug therapy when exposed
      b) Bacteria is spread by respiratory droplets
      c) Mouth-to-mouth or other contact with saliva causes increased risk
      d) Universal precautions are important
         (1) Mask
         (2) Gloves
         (3) Goggles
      e) Risk is quite small but follow-up at hospital is important
   2. Treatment of exposed health care providers must be available

XXI. Approach CNS emergencies and unconsciousness
A. Primary survey **(Slide 7-131)**
   1. Unconscious patients are at risk of airway obstruction
      a) Manual and mechanical techniques should be utilized
      b) Suction should be at the ready
   2. Need for ventilatory support should be quickly established
   3. Patient should be placed in the coma position
B. Secondary survey
   1. History **(Slide 7-132)**
      a) May be primary rationale for treatment
         (1) Diabetes
         (2) Previous stroke

Content

(3) Seizure disorder
b) History of a febrile illness and headaches may suggest meningitis
c) History of present illness **(Slide 7-133)**
(1) Change in mental status rapid or slow?
(2) Was there an abrupt onset?
(3) Any changes in the patient's condition that occurred prior to your arrival?
(4) Is the mental status improving, deteriorating or remaining the same?
(5) Did the therapy you instituted (e.g. oxygen, glucose) make the difference?
(6) Associated complaints
(7) Chronology of events
(8) Similar past experiences
d) Past medical history **(Slide 7-134)**
(1) Big four - heart disease, hypertension, diabetes and C.O.P.D.
(2) Depression or suicide - overdose should not be overlooked
(3) Epilepsy
(4) Stroke
(5) Look for MedicAlert tags
(6) Previous hospitalizations or whether the patient is under a physician's care
(7) Bring medications to the hospital
(8) Allergies

2. Vital signs **(Slide 7-135)**
a) Respirations
(1) Respiratory rate and tidal volume
(2) Abnormal patterns, i.e., Cheyne-Stokes, Kussmaul's
b) Pulse
(1) Character
(2) Rate
(3) Quality
c) Temperature
(1) Infectious causes
(2) Hyperthermia or hypothermia
(3) May be the result of CNS disease
d) Mental status
(1) Orientation
(2) Glasgow coma scale

3. Head-to-toe survey **(Slide 7-136)**
a) Skin color and moisture
(1) Cyanosis, pale skin - hypoxia, shock
(2) Warm, hot, dry skin - heat stroke

Content

b) Abnormal smells on the breath
(1) Alcohol might be noted
(2) A fruity odor would suggest diabetic acidosis
(3) Toxic substances
c) Pupils should be checked for size, equality and reactivity to light
d) Nuchal rigidity (except in trauma)
e) Motor and sensory
f) Reevaluate en route

C. General treatment **(Slide 7-137)**
1. Airway
   a) Manual and mechanical methods
   b) Suction
2. Ventilation and supplemental oxygen as needed
3. Glucose administration
   a) Hypoglycemia as a common cause of altered mental status
   b) If patient is responsive and has gag reflex oral glucose may be administered
   c) Some systems allow EMTs to administer IV glucose or IM glucagon
   d) Never administer an oral agent to an unconscious patient or a patient with no gag reflex
4. Transport decision
   a) Subarachnoid hemorrhage, meningitis, and subdural hematomas require rapid transport
   b) Provide management en route

Chapter 7

CENTRAL NERVOUS SYSTEM EMERGENCIES

Examination

1. The nervous system is structurally divided into two main divisions: the peripheral nervous system and the:

   a. central nervous system
   b. ganglionic nervous system
   c. proximal nervous system
   d. core nervous system

2. The peripheral nervous system is comprised of the:

   a. brain, spinal cord, brain stem
   b. brain, spinal cord, cranial nerves
   c. cranial nerves, brain stem, motor nerves
   d. motor nerves, spinal nerves, sensory nerves

3. The nervous system can also be divided by function which includes autonomic and ____________ divisions.

   a. paravoluntary
   b. voluntary
   c. reflex
   d. ganglionic

4. The two main divisions of the autonomic nervous system are the:

   a. sympathetic and cerebral divisions
   b. parasympathetic and sympathetic divisions
   c. cerebral and peripheral divisions
   d. cerebral and parasympathetic

5. Willful activities, such as throwing a baseball or lifting a suitcase, are examples of functions mediated through the ___________ division of the nervous system.

   a. autonomic
   b. reflex
   c. spinal
   d. voluntary

6. The control of the heart, smooth muscles within organs such as the digestive tract, and the glands are examples of activities mediated through the ____________ division of the nervous system.

   a. autonomic
   b. reflex
   c. spinal
   d. voluntary

7. Which of the following is mediated through the parasympathetic nervous system?

   a. sweating
   b. constriction of pupils
   c. increasing the heart rate
   d. vasoconstriction

8. If complete cessation of oxygen delivery occurs, as in cardiac arrest, the patient will become unconscious in about:

   a. 5 seconds
   b. 1 minute
   c. 4-6 minutes
   d. 10 minutes

9. Approximately how long will it take for irreversible brain damage to occur when the brain is totally deprived of oxygen?

   a. 5-10 seconds
   b. 1-2 minutes
   c. 2-3 minutes
   d. 4-6 minutes

10. The most sensitive indicator of inadequate oxygenation of the brain is aleteration of:

    a. mental status
    b. motor function
    c. sensory function
    d. heart rate

11. A consideration for all patients who present with an altered mental status is:

    a. hyperglycemia and hypocalcemia
    b. hypoglycemia and hypoxia
    c. hyperglycemia and hyperkalemia
    d. hypoglycemia and hyponatremia

12. Nerve cells are very sensitive to:

    a. temperature
    b. high blood cholesterol levels
    c. increased heart rates
    d. pressure

Match the regions of the skull in column B with their related bones in column A (you can use the column B selections more than once).

Column A	Column B
13. mandible	a. cranium
14. frontal	b. face
15. maxilla	
16. temporal	
17. occipital	

18. The brainstem exits the lower skull through an opening called the ______________.

    a. foramen arteriosum
    b. foramen magnum
    c. foramen ovale
    d. foramen minor

19. The space within the adult cranium has about a _______ capacity.

    a. .5 liter
    b. 1 liter
    c. 2 liter
    d. 3 liter

20. If the pressure within the cranium becomes severe, the brain may be forced down through the opening in the base of the skull; this dire emergency is called:

    a. displacement
    b. herniation
    c. pressure syndrome
    d. compression syndrome

Match the number of vertebrae in column B with the type of vertebrae in column A.

Column A		Column B	
21.	cervical	a.	5 (mobile)
22.	lumbar	b.	4 (fused)
23.	coccyx	c.	12
24.	sacral	d.	5 (fused)
25.	thoracic	e.	7

26. Most vertebrae are separated by discs which serve as cushions and are held together by:

    a. ligaments
    b. nerves
    c. bone
    d. tendons

27. The two sites in the skull where the bones do not meet and soft spots are present in newborns are called the anterior and posterior:

    a. meninges
    b. foramen magnum
    c. fontanelles
    d. pressure points

28. The three-layered membranous coverings of the brain and spinal cord which serve to protect the central nervous system are called the:

    a. pleura
    b. periosteum
    c. myelin sheath
    d. meninges

Match the description in column B with the appropriate membranous layer in column A.

Column A		Column B	
29.	pia mater	a.	tough, leathery outer layer
30.	arachnoid	b.	middle layer
31.	dura mater	c.	inner layer

32. The __________ protects and cushions the brain and acts like a liquid shock absorber.

    a. gray matter
    b. ventricles
    c. fontanelles
    d. cerebrospinal fluid

Match the function of the brain in column B with the area of the brain in column A.

Column A		Column B	
33.	occipital area	a.	intellectual functions
34.	temporal area	b.	receives visual stimuli
35.	frontal area	c.	receives smell and hearing
36.	parietal area	d.	control muscles of the eye
37.	brainstem	e.	regulation of vital functions i.e. pulse rate

38. The largest and most superior portion of the brain is called the:

    a. cerebrum
    b. brainstem
    c. cerebellum
    d. diencephalon

39. When the energy processes necessary for the patient's life are compromised, the patient has experienced a(n):

    a. isolated injury
    b. specific injury
    c. metabolic injury
    d. contrecoup

40. A difference when comparing one side of the body to the other, such as unequal pupils, is indicative of a __________ injury:

    a. structural
    b. metabolic
    c. anaerobic
    d. recurrent

41. Complications such as hypoxia, hypotension and hypoglycemia following direct brain injury are termed:

    a. primary complications
    b. secondary complications
    c. structural complications
    d. irreversible complications

42. The most common cause of head injuries in the United States is due to:

    a. falls
    b. motor vehicle accidents
    c. penetrating wounds
    d. diving injuries

43. Ecchymosis (black and blue) over the mastoid bone (behind the ear) is a **late** sign of a:

    a. basilar skull fracture
    b. epidural hematoma
    c. subarachnoid hemorrhage
    d. concussion

44. A patient who sustains a blow to the frontal bone and complains of visual disturbances because the brain continued to move until the occipital lobe struck the inside of the occipital has suffered a __________ injury.

    a. contrecoup
    b. reverse head
    c. lateral head
    d. bilinear head

45. Which of the following are appropriate treatment for scalp lacerations?

    a. use direct gentle pressure to control bleeding, irrigate the wound, distribute the pressure over a wide area if possible
    b. immediately clamp off any arterial bleeding with a hemostat, estimate the degree of blood loss, apply the pressure over the edges of the intact bone if a depressed fracture is suspected
    c. explore the wound to determine depth and extent of injury, irrigate the wound, use direct gentle pressure to control bleeding
    d. use direct gentle pressure to control bleeding, estimate the degree of blood loss, apply pressure over the edges of the intact bone if a depressed fracture is suspected

Match the description in column B with the type of skull fracture in column A.

Column A		Column B	
46.	depressed	a.	a crack in the floor of the skull
47.	basilar	b.	bone fragments that are pressed downward toward the brain
48.	comminuted	c.	a line of non-union along the cranium
49.	linear	d.	multiple cracks radiating outward from the point of impact

50. Cerebrospinal fluid leaking from the ear is indicative of a __________ skull fracture:

    a. depressed
    b. basilar
    c. comminuted
    d. linear

51. Cerebrospinal fluid leaking from the ear should be treated by:

    a. packing the ear to contain fluid
    b. attaching a loose dressing over the ear
    c. doing nothing
    d. positioning the patient on the affected side

52. A transient loss of consciousness or neurological function due to a blow to the brain is called a:

    a. contusion
    b. concussion
    c. compression
    d. contortion

53. Headaches, nausea and vomiting (sometimes projectile) are common signs of ________________ in the conscious head trauma patient.

    a. skull fracture
    b. brain contusion
    c. increased intracranial pressure
    d. infection

54. Which of the following vital sign presentations may signify an increase in intracranial pressure?

    a. decreased pulse rate, increased blood pressure
    b. increased pulse rate, decreased blood pressure
    c. decreased pulse rate, decreased blood pressure
    d. increased pulse rate, increased blood pressure

55. The most sensitive indicator of increasing intracranial pressure is:

    a. decrease of pulse rate
    b. deteriorating level of consciousness
    c. projectile vomiting
    d. increased blood pressure

56. After a severe head injury a patient presents with the arms flexed and the legs extended. This type of posture is called _________ posture:

    a. decorticate
    b. decerebrate
    c. central nervous system
    d. pontine

57. After a severe head injury a patient presents with the arms extended and internally rotated at the shoulders with the wrists and the legs extended. This type of posture is called _________ posture:

    a. decorticate
    b. decerebrate
    c. central nervous system
    d. pontine

58. The type of breathing pattern characterized by slowly increasing then slowly decreasing ventilations in a pattern that is continually repeated with a short interval of apnea best describes:

    a. Ataxic respirations
    b. Biot's respirations
    c. Cheyne-Stokes respirations
    d. Apneustic respirations

59. A patient who presents with a short period of unconsciousness after blunt head trauma, followed by a lucid interval and then a deterioration in the level of consciousness, is indicative of a(n) _________ hematoma:

    a. epidural
    b. pontine
    c. subarachnoid hemorrhage
    d. intercranial

60. High blood pressure and a slow pulse following head injury are referred to as:

    a. Homan's sign
    b. Cushing's reflex
    c. Beck's triad
    d. Cheyne's reflex

61. Epidural hematomas are caused by ______________ bleeding.

    a. arterial
    b. capillary
    c. venous
    d. venule

62. Subdural hematomas are caused by ______________ bleeding.

    a. arterial
    b. capillary
    c. venous
    d. venule

63. The manual airway maneuver of choice for the head-injured patient is:

    a. head tilt-chin lift
    b. head tilt-neck lift
    c. jaw thrust-without head tilt (modified)
    d. triple airway maneuver

64. The Glasgow Coma Scale for a patient who has no verbalizations, does not open his eyes and who is decorticate (abnormal flexion) to painful stimuli is:

    a. 4
    b. 5
    c. 7
    d. 9

65. The first priority in the management of a patient with a severe head trauma is:

    a. performing a neurological exam
    b. establishing an airway and adequate ventilation
    c. applying a cervical collar
    d. control bleeding from the scalp

Match the anatomic sensory area (dermatome) in column B with the appropriate spinal nerve level in column A

Column A	Column B
66. thoracic-4 (T-4)	a. groin
67. cervical-4 (C-4)	b. nipple
68. lumbar-1 (L-1)	c. above clavicle
69. thoracic-10 (T-10)	d. umbilicus

70. The vessels of a patient in neurogenic shock are most likely to be:

    a. constricted
    b. dilated
    c. normal
    d. collapsed

71. The term used to describe a hyperextension injury resulting from a rear end collision is called a ____________ injury:

    a. contrecoup
    b. whiplash
    c. posterior extension
    d. subluxation

Match the mechanisms of injury in column B with the appropriate type of spinal injury force in column A.

Column A	Column B
72. compression	a. face striking the windshield in a front end collision.
73. flexion	b. occipital region striking the bottom of a pool during a dive.
74. extension	c. the superior portion of the skull striking the ground on a direct line with the spinal column.

75. A patient is immobilized on a long spine board and starts to vomit. You should immediately:

a. loosen all the straps and roll the patient on his side
b. do not move the patient but utilize suction to clear the airway
c. tilt the backboard on its side while maintaining spinal immobilization
d. sit the patient up

Match the situation in column B with the approach to immobilization in column A.

Column A		Column B	
76.	short board	a.	unstable passenger in a car
77.	long board	b.	pedestrian struck by a truck
78.	rapid extrication	c.	stable driver of a car

79. A temporary alteration in behavior due to abnormal electrical activity in the brain best defines a:

a. stroke
b. subarachnoid hemorrhage
c. meningitis
d. seizure

Match the definition in column B with the appropriate term in column A.

Column A		Column B	
80.	lethargy	a.	a state of lessened responsiveness
81.	stupor	b.	a lack of responsiveness to the environment
82.	semicoma	c.	sluggishness or sleepiness
83.	coma	d.	a lack of awareness to one's environment from which the patient may be aroused

Match the description or definition in column B to the appropriate term or type of stroke in column A.

Column A		Column B	
84.	cerebral vascular accident	a.	temporary loss of brain function secondary to diminished blood supply
85.	embolus	b.	most common cause of a CVA is from this
86.	thrombus	c.	results from a traveling blood clot
87.	hemorrhage	d.	characterized by neck stiffness
88.	transient ischemic attack	e.	most common structural problem of the brain encountered by the EMT
89.	subarachnoid hemorrhage	f.	highest mortality is due to this type of CVA

90. The most common motor finding in the extremities following a stroke is:

    a. paraplegia
    b. hemiplegia
    c. quadriplegia
    d. normal findings

91. Which of the following pairs of drugs are commonly used in the treatment of epilepsy?

    a. Xylocaine and atropine
    b. epinephrine and isoproterenol
    c. dextrose and reserpine
    d. phenobarbital and Dilantin

Match the descriptions in column B with the phases of a seizure in column A.

Column A	Column B
92. postictal	a. sustained contraction of all voluntary muscles
93. clonic	b. intermittent contractions and relaxations of the skeletal muscles
94. tonic	c. sleepy depressed level of consciousness and confusion

Match the descriptions in column B with the term in column A.

Column A	Column B
95. aura	a. seizure that affects only a portion of the body
96. status epilepticus	b. strange smells or motor events that may herald the onset of a seizure
97. petit mal seizure	c. usually presents with the tonic, clonic and postictal phase
98. grand mal seizure	d. rapid succession of seizures without an intervening period
99. focal seizure	e. more common in children

100. An infection of the brain coverings that may be life threatening and highly communicable is called:

    a. encephalitis
    b. neuritis
    c. duritis
    d. meningitis

Chapter 7

Skill Performance Sheet

Helmet Removal

Student's Name ______________________________ Date __________

Performance Standard	**Performed**	**Failed**
EMT #1		
Maintains in-line immobilization with helmet		
EMT #2		
Cuts or removes chin strap		
Supports occipital area with arm on ground		
Supports mandible along bony margin		
EMT #1		
Laterally spreads and removes helmet (may rotate slightly to clear nose)		
Takes over in-line immobilization (may place towel under occipital area)		

Comments ____

____

____

____

Instructor ____________________ Circle One: Pass Fail

Central Nervous System Emergencies

Skill Performance Sheet

Log Roll Procedure

Student's Name ______________________________ Date __________

Performance Standard	**Performed**	**Failed**
Team leader assumes in-line immobilization		
Cervical collar is applied		
Three rescuers positioned on one side of patient (shoulder, pelvis, legs)		
Spine board positioned on opposite side of patient		
On command from team leader, patient is rolled toward three rescuers		
Board is slid under patient		
On command from team leader, patient is rolled onto board		
Patient is adjusted on board		
Securely attach body then head to spine board		

Comments____

____

____

____

Instructor ____________________ Circle One: Pass Fail

Chapter 8

ABDOMINAL EMERGENCIES

Materials and Equipment for Lesson

1. Anatomy slides, overhead transparencies, drawings or flipcharts
2. Handouts
   - Anatomy and physiology and pathophysiology
   - Abdominal trauma
   - Performance sheets for abdominal skills
3. Slide projector, overhead projector, flipchart and/or blackboard

Section 1

Anatomy, Physiology and Pathophysiology

Objectives
(Slide 8-1)

At the conclusion of the chapter the students will be able to:

1. **Define acute abdomen.**
2. **List 5 types of abdominal emergencies.**
3. **List the borders of the abdominal and pelvic cavities.**
4. **State the difference between visceral and somatic pain.**
5. **List the structures of the digestive system and describe their functions.**
6. **List the structures of the urinary system and describe their functions.**
7. **List the structures of the male and female reproductive systems and describe their functions.**
8. **List 5 signs and symptoms of an acute abdomen.**
9. **List the general steps of treatment for a patient with an acute abdomen.**

Instructor Preparation

Reading preparation for the lesson:

EMT Prehospital Care, Chapter 8, pages 351-378

Optional reading:

Guyton, A.C.: Textbook of Medical Physiology, 8th Ed., W.B. Saunders, Philadelphia, PA 1990

Solomon, E.P., Phillips, G.A.: Understanding Human Anatomy and Physiology. W.B. Saunders, Philadelphia, PA 1987

Suggested Learning Activities
Using a lecture format with the aid of slides, overhead transparencies or charts, provide an overview of abdominal anatomy, physiology and pathophysiology. **Using a manikin or human subject, demonstrate examination of the abdomen.** **When possible, have students palpate structures or monitor activities.**

Content

I. Introduction **(Slide 8-2)**
   A. Abdominal is commonly encountered complaint
   B. Problems with organs - bleeding ulcers or appendicitis
   C. Blunt or penetrating injuries
   D. Diseases outside the abdomen, i.e., MI
   E. Primary concern is the potential for internal hemorrhage
      1. Abdomen contains large vessels including the aorta and vena cava and highly vascular organs
      2. High index for internal bleeding
      3. Be alert for signs of hypovolemic shock
   F. Inflammation of the peritoneal cavity, or peritonitis
      1. "Acute abdomen"
      2. Requires early hospital intervention
   G. Understanding of anatomy and physiology is helpful
   H. Common complaints abdominal problems include: **(Slide 8-3)**
      1. Pain
      2. Bleeding
      3. Nausea and vomiting
      4. Change in eating and bowel habits
      5. Jaundice (a yellowing of the skin or sclera)
   I. Internal bleeding can cause shock without external evidence
   J. Other signs of hypovolemic shock must be searched for
   K. Difficult to diagnose all abdominal emergencies
      1. EMTs will not make a definitive diagnosis **(Slide 8-4)**
      2. Extensive history and physical is counterproductive. EMTs should:
         a) Appreciate the severity
         b) Elicit preliminary findings in the field
         c) Institute shock treatment where appropriate
         d) Concentrate on rapid movement of the patient
         e) Further evaluations take place enroute to hospital

II. Medical emergencies of the abdomen
   A. Overview **(Slide 8-5)**
      1. There are some general categories of medical problems
         a) Hemorrhage
            (1) Most common cause is bleeding from digestive tract
            (2) Aneurysms arising from the abdominal aorta may leak or rupture
         b) Infections
            (1) Infections can involve the digestive, urinary, or reproductive organs
            (2) Tubular structure such as the appendix becomes obstructed
            (3) Large bowel perforates - peritonitis

Content

c) Organ Failure
(1) Abdominal organs may fail to function, due to a variety of reasons
(2) Liver may fail due to the excessive ingestion of alcohol
(3) Dangerous toxins can build up in the blood producing harmful effects to body cells

d) Obstruction **(Slide 8-6)**
(1) Tubular structures may obstruct
(2) Blockage can occur anywhere along the gastrointestinal tract causing back-up
(3) Causes of obstruction include
(a) Twisting of the intestine around a surgical scar
(b) Trapping of the intestine within a hernia
(c) Tumor encroaching upon the lumen of the intestine
(d) Massive swelling secondary to an infection
(4) Blockage of a ureter by a kidney stone will cause backup of urine

e) Perforation
(1) An ulcer can perforate through the GI tract and lead to leakage into peritoneum
(2) Inflammation of the peritoneum (peritonitis) can be life threatening
(3) May also lead to hemorrhage

f) Peritonitis
(1) The peritoneum is the internal lining of the abdominal cavity
(2) Inflammation of lining - peritonitis
(3) Peritonitis is an acute emergency - "acute abdomen"

g) Ischemia
(1) Emboli and thrombi can form in the arteries
(2) Herniation of intestinal tissue can strangulate the blood supply
(3) Organ, loop of bowel or testicle may twist compromising the blood supply
(4) Ischemia represents an emergent problem, requiring prompt surgical attention

III. Anatomy, physiology and pathophysiology
A. The Abdominal cavity, pelvic cavity and peritoneum
1. Abdominal cavity **(Slide 8-7)**.
a) Bordered by the diaphragm above and the pelvic inlet below
b) Organs project under ribs
c) The anterior wall is formed by muscles
d) Sides are formed by muscles and iliac bones
e) Posterior is formed by the lumbar vertebrae, iliac bones, muscles and diaphragm **(Slide 8-8)**
f) Contents include GI tract, liver, pancreas, spleen, kidneys, ureters, adrenal glands and vessels and nerves

Content

2. The pelvic cavity **(Slide 8-9)**
    a) Formed by the pelvic bones
    b) Imaginary plane from the sacrum to the symphysis pubis
    c) Ureters, bladder, sigmoid colon and rectum, internal genitalia
    d) Pelvic bone provides a site of perfuse bleeding when fractured
3. Peritoneum **(Slide 8-10)**
    a) Lining of the inner abdominal cavity
    b) Parietal peritoneum which lines the abdominal and pelvic walls
    c) Visceral peritoneum which covers most of the intra abdominal organs
    d) Space between is called the peritoneal cavity
    e) Folds of tissue called mesentery and omentum
    f) The visceral and parietal peritoneum is innervated with sensory nerves
        (1) Source of the pain associated with abdominal conditions and peritoneal inflammation. Peritonitis can result in diffuse pain due to scope of nerve inervation
    g) The space behind the peritoneum is called the retroperitoneal space
        (1) Kidneys, ureters, adrenal glands, pancreas, intestinal tract, aorta and vena cava
        (2) Bleeding in retroperitoneal space may not be apparent in anterior abdomen exam
4. Abdominal regions **(Slide 8-11)**
    a) Divided by two imaginary lines through the umbilicus into four quadrants
        (1) Left upper quadrant (LUQ)
        (2) Right upper quadrant (RUQ)
        (3) Left lower quadrant (LLQ)
        (4) Right lower quadrant (RLQ)
    b) Allows description of pain or injury
    c) Surface landmarks
        (1) xiphoid and the costal margins
        (2) Iliac crest
        (3) Anterior superior spine
        (4) Inguinal ligament
        (5) Femoral pulse
    d) Other terms **(Slide 8-12)**
        (1) Epigastrium
        (2) Periumbilical
        (3) Suprapubic region

B. Blood Supply **(Slide 8-13)**
1. Primary artery is the abdominal aorta
    a) Behind the peritoneum
    b) In the midline
    c) Common iliac arteries within the pelvic cavity. Aorta is a common source of aneurysms

Content

2. Two major venous drainage systems
    a) Portal venous system
        (1) Brings blood to liver to absorb nutrients, detoxify blood
        (2) Blood is then emptied into the vena cava
    b) Retroperitoneal and pelvic organs feed their returning blood directly into the vena cava, major vein in abdomen.

C. Pain and nerve innervation **(Slide 8-14)**
1. Abdominal pain is transmitted by two distinct pathways
    a) Visceral pathway
        (1) Gives imprecise pain and location
        (2) Innervates the visceral peritoneum and travel via the autonomic nervous system
        (3) Initiated by stretching or distension
        (4) Conditions providing visceral pain
            (a) Intestinal obstruction
            (b) Chemical damage or ischemia
        (5) Pain perceived as diffuse and cramping, aching. Difficult to describe pain
        (6) May feel the pain in another area (referred pain) **(Slide 8-15)**
        (7) Dermatone from which an organ originally developed in embryo
        (8) May be accompanied by autonomic mediated symptoms (nausea, vomiting, sweating)
        (9) Early appendicitis, only the visceral pain fibers may be stimulated
            (a) No RLQ pain
            (b) Periumbilical pain
            (c) Nausea and vomiting
    b) Somatic pathway **(Slide 8-16)**
        (1) Perceived more clearly, sharp quality, and is localized anatomically
        (2) Fibers innervate the parietal peritoneum and abdominal wall through spinal nerves. Occurs when nerve fibers in the parietal peritoneum are stimulated
        (3) Palpation will reveal tenderness and may stimulate guarding
        (4) Thighs flexed to "relax" peritoneum
        (5) Rebound tenderness

D. The digestive system **(Slide 8-17)**
1. Function
    a) Break down foods
    b) Absorb them into the blood stream
    c) Process them into energy, growth, other functions
2. Food is broken down mechanically and chemically
    a) Mechanically by chewing and churning
    b) Chemically broken down by acids and enzymes

Content

3. The mouth
    a) Digestive tract begin with the mouth and teeth
    b) Mechanical breakdown begins during chewing
    c) Salivary glands secrete enzymes and begin the chemical breakdown
    d) Food is directed into the esophagus by the epiglottis
4. The esophagus **(Slide 8-18)**
    a) Travels through chest cavity posterior to trachea
    b) Enters abdominal cavity through the diaphragm
    c) Muscular tube propels food to the stomach
    d) Peristalsis is a muscular action that moves food
        (1) Sequential muscular contractions
        (2) Along esophagus and intestines
        (3) Squeezes food along
        (4) Lower end of esophagus acts as one way valve
    e) Esophageal disorders may cause indigestion or heartburn
        (1) Gastric acid reflux causes irritation of the esophageal wall
        (2) Resulting in a burning or chest pain
        (3) Can be confused with myocardial infarction. Inquire whether relieved with antacids
    f) May also be the site of hemorrhage
        (1) Esophageal varices balloon-like blood vessels which protrude through esophagus
            (a) Severe liver disease
            (b) Heavy alcohol use
            (c) Signs of esophageal bleeding include:
                i) Vomiting blood (hematemesis)
                ii) Black tarry stool with foul odor (melena)
        (2) The esophagus can perforate
            (a) Forceful vomiting or retching
            (b) Ingestion of caustic substances
            (c) Requires surgical intervention
5. Stomach **(Slide 8-19)**
    a) J-shaped organ, in left upper quadrant
    b) Protected by the ribs
    c) When distended, can be palpated in the left upper quadrant
    d) Connects esophagus and the duodenum
    e) Has the ability to expand to ten times size
    f) Stores food and breaks it down mechanically and chemically via strong acids and enzymes
    g) Stomach acid causes melena
    h) Peptic ulcer disease and gastritis **(Slide 8-20)**
        (1) Gastric juices break down lining
        (2) Pain in the epigastric region or back
            (a) Burning
            (b) Indigestion
        (3) Relieved by antacids or milk
        (4) Aggravated by aspirin or coffee

Content

(5) Past medical history of ulcers or gastritis. Common medications
(a) Tagamet
(b) Zantac
(c) Pepcid
(d) Antacids
(6) May bore through a blood vessel and cause massive bleeding (perforation)
(a) Abdominal pain
(b) Hematemesis, melena
(c) Signs of hypovolemic shock

6. Small intestine **(Slide 8-21)**
a) Central abdominal cavity - all four quadrants
b) 10 to 20 feet in length
c) Provides surface area for absorption
d) Divided into three segments
(1) Duodenum
(2) Jejunum
(3) Ileum - ends at the ileocecal junction
e) Small intestine is relatively mobile
f) Duodenum is fixed and subject to tears during deceleration accidents
g) Duodenal ulcers can produce bleeding and symptoms similar to stomach ulcers
h) Obstruction **(Slide 8-22)**
(1) Caused by external compression, internal blockage or twisting or kinking
(2) Ileocecal junction is often the point of blockage
(3) Peritonitis can cause a paralysis of peristaltic movement.
(4) Symptoms of obstruction
(a) Crampy diffuse abdominal pain that comes and goes
(b) Pain becomes steady and severe
(c) Abdominal distension and vomiting
(5) Inquire about last bowel movement or gas
i) Hernias are outpocketings of the peritoneum **(Slide 8-23)**
(1) Inguinal hernia and patients may complain of pain or a swelling in the groin
(2) Incarcerated may result in blockage of blood flow
j) Ischemia to the intestine
(1) Blood supply is compromised by formation of clots or occlusion from emboli
(2) Can be partial or complete leading to intestinal infarction
(3) Sudden pain
(4) Emboli usually come from the heart

7. Pancreas **(Slide 8-24)**
a) Upper abdomen behind the stomach and in front of the spine, in the retroperitoneal space

Content

b) Two general functions
(1) Secretes digestive enzymes
(2) Secretes the hormone insulin to regulate glucose by the body's cells
c) Ulcers from the posterior surface of stomach
d) Pancreatic duct delivers digestive secretions to the duodenum (joins common bile duct)
e) Pancreas produces an odorless, colorless fluid that is rich in enzymes and bicarbonate.
f) Pancreatic insufficiency can lead to malabsorption
g) Pancreatitis - two forms: acute and chronic
h) Pancreatitis can be life threatening
i) Heavy alcohol consumption and gallstones major causes
j) Signs and symptoms
(1) Sudden severe knifelike epigastric, right lower quadrant or left upper quadrant pain which may radiate to the back
(2) Aggravated by lying down and somewhat relieved by sitting up
(3) Eating or drinking may worsen symptoms.
(4) Vomiting, fever and tachycardia
(5) Periumbilical ecchymosis
(6) Hypovolemic shock.

8. Liver **(Slide 8-25)**
a) Large, solid and soft organ located in right lower quadrant below diaphragm partially protected by ribs
b) Functions
(1) Produces bile
(a) Aids in the digestion of fatty foods
(b) Metabolism of carbohydrates, proteins, and fats
(2) Detoxifies drugs, alcohol, and other potentially poisonous substances
(a) When overwhelmed by toxins, liver failure may occur
(b) With chronic alcohol ingestion or by overdose of drugs, i.e., acetaminophen
(3) Produces proteins that play an important role in fluid balance and blood clotting
c) Causes of liver disease **(Slide 8-26)**
(1) Alcohol
(2) Drugs
d) Signs and symptoms of liver disease or failure
(1) Jaundiced (yellow) sclera, skin or mucous membranes (excessive bilirubin) **(Slide 8-27)**
(2) Vomiting
(3) Lethargy and anorexia
(4) Hepatic coma

9. Gallbladder **(Slide 8-28)**
a) Storage organ of bile produced by the liver
b) Right upper quadrant of the abdomen

Content

c) Leaves via common bile duct
d) Obstructed duct may cause inflammation of liver, gallbladder or pancreas
e) Cholecystitis (caused by blockage from gallstones)
(1) RUQ pain initially
(2) Referred to right subscapular region - vomiting
(3) Fever
(4) Jaundice
(5) Tender RUQ

10. Large intestine **(Slide 8-29)**
a) Location
(1) Begins in RUQ (ascending colon)
(2) Transverse colon
(3) Descending colon
(4) Sigmoid colon
b) Function - absorption of water and electrolytes
(1) With constipation - absorbs excess water
(2) With diarrhea - absorbs little water
c) Normally contains bacteria
d) Problems of the colon
(1) Diverticuli **(Slide 8-30)**
(a) Outpouching of inner wall into the muscle layer of the bowel
(b) When occuring near arteries may cause painless bleeding
(c) Majority of cases of massive lower GI bleeds
(d) Diverticuli may become infected - diverticulitis
(e) Signs and symptoms
i) Mild to moderate LLQ pain
ii) Anorexia and nausea
iii) Fever is also common
iv) LLQ tenderness
v) Signs of peritoneal inflammation
(f) Hypovolemia in severe cases
(2) Diarrhea **(Slide 8-31)**
(a) Viral or bacterial infection
(b) Parasitic infections
(c) Ulcerative colitis
(d) Infarction of the large intestine
(e) Dehydration and hypovolemia
(3) Obstruction
(a) Twist, cancerous tumor, fecal impactions are causes of obstruction
(b) Signs and symptoms
i) Pain
ii) Failure to pass gas and stool
iii) Abdominal distension
iv) Vomiting will not usually occur

Content

(4) Intussusception **(Slide 8-32)**
(a) Most often in very young children under the age of 2
(b) Mechanism - peristaltic bowel, telescopes one portion of bowel into the other
(c) Small intestine drags mesentery and blood vessels along
(d) Compression leads to edema, obstruction, increased mucus and capillary bleeding
(e) Signs and symptoms
i) Intermittent, severe pain with legs drawn up
ii) "Sausage-like" mass in RUQ
(5) Appendicitis **(Slide 8-33)**
(a) Most common surgical emergency
(b) Bowel contents become clogged in the lumen of the appendix
(c) Appendix distends
(d) Signs and symptoms
i) Mild vague umbilical pain
ii) Severe pain as distension develops
iii) Loss of appetite, nausea and vomiting
iv) Fever develops
v) Localized to right lower quadrant
(e) Untreated rupture and gangrene develop
(f) Life-threatening emergency
11. Rectum and anus **(Slide 8-34)**
a) Rectum connects the sigmoid colon to the anus
b) Storage container for feces
c) Hemorrhoids
(1) Ballooning of the veins which drain the rectal area
(2) Massive rectal bleeding as the hemorrhoid bursts
(3) Alcoholics, patients with liver disease, pregnant women in whom the venous return is obstructed
d) Foreign bodies
(1) Bottles, light bulbs, and vibrators
(2) Never attempt to remove
(3) Transport in position of comfort and transport
E. The urinary system **(Slide 8-35)**
1. Regulates fluid volume and blood salt concentration, and to filter the blood of toxins
2. Kidneys and ureters
a) Kidneys are located in the retroperitoneum, high up on the posterior abdominal cavity under the diaphragm
b) Connected to the urinary bladder by tubes called ureters
c) Slightly mobile and can move with respiration. Highly vascular organs
d) Renal failure = no urine output **(Slide 8-36)**
(1) Dialysis may be needed

Content

(2) The uremic patient
(a) Decreased or total absence of urine output
(b) Altered mental state
(c) Seizures
(d) Tachycardia
(e) Deep and rapid respirations
(f) Pallor
(g) Congestive heart failure
(h) Pulmonary edema
(i) Uremic frost

e) Pyelonephritis **(Slide 8-37)**
(1) Infection of the kidney which is more common in females but may occur in either sex
(a) Very high fevers
(b) Shaking chills
(c) Abdominal and back pain
(d) Nausea, vomiting
(e) Diarrhea and dysuria
(f) Flank pain
(2) Septic shock may develop

f) Kidney stones **(Slide 8-38)**
(1) Hard stones formed by excessive amounts of certain products in the urine
(2) Renal colic is caused by blockage from a stone in ureters
(3) Spasmodic pain in back or along the path of the urinary system radiating to groin or testicle
(4) Blood in the urine

g) Occurs more often in men than in women (3:1)

3. Urinary bladder and urethra **(Slide 8-39)**
a) Located anteriorly, low in the pelvis
b) Stores urine and releases under voluntary control by sphincter muscles of the urethra
c) Urethra is a tube through which urine is expelled
d) Bladder emergencies may result from infections. Occur more often in females and rarely serious
e) Signs and symptoms of bladder infection **(Slide 8-40)**
(1) Pelvic pain
(2) Difficulty urinating
(3) Blood in the urine
(4) Fever
(5) Suprapubic tenderness
(6) Voluntary guarding
f) Acute urinary retention **(Slide 8-41)**
(1) Caused by obstruction of the urethra
(2) Enlargement or hypertrophy of the prostate
(3) Common in elderly men

Content

(4) Signs and symptoms
(a) Suprapubic pain
(b) Feeling of distress
(c) Distended bladder may be felt suprapubicly
(5) Relief is gained by insertion of a urinary catheter

F. Reproductive System
1. Male reproductive system **(Slide 8-42)**
a) The scrotum is a pouch in which lie the testes and the epididymis
b) Testicles are suspended in the scrotum by the spermatic cord
c) Testicles produce the male hormone testosterone as well as sperm and seminal fluid (semen)
d) Sperm are transported
(1) Via the vas deferens
(2) Up through the spermatic cord
(3) To the ejaculatory duct
(4) Through the prostate
(5) Into the prostatic portion of the urethra
(6) Prostate gland secretes fluid into semen
(7) Through the penis passes the urethra, a tube through which both urine and sperm pass
e) Medical complaints: **(Slide 8-43)**
(1) Acute urinary retention
(2) Testicular torsion
(a) Most common in younger men and adolescents
(b) Testicle can twist in the scrotum about the spermatic cord
(c) Blood supply can be shut off
(d) Gangrene of the testicle can result
(e) Signs and symptoms
i) Swelling in the scrotal area
ii) Marked pain referred to the testicle
iii) Sometimes only abdominal pain
iv) Nausea or vomiting.
(3) Infections **(Slide 8-44)**
(a) Can involve prostate, urethra, bladder, testicles, and epididymis
(b) Signs and symptoms
i) Pain and burning on urination
ii) Dysuria (painful urination), hematuria (blood in the urine), frequency of urination
iii) Discharge of pus
2. Female reproductive system **(Slide 8-45)**
a) Consists of the uterus, ovaries, fallopian tubes, vagina and external genitalia
b) External genitalia
(1) Labia majora
(2) Labia minora

Content

(3) Clitoris
(4) Vaginal orifice
(5) Urethral orifice
(6) Bartholin's glands - mucus-secreting glands
c) The vagina travels upward to surround the cervix of the uterus
d) Uterus is a pear-shaped muscular organ which lies between the bladder and the rectum
e) The cervix of the uterus extends into the vagina
f) Fallopian tubes extend from both sides of the uterus to receive ovum from the ovaries
g) Hormones, estrogen and progesterone, are produced by ovary and control menstruation
h) Major medical emergencies
(1) Ectopic pregnancy **(Slide 8-46)**
(a) Defined - implantation of the fertilized ovum in an area outside the uterus
(b) Outgrows the tube and ruptures
(c) Signs and symptoms
i) Abdominal pain
ii) Amenorrhea
iii) Abdominal tenderness
iv) Signs of shock
v) Vaginal bleeding
(2) Infections **(Slide 8-47)**
(a) Pelvic inflammatory disease (PID)
i) Bacterial infection of reproductive organs
ii) Signs and symptoms
1) Fever
2) Abdominal or pelvic pain
3) Peritonitis
(3) Vaginal bleeding **(Slide 8-48)**
(a) Can occur for multiple reasons
i) Severe menstrual bleeding
ii) Endometriosis
iii) Threatened abortion
iv) Miscarriage
(b) Treat for shock
(c) Do not pack vagina

G. The endocrine system **(Slide 8-49)**
1. Consists of many hormone-secreting organs throughout the body
a) Adrenals
b) Pancreas
c) Ovaries
d) Testicles
2. Plays an important role in regulation, i.e., adrenalin

H. Spleen
1. Highly vascular organ
2. Left upper quadrant and protected by the ribs

Content

3. Main concern if injured is fatal hemorrhage
4. Filters RBCs
5. Can live without spleen

I. Abdominal aortic aneurysm **(Slide 8-50)**
1. Caused by atherosclerosis
2. Can leak and rupture
3. Life-threatening hemorrhage
4. Signs and symptoms
    a) Tearing abdominal pain and/or back pain
    b) Palpable pulsating mass in the midline
    c) Avoid deep palpation
5. Rapid transport is essential

J. Other causes of abdominal pain **(Slide 8-51)**
1. Pneumonia
2. Myocardial infarction
3. Muscular strains
4. Diabetic ketoacidosis
5. Sickle cell crisis
6. Toxins

K. Fluid shifts and hypovolemia in abdominal pain **(Slide 8-52)**
1. Obstruction and peritonitis may shift fluid to the abdomen
2. Loss of circulating blood volume and hypovolemia
3. Need volume replacement
4. Rapid transport
5. Vomiting and diarrhea will also produce hypovolemia

IV. The acute abdomen **(Slide 8-53)**

A. Unremitting abdominal pain of recent onset

B. Others reserve term for peritonitis

C. Signifies the importance of early diagnosis of these patients

D. Signs of an acute abdomen
1. Lying still
2. Knees drawn up
3. Breathing shallow breaths
4. Abdominal pain
5. Local or diffuse abdominal tenderness
6. Guarding
7. Hypovolemia
8. Rapid pulse
9. Perhaps lowered blood pressure

V. Approach to the patient with abdominal pain **(Slide 8-54)**

A. Difficult to diagnose in the field

B. Timely hospital interventions

C. Identifying life threatening conditions

D. Requires rapid surgical intervention

E. Primary survey **(Slide 8-55)**
1. Airway and oxygen
2. Shock present, rapid transport

Content

3. Position determined by mental status, comfort, and airway to prevent aspiration
4. Consider MAST

F. History **(Slide 8-56)**

1. Chief complaints
   a) Pain or bleeding
   b) Weakness
   c) Vomiting
   d) Change in bowel habits
   e) Inability to urinate
2. History of present illness **(Slide 8-57)**
   a) Abdominal pain
      (1) Location
      (2) Quality
      (3) Duration
      (4) Aggravating and relieving factors
         (a) Antacids
         (b) Eating
         (c) Position
   b) Bleeding
      (1) Mouth
      (2) Rectum
      (3) Urinary tract
      (4) Vagina
   c) Jaundice **(Slide 8-58)**
   d) Nausea and vomiting
   e) Anorexia
   f) Diarrhea and constipation
   g) Chills and fever
   h) Urinary symptoms
   i) Cardiorespiratory
3. Past medical history **(Slide 8-59)**
   a) Heart disease, C.O.P.D., hypertension and diabetes
   b) History of abdominal disease
   c) Abdominal surgery
   d) Abdominal aneurysm
   e) Similar episodes in the past
4. Medications and allergies

G. Physical exam **(Slide 8-60)**

1. Vital signs
2. Jaundice
3. Signs of dehydration
4. Any unusual odors
5. Position
6. Inspect **(Slide 8-61)**
7. Palpation **(Slide 8-62)**

Content

VI. Treatment of medical abdominal emergencies **(Slide 8-63)**
- A. Maintain an airway
- B. Give high concentration oxygen
- C. Treat shock if present
- D. Maintain body temperature
- E. Elevate legs
- F. Consider the MAST
- G. Transport in position of comfort
- H. Give nothing by mouth
- I. Complete exam en route
- J. Record your findings
- K. Notification

Chapter 8

Section 2

Trauma to the Abdomen

Objectives
(Slide 8-64)

At the conclusion of the chapter the students will be able to:
1. Demonstrate care of patient with the following trauma to the abdomen: **Evisceration** **Impaled object** **Blunt abdominal trauma** **2. Describe emergency care of injuries to male and female genitalia.** **3. List the basic steps in the management of a victim of sexual assault.**

Instructor Preparation

Reading preparation for the lesson:

EMT Prehospital Care, Chapter 8, pages 378-385

Optional reading:

Prehospital Trauma Life Support Committee of The National Association of EMTs: Pre-Hospital Trauma Life Support. 2nd Ed., Emergency Training. Akron, Ohio, 1990.

Suggested Learning Activities
Using a lecture format with the aid of slides, overhead transparencies or charts, provide a presentation of abdominal trauma. **Using a manikin or human subject, demonstrate the proper transport position for a patient with abdominal trauma.** **Provide case histories that illustrate different types of abdominal trauma.**

Content

VII. Trauma to the abdomen
- A. Overview **(Slide 8-65)**
  1. Bleeding main problem
  2. Abdomen can hold entire blood volume
  3. Mechanism of injury is important
  4. Maintain high index of suspicion
  5. Automobile accidents and pedestrians most common
- B. Goal of prehospital care **(Slide 8-66)**
  1. Quickly recognize life threatening injuries
  2. Rapid transport
  3. Essential life support enroute
  4. Identify trauma center candidates
- C. Mechanism of injury **(Slide 8-67)**
  1. Determining the severity of intrabdominal injuries
  2. Blunt abdominal trauma
     - a) Compression injuries **(Slide 8-68)**
       - (1) Two opposing forces compress organs
       - (2) Contusions, tears or rupture
       - (3) Steering wheel common example
       - (4) Fragile organs, i.e., liver, spleen
       - (5) Diaphragm may rupture
     - b) Deceleration **(Slide 8-69)**
       - (1) Organs or vessels tear at a point of attachment during deceleration
         - (a) Car hits a wall
         - (b) Organs continue to move
         - (c) Shearing forces tear and rupture organs
         - (d) Liver (ligamentum teres)
         - (e) Kidneys (vascular pedicle) **(Slide 8-70)**
         - (f) Intestines
         - (g) Spleen
       - (2) Deceleration injuries can be deceiving
     - c) Seatbelt injuries **(Slide 8-71)**
       - (1) Properly applied seatbelt - iliac spine and the femur at a 45 degree angle
       - (2) Bony pelvis will protect soft organs within
       - (3) Improper position - can transmit to the abdominal organs
  3. Penetrating injuries
     - a) Stab wounds **(Slide 8-72)**
       - (1) Can range in severity
         - (a) Superficial punctures and lacerations of skin
         - (b) Through penetration of organs and vessels
       - (2) Severity determined by location organs or structures
       - (3) Bring weapon to hospital when possible
       - (4) Maintain high index of suspicion

Content

b) Missile Injuries **(Slide 8-73)**
(1) Muzzle velocity is the major factor
(a) Handguns - 500-1500 feet per second
(b) Large rifles - 2000 to 3000 feet per second
i) Kinetic energy is displaced to the surrounding tissues
ii) Zone of injury
iii) Greater velocity, greater kinetic energy, larger zone of injury
(2) Other factors **(Slide 8-74)**
(a) Distance
(b) Location
(c) Secondary missiles (bone)
(d) Deformity of the bullet

D. Patient assessment **(Slide 8-75)**
1. Mechanism of injury
2. Signs of hypovolemia
3. Patient's complaints
a) Early bleeding may not cause peritoneal signs
b) Nausea or vomiting
c) Pain, referred pain
d) Position of the patient
e) Entrance and exit wounds
f) Bruises, tire marks, seatbelt marks on the abdominal wall
g) Alcohol may mask signs
h) Broken bones
4. Ample history **(Slide 8-76)**
a) Allergies
b) Medications
c) Past history
d) Last meal
e) Events leading up to injury
5. Physical exam **(Slide 8-77)**
a) Palpate
b) Inspection
c) Signs of hypovolemia

E. Special considerations
1. Evisceration **(Slide 8-78)**
a) Intestines protruding through a laceration **(Slide 8-79)**
b) Occurs with slash injury
c) Moist dressing or airtight dressing **(Slides 8-80 to 85)**
d) Position with legs flexed
2. Urinary tract injuries **(Slide 8-86)**
a) Male injuries
(1) Bruises over the flank
(2) Blood in the urine
(3) Blood at the penile meatus or a scrotal hematoma
(4) Black or bluish discoloration of the scrotum

Content

(5) Lacerations, bruising, avulsion or even amputation
(a) Direct pressure (moisten dressings)
(b) Bring avulsed or amputated parts
(6) Zipper injuries
b) Female genitalia injuries **(Slide 8-87)**
(1) Direct trauma or straddle injuries
(2) Do not place dressings within the vagina
(3) Triangular bandage
c) Foreign bodies **(Slide 8-88)**
(1) Left in place
(2) Penetrating objects left in place
(a) Stabilize
(b) Stacked dressing

F. Treatment of traumatic abdominal injuries **(Slide 8-89)**
1. Treat the whole patient
2. Maintain the airway
3. Give high-concentration oxygen
4. Control external bleeding
5. Secure penetrating objects
6. Treat for shock
a) Maintain body temperature
b) Elevate legs
c) Consider the MAST
7. Position the patient
8. Give nothing by mouth
9. Complete exam en route
10. Record your findings
11. Select hospital by local protocols

G. Sexual assault and rape **(Slide 8-90)**
1. Rape defined as sexual intercourse against the will of the victim
2. Need for psychological support
3. Preservation and collection of medical legal evidence
4. May be accompanied by other injuries
5. Prioritize the medical response
6. Professional attitude **(Slide 8-91)**
7. Psychological considerations
a) Loss of control
b) Maintain privacy
8. Medical-legal considerations
a) May refuse to press charges
b) Try to maintain evidence
(1) Clothes
(2) Semen-soaked objects

Content

c) Guidelines may assist your response. **(Slide 8-92)**

(1) Preserve the patient's privacy
(2) Questions should be medical
(3) Record the patient's statements
(4) Ask the victim to come to the hospital
(5) Do not shower or douche
(6) Collect clothing with minimal handling
(7) Maintain a chain of custody
(8) Interfere as little as possible with scene. Impaled objects removed in the hospital
(9) Respect patient's wishes

Chapter 8

ABDOMINAL EMERGENCIES

Examination

1. The internal lining of the abdominal cavity is called the:

   a. pleura
   b. peritoneum
   c. ileum
   d. colon

2. The mesentery and omentum are:

   a. structures used for digestion
   b. responsible for the secretion of bile
   c. ligaments and folds of tissue which suspend abdominal organs from the walls of the abdominal cavity
   d. tubular structures through which nutrients and waste products pass

3. The abdomen is divided into _____ quadrants which allow us to describe areas of pain:

   a. 2
   b. 4
   c. 6
   d. 8

4. A patient is complaining of pain just above the groin. This region is called the:

   a. epigastric region
   b. periumbilical region
   c. suprapubic region
   d. superpubic region

5. The abdominal aorta is:

   a. the primary artery within the abdomen
   b. located on the left flank behind the spleen
   c. located on the right flank behind the appendix
   d. the primary vein within the abdomen

6. Abdominal pain transmitted by the ________ pathway gives perceptions that are imprecise as to both the quality of the pain and its actual location.

   a. somatic
   b. visceral
   c. gastric
   d. intrinsic

7. Pain which is caused by an injury to the spleen and described by the patient as pain in his left shoulder is called:

   a. transmitted pain
   b. psychogenic pain
   c. somatic transmitted pain
   d. referred pain

8. The digestive tract begins with the:

   a. esophagus
   b. stomach
   c. small intestine
   d. mouth and teeth

9. Food enters the stomach at the esophagus and exits the stomach at the:

   a. large intestine
   b. duodenum
   c. ileum
   d. jejunum

10. Outpocketing of the peritoneum into abnormal openings in the abdominal wall is called a(n):

   a. aneurysm
   b. peptic ulcer
   c. hernia
   d. obstruction

11. The initial symptom of an abdominal obstruction is:

   a. nausea
   b. intermittent crampy abdominal pain
   c. rectal bleeding
   d. diarrhea

12. The organ which secretes the hormone insulin is the:

    a. gallbladder
    b. appendix
    c. liver
    d. pancreas

13. The organ responsible for the detoxification of drugs, alcohol, and other potentially poisonous substances is the:

    a. gallbladder
    b. appendix
    c. liver
    d. pancreas

14. The organ that stores and concentrates bile is the:

    a. gallbladder
    b. appendix
    c. liver
    d. pancreas

15. The large intestine is comprised of several segments. Digestive contents travel through the large intestine in the following order:

    a. cecum, ascending colon, descending colon, sigmoid colon, transverse colon
    b. ascending colon, transverse colon, cecum, descending colon, sigmoid colon
    c. transverse colon, ascending colon, descending colon, sigmoid colon, cecum
    d. cecum, ascending colon, transverse colon, descending colon, sigmoid colon

16. The most common surgical emergency is:

    a. tonsillitis
    b. pancreatitis
    c. hernia
    d. appendicitis

17. The term melena refers to:

    a. black tarry stool
    b. a malignancy in the digestive tract
    c. the junction of the kidneys and ureters
    d. skin pigmentation

18. Dialysis patients who fail to receive their dialysis treatment may exhibit signs of:

    a. increased urinary output
    b. uremia
    c. pyelonephritis
    d. kidney stones

19. Urine enters the bladder through the ureters and leaves through the:

    a. fallopian tubes
    b. urinary catheter
    c. urethra
    d. urinary vesicle

20. The following are all parts of the male reproductive system:

    a. testicles, prostrate gland, urethra, and ureter
    b. prostrate gland, urethra, scrotum, and vas deferens
    c. epididymis, seminal vesicle, penis, and ureter
    d. seminal vesicle, epididymis, vas deferens, and ureter

21. The pear-shaped muscular organ in the woman that lies between the bladder and rectum is the:

    a. vagina
    b. fallopian tubes
    c. cervix
    d. uterus

22. An implantation of the fertilized ovum in an area outside the uterus is defined as (an):

    a. ectopic pregnancy
    b. breech pregnancy
    c. cephalic presentation
    d. external pregnancy

23. The adrenal glands which are responsible for the secretion of epinephrine are located:

    a. behind the liver
    b. attached to the gallbladder
    c. attached to the kidneys
    d. attached to the pancreas

24. The highly vascular organ located in the left upper quadrant which is easily injured is the:

    a. liver
    b. spleen
    c. pancreas
    d. gallbladder

25. Abdominal aortic aneurysms are usually caused by:

    a. blunt trauma
    b. penetrating trauma
    c. intestinal obstructions
    d. atherosclerosis

26. A patient with abdominal pain, lying still, knees drawn up, shallow breaths, with local or diffuse abdominal tenderness and/or guarding; and with hypovolemia, rapid pulse and perhaps lowered blood pressure best describes:

    a. acute urinary retention
    b. an acute abdomen
    c. acute pyelonephritis
    d. acute cystitis

27. A patient is complaining of sharp abdominal pain in the right lower quadrant. When you palpate the abdomen you will palpate which quadrant last?

    a. left upper quadrant
    b. left lower quadrant
    c. right upper quadrant
    d. right lower quadrant

28. Jaundice, a yellowish tinge to the sclera of the eyes or skin, is indicative of:

    a. kidney failure
    b. acute urinary retention
    c. an acute abdomen
    d. liver disease

29. A small puncture wound to the abdomen from an ice pick:

    a. is usually a benign injury
    b. does not necessitate transportation to the hospital
    c. may have caused a significant injury
    d. contraindicates the use of the PASG

30. Early signs of shock include:

a. hypotension, delayed capillary refill, and rapid breathing
b. altered mental status, rapid breathing, and pale skin
c. pale and sweaty skin, delayed capillary refill, and hypovolemia
d. delayed capillary refill, rapid breathing, and tachycardia

31. The presence of the intestines through an abdominal laceration is called a(n):

a. intestinal obstruction
b. evisceration
c. denuded injury
d. avulsion

32. A patient presents with a knife impaled in the abdomen. You should:

a. leave the knife alone
b. carefully remove the knife
c. stabilize the knife in place
d. saw off the knife at skin level

33. If a rape patient should desire to take a "quick" shower prior to coming to the hospital, you should:

a. advise against it to preserve evidence
b. respect her wishes and wait for the patient
c. advise her to shower but not to use soap
d. forcibly restrain her to preserve evidence

34. The retroperitoneal space contains the:

a. kidneys, ureters, pancreas, and stomach
b. pancreas, adrenal glands, spleen, and abdominal aorta
c. kidneys, liver, pancreas, and adrenal glands
d. kidneys, ureters, adrenal glands, and abdominal aorta

35. Peristalsis is the:

a. muscular action that causes guarding of the abdomen
b. muscular action that moves food in the digestive system
c. fluid wave that can be palpated in patients with ascites
d. a voluntary act of digestion

36. Hematemesis is the:

a. coughing up of blood
b. passing of bloody stool

36. Hematemesis is the:

    a. coughing up of blood
    b. passing of bloody stool
    c. vomiting up of blood
    d. passing of blood in the urine

37. Scarring of the liver is called:

    a. hepatitis
    b. varices
    c. cirrhosis
    d. alcoholic gastritis

38. Diverticula, an outpouching of the inner wall of bowel tissue, most commonly occurs:

    a. on the left side of the large intestine
    b. on the left side of the small intestine
    c. on the right side of the large intestine
    d. on the right side of the small intestine

39. Intussusception most commonly occurs in:

    a. males over age 60
    b. teenagers
    c. women
    d. children under 2

40. Ballooning of the veins that drain the rectal area is called:

    a. rectal aneurysm
    b. berry aneurysm
    c. hemorrhoids
    d. rectal polyps

41. The kidneys, ureters, urinary bladder, urethra and external genitalia make up the ________ system:

    a. reproductive
    b. digestive
    c. urinary
    d. adrenal

42. A severe infection of the kidneys is called:

    a. pyelonephritis
    b. urinary sepsis
    c. pelvic inflammatory disease
    d. septicemia

43. Acute urinary retention is most commonly caused by:

   a. an obstruction of the ureter
   b. a kidney stone
   c. an obstruction of the urethra
   d. urinary polyps

44. The opening of the uterus which permits menstrual blood flow and dilates during delivery of a baby is the:

   a. vagina
   b. fallopian tube
   c. ovary
   d. cervix

45. A patient complains that he has an urge to urinate more frequently than normal. This is called:

   a. polyuria
   b. auria
   c. dysuria
   d. hematuria

46. If parts of the male and female genitalia are completely avulsed or amputated in an assault you should:

   a. leave them on the scene for evidence
   b. wrap in gauze and plastic bag and place on ice
   c. place in saline solution
   d. reattach them in their normal position

47. Patients with severe diarrhea will develop:

   a. bowel obstruction
   b. necrosis of the colon
   c. ischemia of the bowel
   d. dehydration and hypovolemia

48. Absence of urine output, altered mental state, seizures, tachycardia, deep and rapid respirations, pallor, congestive heart failure and pulmonary edema best describe:

   a. acute urinary retention
   b. renal failure
   c. pyelonephritis
   d. cystitis

49. The process in which organs or vessels continue to move forward and tear at a point of attachment, during a sudden cessation of motion in a fall or auto collision, best describes what mechanism of injury?

    a. contrecoup
    b. deceleration
    c. penetrating
    d. velocity tears

50. The factor that will most affect the extent of injury due to gunshot wounds is the:

    a. mass of the bullet
    b. velocity of the bullet
    c. shape of the bullet
    d. material that the bullet is made of

Chapter 8

Skill Performance Sheet

Applying an Evisceration Dressing and Bandage

Student's Name________________________ Date_________

Performance Standard	**Perform**	**Failed**
MOISTENED DRESSING TYPE		
Moisten multitrauma dressing		
Apply to exposed bowel		
Cover with dry dressing		
Tape in place		
SARAN WRAP OR ALUMINUM FOIL TYPE		
Apply wrap to bowel		
Tape border completely to create airtight seal		

Comments____

____

____

____

Instructor ________________ Circle One: Pass Fail

Chapter 9

SOFT TISSUE INJURIES

Materials and Equipment for Lesson

1. Anatomy slides, overhead transparencies, drawings or flipcharts
2. Handouts
   - Soft tissue injuries
   - Injuries to the face, head and neck
   - Performance sheets for bandaging skills
3. Slide projector, overhead projector, flipchart and/or blackboard

Section 1

Anatomy, Physiology and Wounds

Objectives
(Slide 9-1)

At the conclusion of the chapter the student will be able to:

1. List the locations and functions of the layers and major structures of the skin.

2. Describe the differences between open and closed wounds.

3. Describe the appearance of the following types of wounds:

Contusion	**Abrasion**
Laceration	**Avulsion**
Puncture	**Amputation**
Crush injury	

4. Describe the management of the following types of soft tissue injuries:

Amputation	**Avulsion**
Impaled objects	

5. Describe the steps for applying a pressure bandage.

Chapter 9

Instructor Preparation

Reading preparation for the lesson:

EMT Prehospital Care, Chapter 9, pages 387-402

Optional reading:

Guyton, A.C.: Textbook of Medical Physiology. 8th Ed., W.B. Saunders, Philadelphia, PA 1990

Solomon, E.P., Phillips, G.A.: Understanding Human Anatomy and Physiology. W.B. Saunders, Philadelphia, PA 1987

Suggested Learning Activities
Using a lecture format with the aid of slides, overhead transparencies, or charts, provide an overview of anatomy, physiology, and pathophysiology of soft tissues. **Display and distribute different types of dressings and bandages to students during lecture.** **When possible, have students palpate structures on self or other students and monitor activities.**

Content

I. Integumentary system **(Slide 9-2)**

A. Overview

1. The largest organ of the body providing a protective covering and insulation
2. Separates the internal from the external environment
3. Barrier to infection and loss of body fluids
4. Important for regulation of body temperature

B. Layers of the skin **(Slide 9-3)**

1. The Epidermis
   a) Surface or outermost layer
   b) Nonvascular and made up of four separate sublayers
   c) Impermeable to microorganisms
   d) Prevents water loss from the cells underneath
   e) Superficial layer is dead tissue that is flaked away and replaced from living cells beneath
   f) Filled with a protein called keratin as they move upward toward the skin surface
      (1) Partially responsible for impermeable barrier
   g) Responsible for the color of the skin
      (1) Pigment called melanin, which helps protect us from the sun's radiation
      (2) Contributes to the color of the skin
      (3) Produced deep within the layers of the epidermis
      (4) Color also affected by blood in the dermis
2. The Dermis
   a) Composed of dense connective tissue that contains
      (1) Nerves
      (2) Blood vessels
      (3) Sweat and sebaceous glands
      (4) Hair follicles
      (5) Connective tissue serves to anchor and support the other structures
   b) Nerves in the dermis terminate in specialized endings
      (1) Perceive pressure, vibration, pain, warmth and cold, etc.
      (2) If damaged (i.e., third-degree burns), there will be no sensory perception
   c) Blood vessels play important role in temperature regulation
      (1) Constrict to prevent heat loss
      (2) Dilate to give off heat
   d) Sweat glands play an important role in body temperature regulation
      (1) Cooling hot environments
      (2) Loss of internal heat production (exercise)
   e) Sebaceous glands secrete sebum
      (1) Moisturizes skin
      (2) Located near hair follicles, which guide the sebum to the surface

Content

- f) Hairs grow from hair follicles
    - (1) Hair follicles and sweat glands allow for regrowth of new skin
    - (2) Burns that destroy all structures within the dermis will require skin grafting
- 3. Mucous Membranes **(Slide 9-4)**
    - a) Continue into a body orifice
    - b) Keratinized layer of the epidermis is replaced by mucous membranes
    - c) Line the internal surface, i.e. intestine
        - (1) Pharynx
        - (2) Ureters
        - (3) Bladder
        - (4) Lungs
        - (5) Intestines
    - d) Rich in mucous glands
    - e) Protect the body from invading organisms
- 4. Subcutaneous Tissue **(Slide 9-5)**
    - a) Layer of fat and connective tissue beneath skin
    - b) Serves as insulator and for energy storage
    - c) Beneath SQ is the fascia
        - (1) Fibrous membrane
        - (2) Separates SQ from skeletal muscles

II. Wounds **(Slide 9-6)**

- A. Closed wounds
    - 1. Blunt or compression forces
    - 2. Capillaries or larger vessels may leak or rupture
    - 3. Slight swelling from leakage of plasma (edema) into injured area
    - 4. Tenderness or pain at the site of injury
    - 5. Commonly referred to as bruises or contusions
    - 6. Leakage of blood from injured vessels
        - a) Visible under the skin as a black and blue area (ecchymosis) **(Slide 9-7)**
        - b) Changes to greenish brown and then to yellow over time
        - c) Hematoma - blood beneath the skin **(Slide 9-8)**
- B. Open wounds
    - 1. Any wounds that result in a break of the skin
    - 2. Abrasion **(Slide 9-9)**
        - a) Scraping of the surface of the skin or mucous membrane
        - b) Causes an oozing of blood at the skin's surface
        - c) Very painful but does not usually result in significant blood loss
        - d) Subject to infection as are other open wounds
    - 3. Laceration **(Slide 9-10)**
        - a) A tearing of the skin or other soft tissues
        - b) Result of a blunt tearing force or from a sharp object
        - c) Extent of tissue damage is a function of the mechanism of injury

Content

4. Avulsion **(Slide 9-11)**
    a) A tearing away of the skin's surface
    b) Complete vs incomplete
        (1) Incomplete attached with pedicle
        (2) Should be left in place
5. Puncture **(Slide 9-12)**
    a) Sharp instrument is driven through the skin's outer layer
    b) Can be very deceiving
    c) Small puncture (i.e., ice pick) may result in significant injury
    d) Object may be impaled **(Slide 9-13)**
6. Amputation **(Slide 9-14)**
    a) Cutting away from the body of a limb or protruding structure
    b) Tearing, cutting, or crushing forces
    c) Time to surgical intervention is essential
7. Crushing **(Slide 9-15)**
    a) May result in both open and closed wounds
    b) Result of a severe compressing force
    c) Damages soft tissues and underlying structures

C. Severity and complications **(Slide 9-16)**
1. Dependent on the mechanism, site, and extent of injury
2. Introduction of foreign bodies or contamination into the wound
3. Consider damage to underlying blood vessels, nerves, ligaments and bones, joints, and organs
4. Common complications **(Slide 9-17)**
    a) Bleeding
    b) Infection
    c) Nerve damage
    d) Fractures and injury to muscles, tendons, and ligaments

D. Assessment **(Slide 9-18)**
1. Mechanism of injury
2. Life-threatening conditions take priority
    a) Airway
    b) External hemorrhage
3. Location may suggest underlying organ damage or internal bleeding
4. Missile wounds - look for exit wounds
5. Loss of function - damage to bones, muscles, nerves, and vessels
6. Check for neurovascular function

E. Management **(Slide 9-19)**
1. Bleeding control
    a) Direct pressure
        (1) Manual
        (2) Pressure dressing
        (3) Pressure devices (i.e., BP cuff)
    b) Elevation
    c) Pressure points
    d) Tourniquets

Content

2. Care of closed wounds
    a) Large contusions or hematomas may require counterpressure via pressure dressings or PASG
    b) Ice or cold packs and elevation may reduce further swelling
    c) Splinting may be appropriate with pain on movement
3. Infection
    a) All open wounds are subject to infection
    b) Sterile dressings are applied when possible
    c) Wounds should not be washed or irrigated in the field, except
        (1) Superficial abrasions that are very dirty
        (2) Gross contamination of avulsions
4. Immobilization
    a) Immobilization will minimize blood flow swelling
    b) Elevation may be utilized to reduce swelling
5. Preservation of avulsed or amputated parts **(Slide 9-20)**
    a) Can often be reattached
    b) Proper handling will increase chances of reattachment
    c) Avulsed flaps that remain attached must be handled gently to preserve blood supply
        (1) Irrigate gross debris with saline
        (2) Return to normal anatomic position
    d) Handling of amputated or complete avulsions
        (1) Remain viable for a few hours at room temperature
        (2) Cooled part can remain viable for up to 18 hours
            (a) Parts can suffer frostbite
            (b) Never place directly on ice
        (3) Gross contamination should be rinsed with sterile saline or water
        (4) Covered with a sterile dressing
        (5) Placed in a watertight plastic bag
        (6) Bag should be placed in container with ice or ice and water
        (7) Labeled, and transported with the patient
6. Impaled Objects **(Slide 9-21)**
    a) May cause injury to underlying structures if moved
    b) May be occluding flow from a severed blood vessel
    c) Removal may precipitate active hemorrhage
    d) Should be stabilized in place
        (1) Large objects may be shortened for transport
        (2) Object in cheek may be removed to assure adequate ventilation and airway
7. Special considerations **(Slide 9-22)**
    a) Wounds to the veins of the neck
    b) May lead to air embolism
    c) Changes in intrathoracic pressure may suck air in through wound opening
    d) Air embolism may block blood flow
    e) Wound should be covered with an occlusive dressing
    f) Patient should be transported supine or with leg elevated

Content

g) Chest wounds are also covered with occlusive dressing to prevent air from entering pleura

III. Dressings and Bandages **(Slide 9-23)**
  A. Dressing is any material that covers a wound
    1. Prevents further contamination
    2. Aids in bleeding control
    3. Sterile dressing should be used when possible
  B. Bandage is material used to secure a dressing in place
    1. Provides pressure over the dressing to aid in the control of bleeding
    2. Several types are available
  C. Dressings **(Slide 9-24)**
    1. Gauze 4x4
      a) Most punctures or lacerations can be effectively covered with a 4x4 gauze dressing
      b) Simple nonadherent material
    2. Occlusive or airtight dressings
      a) Sterile plastic wrap
      b) Aluminum foil
      c) Petroleum-impregnated gauze
    3. Multitrauma
      a) Large dressing for wide abrasions
      b) Thick absorbent material, measuring 9 x 36 inches in size
      c) Useful to cover large areas such as abrasions, burns or as a pressure dressing over long open wounds
      d) Also useful as a padding for splints
  D. Bandages **(Slide 9-25)**
    1. Self-Adherent Bandages
      a) Rolls of slightly elastic, gauzelike material
      b) Easy to work with which allows for their rapid application
      c) Elastic quality helps in applying pressure to control arterial hemorrhage
    2. Ace Bandages
      a) Used to support joints and attach splints
      b) Should not be confused with self-adherent bandages
      c) Much more elastic and may obstruct distal blood flow and pressure on local nerves
    3. Gauze Roller Bandage
      a) Cotton and relatively nonelastic roller bandage
      b) Comes in various widths
      c) Commonly used for extremity and head dressing applications
    4. Triangular Bandage
      a) Most versatile of all bandages
      b) Formed from cutting a 36- to 42-inch square of cloth (usually muslin) diagonally
      c) Multiple uses
        (1) Allows for rapid application of direct pressure and/or support
        (2) Used as a sling in the triangular form
        (3) May be folded and utilized as a cravat-type bandage
        (4) Commonly used as tourniquet

Content

5. Adhesive Tape
   a) Utilized to secure bandages and dressings in place
   b) Care should be used when applied circumferentially to an extremity to avoid obstruction of blood flow
6. Air Splints **(Slide 9-26)**
   a) Inflatable cylindrical tube
   b) For wounds associated with fractures
   c) May be applied over a dressing and bandage
   d) Available in various sizes to adapt to upper and lower extremities
   e) PASG may be used in a similar fashion over the lower extremities and pelvis
7. Blood Pressure Cuffs
   a) Used for added pressure needed to control hemorrhage
   b) Pressure of the cuff can be inflated until arterial bleeding is controlled
   c) Careful attention should be paid to distal blood flow
8. Applying a pressure dressing **(Slide 9-27)**
   a) Apply dressing and direct pressure until bleeding is controlled **(Slide 9-28)**
   b) Continue to apply pressure and attach a self-adherent or roller bandage **(Slide 9-29)**
   c) Just enough pressure to control bleeding
   d) Reinforce dressing when necessary
   e) If bleeding recurs, additional dressings and bandages may be applied
   f) Evaluate distal blood flow with pulse and capillary refill
   g) Immobilize and elevate injured part
9. Basic methods of applying a roller bandage **(Slide 9-30)**
   a) Work at a steady pace
   b) Spread the bandage evenly over the body surface
   c) Maintain a uniform pressure
   d) Avoid clumping of the bandage material
   e) Roll with the bulk of the bandage facing up and held close to the body surface
   f) After encircling body part once, anchor in place
   g) Overlap approximately halfway over the previous layer
   h) Should be tight enough to control bleeding but loose enough to allow distal blood flow
   i) Once in place attach by adhesive tape
10. Head Bandage **(Slide 9-31)**
   a) Encircle circumference of head
   b) Anchor below the occipital protuberance **(Slide 9-32)**
   c) Circle head completely once or twice **(Slide 9-33)**
   d) Traverse the bandage back and forth across the **(Slide 9-34)** top of the head until dressing is completely covered
   e) Secure the bandage in place **(Slide 9-35)**

Content

11. Bandage for chest and back **(Slide 9-36)**
    a) Most dressing to the chest and back can be done with tape
    b) Cravats may also be used to traverse area
12. Bandage for knee or elbow
    a) Figure-eight bandage secures a dressing over a joint while allowing for mobility **(Slide 9-37)**
    b) Start the roller bandage above the joint and anchor it in place **(Slide 9-38)**
    c) Traverse the bandage diagonally across the joint over the dressing **(Slide 9-39)**
    d) Circle the bandage below the joint **(Slide 9-40)**
    e) Circle the distal portion, traverse upward to form an "x" over the dressing on the joint **(Slide 9-41)**
    f) Continue this pattern until the bandage is complete **(Slide 9-42)**
13. Impaled object
    a) Place a dressing around the impaled object **(Slide 9-43)**
    b) Place bulky pads around the object
    c) Bandage them securely in place **(Slide 9-44)**
    d) Should be sufficient to limit any movement of the impaled object
    e) If impaled in the thoracic cavity, an occlusive dressing should be utilized around object

Section 2

Injuries to The Face, Head and Neck

Objectives
(Slide 9-45)

At the conclusion of the chapter the student will be able to:

1. **List the major structures of the eye and their functions.**
2. **Describe the management of the following eye injuries:**

Foreign bodies	**Corneal abrasions**
Chemical injuries	**Light injuries**
Lacerations	**Contusions**
Extruded eyeball	**Fracture of the orbit**

3. **List the major structures of the ear and their functions.**
4. **Describe the management of the following ear emergencies:**

Avulsions	**Foreign bodies**
Barotrauma	**Infections**

5. **List the major bones of the face.**
6. **Describe the assessment and management of facial fractures.**
7. **Describe the management of airway compromise secondary to fractures of the mandible.**
8. **Describe the management of the following types of face and neck emergencies:**

Esophageal injuries	**Avulsions**
Impaled objects	**Nosebleeds**
Tracheal injuries	**Vascular injuries**

Instructor Preparation

Reading preparation for the lesson:

EMT Prehospital Care, Chapter 9, pages 402-427

Optional reading:

Prehospital Trauma Life Support Committee of The National Association of EMTs: <u>Pre-Hospital Trauma Life Support</u>. 2nd Ed., Emergency Training. Akron, Ohio 1990

Suggested Learning Activities

Using a lecture format with the aid of slides, overhead transparencies or charts, provide a presentation of head, face and neck trauma.

Provide case histories that illustrate different types of head, face and neck trauma.

Content

IV. Injuries to face, head and neck
  A. Overview **(Slide 9-46)**
    1. Airway is first concern
    2. Facial bones give structural support to airway
    3. Loss of integrity can compromise airway patency
    4. Bleeding, foreign bodies, broken teeth, vomitus, etc. can obstruct the air passage
    5. Face has a rich blood vessel supply, and injuries can cause extensive bleeding
    6. Face offers protection to the brain **(Slide 9-47)**
      a) Trauma can cause injury to the brain
      b) Search for signs of injury to the brain and the cervical spine
    7. Facial bones also offer protection to the eye and ear
    8. Special handling is needed for these sensitive organs
  B. Anatomy
    1. Neck **(Slide 9-48)**
      a) Many vital structures are closely packed
        (1) Larynx and trachea
        (2) Major arteries and veins
        (3) Esophagus and cervical spine
      b) Organs and structures are prone to injury
      c) Patient can form an air embolism from a laceration of a major vein
    2. Face
      a) Bones of the face **(Slide 9-49)**
        (1) Maxilla forms the upper jaw
        (2) Mandible forms the lower jaw
        (3) Zygoma connects maxilla, frontal and temporal bones
        (4) Orbit - bones of the eye socket
        (5) Nasal bones consist of cartilage and soft tissues, which make up the nose
      b) Soft tissues **(Slide 9-50)**
        (1) Face is rich in soft tissue structures, blood vessels and nerves
          (a) Bleeding is often brisk
          (b) Usually easily controlled with direct pressure
          (c) Nerves exit through foramen or small openings in the skull
          (d) Salivary glands secrete saliva
          (e) Facial muscles over entire face
  C. Injuries to face **(Slide 9-51)**
    1. Maintaining a clear airway in the presence of bleeding and foreign bodies is often difficult
    2. May require use of many techniques
      a) Manual extraction of foreign bodies
      b) Control of bleeding
      c) Suctioning
      d) Appropriate airway techniques
      e) Positioning of the patient to permit drainage

Content

3. Fractures and airway compromise **(Slide 9-52)**
    - a) When the facial bones collapse traditional airway maneuvers may need to be modified
    - b) Standard techniques rely on the structural integrity of the facial bones
    - c) Tongue-jaw lift maneuver and oropharyngeal or nasopharyngeal airways may be needed
    - d) Head tilt is contraindicated if cervical spine fracture is suspected
    - e) Advanced airway maneuvers may be needed to secure airway
4. Recognition of facial fractures **(Slide 9-53)**
    - a) Force
        - (1) Less force is needed to fracture facial bones than the frontal bone of the cranium
        - (2) Nasal bones most common fracture other than wrist
        - (3) Zygomas, mandible, and maxilla require more energy to fracture
        - (4) Frontal bones of the cranium require a significantly greater blow
        - (5) Force absorbed by collapsing face helps prevent brain injury
    - b) Common sites of fractures **(Slide 9-54)**
        - (1) Maxilla
            - (a) Broken in high-speed impact accidents
            - (b) Face is thrown forward onto dashboards, windshields or steering wheel
            - (c) Common sites described by Le Forte in 1900
                - i) Le Forte I- a transverse fracture
                    - i) Above the roots of the teeth
                    - ii) Instability of the upper teeth and upper palate
                - ii) Le Forte II - fractured triangular segment
                    - i) Nasal bones
                    - ii) Frontal process of the maxilla
                    - iii) Instability of the nose and upper teeth
                - iii) Le Forte III
                    - i) Maxilla, nasal bones and zygomas
                    - ii) Instability of the entire midface
            - (d) Inspection of midface fractures **(Slide 9-55)**
                - i) May appear elongated
                - ii) Swelling and periorbital ecchymosis and edema
            - (e) Palpation **(Slide 9-56)**
                - i) Tenderness and crepitus
                - ii) Deformity
                - iii) Asymmetry
                - iv) Can be assessed by gentle palpation

v) Midface fractures are associated with damage to base of the skull
vi) Use of the nasopharyngeal airway should be contraindicated

(2) Mandible **(Slide 9-57)**
(a) Fractures can cause severe airway problems
(b) Often breaks at more than one site following injury
(c) Pain in the jaw
(d) Inspection
i) Problems with alignment of the teeth
ii) Not able to close the jaw
iii) Collapse of the airway
iv) Tongue-jaw lift and oral airways may be needed
v) Palpation should be gentle

(3) Orbits **(Slide 9-58)**
(a) Fractures of the orbits may be isolated or as part of a midface fracture
(b) Fractures of the lower rim can cause entrapment of muscles

5. Bleeding from facial injuries **(Slide 9-59)**
a) Blood or other foreign bodies should be removed with finger sweep and/or suction
b) Conscious patient may be allowed to sit if no cervical spine injury is suspected
c) Unconscious patients are placed in the lateral recumbent position
d) With possible cervical spine injury
(1) Maintain cervical alignment
(2) Provide for airway clearance by rotating spine board
(3) Swelling and hematomas may cause obstruction
(a) May require surgical airway
(b) Forced positive pressure may be needed
e) External or oral cavity bleeding should be controlled with direct pressure
f) Avulsions **(Slide 9-60)**
(1) Place moistened with sterile saline directly over the wound to prevent drying
(2) Bandage should be applied over the moistened dressing
(3) Avulsed parts
(a) Rinsed of gross debris
(b) Placed in dressing
(c) Inserted in watertight plastic bag
(d) Transported on ice or ice and water
(e) Broken denture fragments should be transported
g) Impaled objects **(Slide 9-61)**
(1) Should be removed from cheek
(2) Interfere with respiration

Content

(3) Gently pull the object back through the wound
(4) Control bleeding
(5) Position the patient to allow for drainage if necessary

D. Injuries to nose **(Slide 9-62)**

1. Nosebleeds are one of the most common findings following nasal fractures
2. Relationship of anatomy to bleeding control
    a) Nose is mostly cartilage, which extends from the nasal bones
    b) Septum divides the nose into halves
    c) Inner surface is lined by a thin mucosal membrane
    d) Main blood vessels are contained within the mucous membrane along bone and cartilage
    e) Conditions with cool, dry air and upper respiratory infections cause nosebleeds
    f) Anterior nosebleeds **(Slide 9-63)**
        (1) 90% occur in a region known as Kiesselbach's plexus
        (2) Along the nasal septum within 2 centimeters from the nasal tip
        (3) Direct pressure can be applied to this general area by pinching the nostrils **(Slide 9-64)**
        (4) Pressure point **(Slide 9-65)**
            (a) Applied to artery between the upper lip and the gums **(Slide 9-66)**
            (b) Gauze is placed between inner lip and gum to focus pressure
    g) Posterior nosebleeds **(Slide 9-67)**
        (1) 10% of nosebleeds are considered posterior
        (2) Can not be distinguished in the field
        (3) Can bleed extensively
        (4) Not controlled with maneuvers in the field
        (5) Require packing and internal pressure to control
3. Causes of nosebleeds **(Slide 9-68)**
    a) Traumatic Causes
        (1) Fractures of the nose
        (2) Leakage of cerebrospinal fluid
            (a) Fractures to the base of the skull
            (b) Cerebrospinal fluid or blood
            (c) Damming up may predispose the patient to infection and increased intracranial pressure
            (d) Other signs
                i) Raccoon's sign
                ii) Battle's sign
        (3) Digital trauma
            (a) The most common cause of nosebleeds is self-exploration of the nostrils
            (b) Bleeding is usually minor and can be controlled with the nasal pinch
    b) Nontraumatic Causes **(Slide 9-69)**
        (1) Drying and congestion of the mucous membranes
        (2) Associated with anterior nosebleeds

Content

(3) Foreign bodies should be suspected in children
(4) Arteriosclerosis
(5) Inherited bleeding disorders
(6) Patients taking anticoagulants or "blood thinners"
(7) Hypertension may or may not cause nosebleeds

4. Management of nosebleeds **(Slide 9-70)**
a) Direct pressure as discussed earlier to control bleeding
b) Continue pressure for 5 minutes to allow clotting to take place
c) Repeat if bleeding continues
d) Hypovolemic shock **(Slide 9-71)**
(1) Excessive bleeding can occur from posterior nosebleeds
(2) Difficult to estimate owing to swallowed blood
(3) Observe for signs of shock
(a) Pale, cool, clammy skin
(b) Tachycardia
(c) Orthostatic hypotension
(d) Hypotension
(e) Altered mental status
(4) Should receive the same urgency as any patient with severe internal bleeding

E. Eye injuries **(Slide 9-72)**
1. Anatomy and physiology
a) Delicate organ whose unique structure demands special handling
b) Improper handling may result in further damage and loss of vision
c) Globular structure filled with a jell-like fluid called the vitreous humor
d) Eye rotates within the bony orbit under action of the orbital muscles
e) Sclera is outer layer of fibrous, opaque protective membrane except anterior portion
f) Cornea is transparent so that light rays can enter the opening of the eye (pupil)
g) Iris is the pigmented or colored portion of the eye surrounding pupil **(Slide 9-73)**
(1) Circular muscular structure
(2) Controls the amount of light that enters the eye through the pupil
(3) Made of constricting and dilating muscles
(4) Pupil constricts in response to bright light and dilates in dim light
(5) Changes in size when one focuses on near or far objects
(6) Pupil used to evaluate the effect of drugs and other conditions upon the central nervous system
h) Lens focuses light onto the posterior wall of the eye or the retina
i) Ciliary muscles are attached to the lens to change its shape
j) Retina is composed of sensory receptors, which convert light into nervous impulses

Content

k) Optic nerve transmits impulses to the brain for interpretation as a visual image

l) Chambers of the eye
- (1) Eye can be divided into an anterior and a posterior chamber by the lens
  - (a) Anterior chamber is filled with a fluid called the aqueous humor
  - (b) Posterior chamber is filled with a firmer jelly called the vitreous humor
  - (c) Aqueous and vitreous humors give shape and firmness to the eye
- (2) Importance of humors
  - (a) Aqueous humor continuously formed from special capillaries
  - (b) Circulate in the anterior chamber and drained
  - (c) Reabsorbed into other capillaries
  - (d) When drainage is obstructed, pressure builds up (glaucoma)
  - (e) If not corrected the nerves can be damaged resulting in loss of vision
  - (f) Vitreous humor is not formed or drained
  - (g) Cannot be lost without permanent damage
  - (h) Loss of the vitreous humor can result in permanent loss of shape and function
  - (i) Direct pressure must never be applied to an injured eyeball
- (3) Protection **(Slide 9-74)**
  - (a) Eye is set deep within bony orbits or sockets formed by many bones
  - (b) Protected in front by the eyelids
    - i) Can blink quickly to protect the eye from oncoming objects
    - ii) Eyelashes aid as filters to prevent small particles from entering eye
  - (c) Conjunctiva lines interior surface of lids and anterior surface of the eye
    - i) Changes its composition as it extends over the sclera and cornea
    - ii) When irritated vessels become prominent and pink - conjunctivitis **(Slide 9-75)**
  - (d) Lacrimal glands secrete tears
    - i) Located at the superior lateral surface of each eyeball
    - ii) Continuously secreted, serve to moisten, clean and lubricate
    - iii) Drained through lacrimal canals at the medial portion of each eyeball

(e) Layer of fat behind eye serves as an additional cushion
(f) Loss of this fat during starvation explains why eyes may appear sunken

2. Specific injuries **(Slide 9-76)**
    a) Principles when caring for eye injuries
        (1) Avoid pressure to avoid leakage of humors
        (2) Cover both eyes to limit movement
        (3) Gain patient's cooperation
    b) Foreign bodies **(Slide 9-77)**
        (1) Very irritating and cause considerable pain
        (2) May be on the eyeball, lower or upper eyelid
        (3) Upper lid foreign body may be felt by the patient during blinking
        (4) May be superficial or deeply embedded and require eye surgery
        (5) Inspection **(Slide 9-78)**
            (a) Lower lid and most of the eyeball are easily visualized
            (b) Have the patient look to either side and up and down to inspect most of eye
            (c) To inspect upper lid
                i) Patient must look downward
                ii) Evert the upper lid using a cotton-tipped applicator as a fulcrum
                iii) Grasp the eyelashes with your thumb and finger
                iv) Pull lid forward and up, causing it to fold back over applicator
        (6) Removal
            (a) With lid everted, rinse a foreign body away with irrigating solution **(Slide 9-79)**
                i) Irrigate gently from medial to lateral side
                ii) Use saline or sterile water
                iii) Coach patient to keep eye open
            (b) Gently remove it with a moistened cotton-tipped swab if irrigation is unsuccessful
            (c) Patch eye after removal
    c) Corneal abrasions **(Slide 9-80)**
        (1) Cornea is particularly sensitive
        (2) Scratches are very painful
        (3) Feeling may persist even after a foreign body is removed
        (4) Patching the eye may give some pain relief
    d) Impaled objects **(Slide 9-81)**
        (1) Never remove impaled object
        (2) Loss of the vitreous humor and permanent damage to the eye

Content

(3) Stabilize the object with dressing built around the impaled object **(Slide 9-82)**
(a) Cover the dressing with a paper cup or piece of cardboard
(b) Patch other eye

e) Chemical burns **(Slide 9-83)**
(1) Damage depends on the nature of the chemical and the length of time
(2) Alkaline and acid materials are particularly deleterious
(3) Other toxic chemicals can have variable effects
(4) Immediately flush the eye with clean water or other irrigating solution
(5) Intravenous is effective to direct the flow over the eyeball
(6) Irrigate from medial to lateral
(7) Hold the eyelids open with your fingers. Continue irrigation for at least 20 minutes
(8) Longer for alkaline agent
(9) If irrigating solution is not available, use tap water
(10) Topical anesthetic is used by some systems to help keep eye open
(11) Irrigation should continue throughout transport

f) Light injuries **(Slide 9-84)**
(1) Injury due to sun or from arc welding without protective goggles
(2) Can result in painful burns to the cornea
(3) Pain usually occurs a few hours after exposure
(4) Cover the eyes with moist patches and transport

g) Burned eyelids **(Slide 9-85)**
(1) Exposure to fire and intense heat can cause burns to the eyelids
(2) Cover the eyelids with a moist sterile dressing and transport

h) Eyelid lacerations **(Slide 9-86)**
(1) Can cause brisk bleeding because of the rich blood supply
(2) Check for accompanying damage to the eye
(3) Use gentle and direct pressure to control bleeding from the eyelid
(4) Avoid transmitting pressure to the eye
(5) Eye lacerations, cover both eyes with loose dressings and transport

i) Contusions **(Slide 9-87)**
(1) Contusions can result in bleeding within eye or on surface
(2) Subconjunctival hematoma may be noted but is usually not serious **(Slide 9-88)**
(3) Bleeding is sometimes visible between the iris and the cornea **(Slide 9-89)**
(4) Cover the eye and transport the patient in the supine position

Content

j) Traumatic iritis **(Slide 9-90)**

(1) Trauma to eye can cause spasm of iris and inflammation of the conjunctiva

(2) Pupil may appear fixed in mid position or slightly dilated

(3) May be unresponsive to light

(4) May be confused with pupil changes related to CNS injury

k) Extruded eyeball **(Slide 9-91)**

(1) If eyeball is extruded, do not attempt to replace it

(2) Place 4x4's with a hole cut out of the center

(3) Moisten with sterile saline around the extruding eyeball

(4) Attach a cup or cone shaped from cardboard

(5) Cover the opposite eye and transport

l) Fracture of the orbit **(Slide 9-92)**

(1) Significant blows can fracture orbit

(2) Signs and symptoms

(a) Pain and tenderness

(b) Soft tissue trauma along the orbital ridge

(c) Impairment of eye movement and visual disturbance **(Slide 9-93)**

i) Muscles become entrapped in the fracture

ii) Patient may not be able to move both eyes symmetrically

iii) Can experience double or impaired vision

3. Nontraumatic eye pain **(Slide 9-94)**

a) Severe eye pain not associated with injury

b) Blockage of outflow of the aqueous humor can cause build up of pressure (glaucoma)

c) Other signs and symptoms

(1) Visual disturbance such as halos around lights

(2) Headache, nausea and vomiting

(3) Cornea may appear hazy and steamed

(4) Pupil stuck in mid position and not responsive to light

(5) Sclera may appear pink and inflamed

(6) Rapid transport is essential

F. Ear Injuries

1. Anatomy and physiology **(Slide 9-95)**

a) Overview

(1) Functions include hearing, position sense and balance

(2) Movement changes body position and causes fluid-filled structures to detect movement

(3) Movement is relayed as nerve impulses to different parts of the brain

(4) Blood extruding from the ear after trauma is a sign of possible skull fracture

(5) Ear infections are a potential cause of meningitis

Content

b) External ear
   (1) Comprised of the auricle or pinna which is the outer visible ear flap
   (2) External auditory canal leads through the temporal bone to the tympanic membrane
   (3) Auricle made up of skin and cartilage
      (a) Provides protection to the opening
      (b) Directs sound waves into the auditory canal
   (4) Auditory canal is lined with modified sweat glands
      (a) Secrete earwax or cerumen
      (b) Trap particles and bacteria that may enter the ear

c) Middle ear
   (1) Air-filled cavity transmits sound waves to the inner ear
   (2) Begins at the tympanic membrane or eardrum and ends at the oval window
   (3) Communicating across from the eardrum are three tiny bones
      (a) Malleus (hammer), Incus (anvil), Stapes (stirrup)
      (b) Transmit sound waves collected at the eardrum to the inner ear
      (c) Attached to each other acting as a series of levers
   (4) Middle ear communicates with the nasopharynx via the eustachian tube
      (a) Allows equalization of air pressure between middle ear and atmosphere
      (b) Infections of the pharynx can travel up and cause middle ear infections

d) Inner ear
   (1) Encased within the skull
   (2) Contains coiled, looped tubes filled with fluid
   (3) Lined with sensory cells
   (4) Three structures within
      (a) Vestibule and semicircular canals at right angles to each other
      (b) Cochlea a spirally wound tube resembling a snail shell
      (c) Lined with receptor cells
      (d) Vestibule and semicircular canals are concerned with position sense
      (e) Cochlea is concerned with hearing
      (f) Nerve fibers from receptor cells travel to brain

Content

e) Hearing
(1) Sound waves are physical vibrations of air
(2) They have amplitude and frequency characteristics
(a) Amplitude or size and energy of the waves is related to loudness
(b) Frequency (or cycles) per second is related to the pitch of the sound
(3) As sound waves hit tympanic membrane they set the ossicles in motion
(4) Ossicles are connected to the oval window of the inner ear
(5) Transmitting sound waves from the tympanic membrane to the inner ear
(6) Waves cause an inward and outward motion of the oval window
(7) Movement causes a movement of fluid within the cochlea
(8) Movement is sensed by the receptor cells within
(9) Receptor cells initiate nerve impulses which are sent to the brain
(10) Muscles connected to ossicles dampen sound waves if they are excessive
(a) Sudden explosions may still damage the hearing mechanisms
(b) As can continued and unprotected exposure to loud noises

f) Balance and position
(1) Fluid in semicircular canals and vestibule is set in motion by head movement
(2) Sensitive hair cells detect the effect of movement and gravitation on the fluid
(3) Hair cells send impulses through vestibular nerve to cerebrum and cerebellum
(4) Aid in determination of position and balance

2. Injuries to ear
a) Blunt trauma **(Slide 9-96)**
(1) Can cause contusions and hematoma of the auricle
(2) Severe blows can damage the eardrum with resulting pain and/or bleeding
(3) Blood or fluid from ear should always be considered as sign of possible skull fracture
(4) Loose sterile dressing should be applied

b) Lacerations and avulsions of auricle **(Slide 9-97)**
(1) Auricle is susceptible to laceration, avulsions, and complete amputation
(2) If possible remove gross contamination and apply a sterile dressing
(3) Bulky dressing should be applied around the pinna before bandaging

Content

(4) Treat incomplete avulsed parts by approximating their anatomic position
(5) Treat completely avulsed or amputated parts as you would any other
(6) Keep the part cool by placing it over ice or in water with ice added

c) Foreign bodies **(Slide 9-98)**
(1) Foreign bodies lodged in auditory canal should be removed in emergency department
(2) Eardrum is sensitive and may be painful if punctured and can cause bleeding
(3) Be careful not to obstruct blood flow from the auditory canal

d) Barotrauma **(Slide 9-99)**
(1) Caused by changing environmental pressures (flying or diving)
(2) Middle ear maintains equal pressure via air movement through the eustachian tubes
(3) Changes in pressure before equalization cause distortion and rupture of eardrum
(4) Balloon and diver example **(Slide 9-100)**
(a) As balloon or diver descends atmospheric pressure increases
(b) Filled balloon at surface is compressed as it descends
(c) Caused by increased pressure from the water on all sides
(d) Tympanic membrane is also subject to these pressures
(e) Normally pressure on inside of tympanic membrane matches outside
(f) If diver cannot equalize pressure owing to blockage of the eustachian tube
(g) Rupture of the eardrum can result
(5) Patients with barotrauma of ear present with pain and/or hearing loss
(6) Upper respiratory infections may predispose patients to barotrauma
(7) No prehospital treatment for barotrauma of the ear

3. Middle ear infections **(Slide 9-101)**
a) Infections of upper respiratory tract can invade middle ear through eustachian tube
b) Tend to be painful and associated with high fever
c) Children are more prone to infection because of short and straight eustachian tube
d) Fluid builds up against the tympanic membrane, pressure causes intense pain
e) Tympanic membrane may burst

f) Rupture usually results in relief of pain
g) Drainage is usually bloody, purulent (puslike) fluid
h) Middle ear infections can lead to infection of the meninges of the brain, or meningitis

G. Neck injuries **(Slide 9-102)**

1. Major causes of death from neck injuries are airway obstruction and hemorrhage
2. Signs of airway distress and exsanguinating hemorrhage dictate rapid intervention
3. Precautions are taken for potential cervical spine injuries
4. Anatomy
    a) Respiratory components
        (1) Pharynx, larynx and trachea
            (a) Larynx and the trachea are anterior and are palpable
            (b) Formed of cartilage and subject to fracture and collapse
            (c) Larynx contains the vocal cords
            (d) Epiglottis is located at the superior portion of the larynx
        (2) Major circulatory vessels
            (a) Common carotid arteries
                i) Lateral to the larynx and trachea
                ii) Medial (upper) and posterior (lower) to sternocleidomastoid muscles
            (b) Internal and external jugular veins
                i) Externals are on anterolateral aspect of the neck and are quite superficial
                ii) Externals extend from angle of the jaw down to the clavicle
                iii) Internal jugulars are located lateral and posterior to the carotid arteries
            (c) Posterior to the larynx and trachea is the esophagus
            (d) Posterior portion of the neck is made up of the cervical vertebrae
            (e) Major peripheral nerves also pass through the neck
            (f) Nerves innervate important structures such as the vocal cords and diaphragm
5. Mechanisms of injury
    a) Blunt **(Slide 9-103)**
        (1) Motor vehicle accidents where anterior neck impacts on steering wheel or dashboard
        (2) Hyperflexion and hyperextension injuries may injure soft tissues and spine
        (3) Other causes of blunt injuries
            (a) Strangling
            (b) Hanging
            (c) "Clothesline" injuries during sports

Content

- (d) Snowmobile accidents where the driver fails to see a chain across the road
- (e) Assaults

(4) Blunt injuries often result in airway obstruction owing to fracture and collapse

b) Penetrating **(Slide 9-104)**

(1) Can result from missile or stab wounds
(2) Depending on location, any of structures can be affected
(3) Most common cause of death is hemorrhage
(4) Airway may be penetrated directly or may be compressed owing to expanding hematoma
(5) Interruption of carotid flow may result in signs of stroke
(6) Laceration to the jugular veins may lead to air embolism

6. Specific injuries

a) Respiratory injuries **(Slide 9-105)**

(1) Larynx and trachea can fracture, tear, or collapse
(2) Air can escape into the soft tissues resulting in subcutaneous emphysema
(3) Complete obstruction
- (a) Signs of respiratory efforts with little or no air movement
- (b) Respiratory arrest with inability to ventilate

(4) Partial obstruction **(Slide 9-106)**
- (a) Stridor may be heard
- (b) Dyspnea and increased work of breathing
- (c) Respiratory rate may be increased
- (d) Accessory muscles active on inspection
- (e) Hemoptysis
- (f) Subcutaneous emphysema **(Slide 9-107)**
- (g) Evidence of deformity of larynx noted on gentle palpation
- (h) Hoarse voice quality
- (i) Pain swallowing, coughing, talking, and during neck movement

b) Penetrating injuries **(Slide 9-108)**

(1) Wounds may penetrate the airway structures
(2) Characterized by bubbling blood over the skin wound and a false airway
(3) Extreme care must be taken when evaluating and managing patients
- (a) Palpation should be gentle
- (b) Avoid manipulation and further disruption of the air passage
- (c) Opening in airway structure may be primary means of ventilation
- (d) Manipulation may cause complete obstruction

(4) Wounds should be dressed with sterile 4x4's

Content

(5) Attention must be paid to prevent blood from entering the air passage

(6) Management **(Slide 9-109)**

(a) Open the airway with manual maneuver

(b) Assess and provide positive-pressure ventilation if needed

(c) If resistance is noted and there is no chest excursion:

i) Readjust the airway

ii) Attempt ventilations again

(d) If still unsuccessful

i) Consider foreign body airway obstruction

ii) Initiate the appropriate procedures

(e) If evidence of airway injuries exists (e.g., flattening of larynx or subcutaneous emphysema):

i) Access advanced airway procedures

ii) Provide forced positive-pressure ventilation

(f) Patients with partial obstruction

i) Positive-pressure ventilations (if indicated)

ii) Supplemental oxygen

iii) With good air exchange administer oxygen via a nonrebreather mask

(g) Suction should be readily available

c) Vascular injuries **(Slide 9-110)**

(1) Major problem is hemorrhage (leading to hypovolemic shock)

(2) Airway compromise secondary to an expanding hematoma

(3) Air embolism

(4) Ischemia of the brain secondary to loss of carotid blood flow

d) Arterial bleeding **(Slide 9-111)**

(1) Arterial bleeding in the neck must be controlled with direct pressure

(2) With massive hemorrhage, use of a pressure point carotid artery

(3) This is the only time one uses the carotid artery as a pressure point

(4) Pressure must be maintained manually en route to the hospital

e) Venous bleeding **(Slide 9-112)**

(1) Should be covered with an occlusive dressing to prevent air embolism

(2) Laying the patient in head-down position will increase venous pressure

(3) Reduces chance of an air embolism

f) Neurologic symptoms **(Slide 9-113)**

(1) Neurologic symptoms (hemiparesis, facial droop, etc.)

(2) Suggest obstruction of carotid blood flow

Content

g) Cervical spine injuries **(Slide 9-114)**
   (1) Assumed when patients suffer severe blunt trauma to the neck
   (2) Penetrating injuries injure cervical spine as well
   (3) Head should be maintained in the neutral in-line position
   (4) Appropriate immobilization techniques should be used to maintain position

h) Esophageal injuries **(Slide 9-115)**
   (1) Perforation of the esophagus can result in bleeding and the vomiting of blood
   (2) May lead to subcutaneous emphysema
   (3) Pain on swallowing (dysphagia)
   (4) Bleeding from the mouth can be aspirated

i) Chest **(Slide 9-116)**
   (1) Penetrating wounds to neck may be directed from above in a downward direction
   (2) Maintain a high suspicion of pneumothorax, hemothorax or tamponade

Chapter 9

SOFT TISSUE INJURIES

Examination

1. The two major layers of the skin are the:

   a. fascia and epidermis
   b. dermis and subdermis
   c. epidermis and subdermis
   d. dermis and epidermis

2. The structure contained in the skin that plays an important role in the regulation of body temperature is called the:

   a. sebaceous glands
   b. sweat glands
   c. hair follicles
   d. keratin

Match the description in column B with the type of wound in column A:

Column A			Column B	
3.	____	puncture	a.	a tearing of the skin or other soft tissue.
4.	____	laceration	b.	a wound caused by a sharp instrument being driven through the skin.
5.	____	abrasion	c.	cutting away from the body of a limb or protruding structure.
6.	____	avulsion	d.	a tearing away of the skin's surface.
7.	____	contusion	e.	bruising of the skin.
8.	___	amputation	f.	scraping of the surface of the skin or mucous membrane.
9.	____	crushing	g.	an injury caused by the severe compressing force that damages and sometimes tears the soft tissues and underlying structures.

10. Control of bleeding should be accomplished in the following order:

    a. elevation, direct pressure, use of pressure points, and the application of a tourniquet
    b. use of pressure points, elevation, direct pressure, and the application of a tourniquet
    c. direct pressure, elevation, use of pressure points, and the application of a tourniquet
    d. direct pressure, use of pressure points, elevation, and the application of a tourniquet

11. Infants have a blood volume of _________ ml per kilogram of body weight:

    a. 50-70
    b. 80-100
    c. 110-130
    d. 140-160

12. In general, impaled objects should be left in place because:

    a. the physician can then determine how far in the object went
    b. if you remove the object a portion may break off necessitating surgery to remove it
    c. the object may be implanted in such a way as to be actually occluding blood flow from a severed blood vessel
    d. the risk of infection is reduced if the object is removed in the hospital

13. What blood vessels, when severed, may lead to an air embolism?

    a. arteries in the chest
    b. veins in the neck and upper chest
    c. capillaries in the chest
    d. arteries in the head

14. The _________ connects the maxilla, frontal and temporal bones:

    a. mandible
    b. zygoma
    c. frontal
    d. maxilla

15. The _________ is the bone of the lower jaw:

    a. mandible
    b. zygoma
    c. frontal
    d. maxilla

Match the description in column B with the type of bandage or dressing in column A:

Column A			Column B	
16.	____	occlusive	a.	used as a sling or cravat bandage
17.	____	self-adherent	b.	aluminum foil, Saran wrap or petroleum gauze
18.	____	air splint	c.	large dressing used for massage of abrasions or burns
19.	____	multitrauma	d.	allows elastic pressure for arterial bleeding
20.	____	triangular	e.	an inflatable cylindrical tube

21. The primary concern for patients with facial injuries is:

    a. damage to the teeth
    b. facial disfigurement
    c. patency of the airway
    d. permanent loss of vision

22. Fractures of the jaw may cause collapse and obstruction of the airway. If this is encountered, you should:

    a. perform a head tilt-neck lift
    b. pull the tongue and lower jaw forward
    c. perform a tracheostomy
    d. administer oxygen via a nasal cannula

23. The categorization of facial fractures into three groups in relation to the level and instability of the facial bones is called:

    a. Le Forte fractures
    b. Cushing's fractures
    c. Colles's fractures
    d. Homan's fractures

24. When the teeth are not aligned properly or the patient is unable to close his mouth it may suggest a fracture of the:

    a. zygoma
    b. frontal bone
    c. orbit
    d. mandible

25. Complete and deep avulsions of the facial skin should be treated by placing a ________________ dressing directly over the wound.

    a. Vaseline
    b. aluminum foil
    c. moistened
    d. surgipad

26. In addition to direct pressure to control nosebleeds, pressure over the __________ artery may be useful:

    a. facial
    b. carotid
    c. septal
    d. labial

27. The nose is divided into halves by the cartilaginous structure called the:

    a. nares
    b. palate
    c. septum
    d. pharynx

28. Ten percent of all nosebleeds occur in the ___________ portion of the nose.

    a. anterior
    b. middle
    c. posterior
    d. external

29. The eye contains vitreous humor, which is:

    a. a jell-like fluid
    b. the pigmented portion of the eye
    c. a tough, fibrous protective membrane
    d. the nerve connecting the optic and cranial nerves

30. An injury to the eye should be treated with:

    a. direct pressure and bandaging of the injured eye
    b. avoiding pressure and bandaging of the injured eye
    c. direct pressure and bandaging of both eyes
    d. avoiding pressure and bandaging of both eyes

31. A chemical burn to the eye should be treated with irrigation for a minimum of:

    a. 5 minutes
    b. 10 minutes
    c. 15 minutes
    d. 20 minutes

32. The collection of bones that surround the eye is commonly called the:

    a. ocular bones
    b. orbit
    c. periocular bones
    d. acetabular bones

33. The pigmented or colored portion of the eye that regulates the diameter of the pupil is called the:

    a. retina
    b. iris
    c. cornea
    d. macula

34. Blockage of the outflow of aqueous humor can cause a buildup of pressure and causes a condition known as:

    a. retinitis
    b. glaucoma
    c. cataracts
    d. aqueous tension

35. The lacrimal glands are responsible for:

    a. secretion of vitreous humor
    b. secretion of tears
    c. secretion of aqueous humor
    d. drainage of aqueous humor

36. The best method for removing foreign bodies of the eye in the field is:

    a. with the use of suction cups
    b. irrigation
    c. with the use of a cotton-tipped applicator
    d. by rapid eyelid movement

37. An extruded eyeball should be managed by:

    a. replacing it in the eye socket
    b. covering it with a dry 4x4 and a patch
    c. covering it with a moist dressing and a cup
    d. irrigation during transport

38. The ear is composed of three sections called the:

    a. external, middle, and inner ears
    b. anterior, posterior, and cephalad ears
    c. middle, inner, and translumen ears
    d. middle, anterior and posterior ears

39. The malleus, incus and stapes are three:

    a. nerves in the ear
    b. glands in the ear
    c. ducts in the ear
    d. bones in the ear

40. The cochlea, a spirally wound tube, is part of the:

    a. anterior ear
    b. middle ear
    c. inner ear
    d. posterior ear

41. Sound waves, the physical vibrations of air, have __________ and __________ characteristics:

    a. amplitude, frequency
    b. duration, frequency
    c. capacitance and duration
    d. tympanic and harmonic

42. The middle ear communicates with the nasopharynx via the:

    a. semicircular canal
    b. cochlea
    c. eustachian tube
    d. vestibule

43. The inner ear contributes to control of:

    a. voice transmission
    b. heat exchange
    c. balance and position
    d. fluid excretion

44. Rupture of the eardrum due to changes in pressure is called:

    a. tympanic syndrome
    b. barotrauma
    c. the bends
    d. pneumotympanic rupture

45. The membrane that separates the external and middle ear that vibrates in response to sound waves is called the:

a. auricle
b. lacrimal membrane
c. tympanic membrane
d. eustachian membrane

46. Blood or clear fluid flowing from the ear should always be considered as a possible sign of:

a. skull fracture
b. eardrum rupture
c. cochlear injury
d. overhydration

47. The structure in the neck that contains the vocal cords is the:

a. esophagus
b. trachea
c. pharynx
d. larynx

48. Tearing or fractures of the airway may cause:

a. barotrauma
b. subcutaneous emphysema
c. air embolism
d. chronic lung disease

49. It is assumed that any patient who suffers blunt trauma to the neck has __________:

a. a fractured larynx
b. a partial airway obstruction
c. cervical spine injuries
d. a complete airway obstruction

50. When a neck vein is severed and no cervical injury is suspected you should:

a. apply a Teflon dressing and sit the patient upright
b. apply an airtight dressing and place the patient supine
c. apply a saline dressing and place the patient on their side
d. apply a multitrauma dressing and place the patient prone

Basic Bandage Application

Student's Name________________________ Date________

Performance Standard	Performed	Failed
Universal precautions (gloves, goggles)		
Apply dressing over wound		
Circle area and anchor bandage		
Begin circular attachment of bandage covering the previous layer by 50% each time		
Continue past the dressing and secure bandage in place		
Elevate the affected part		
Check distal pulse		

Comments____

____

____

____

Instructor ______________ Circle one: Pass Fail

Chapter 9

Skill Performance Sheet

Stabilizing an Impaled Object

Student's Name______________________________ Date__________

Performance Standard	Performed	Failed
Universal precautions (gloves, goggles)		
EMT #1 stabilizes object with hand		
Place stacked multitrauma dressing on both sides of the object approximately halfway up		
Tape across the dressings in both directions to provide support		
Check to establish stability		
Reinforce as needed		

Comments____

____

____

____

Instructor ___________________ Circle one: Pass Fail

Chapter 10

MUSCULOSKELETAL INJURIES

Materials and Equipment for Lesson

1. Anatomy slides, overhead transparencies, drawings or flipcharts
2. Skeleton
3. Handouts
   - Anatomy and physiology
   - Musculoskeletal injuries
   - Performance sheets for splinting skills
4. Slide projector, overhead, flipchart and/or blackboard
5. Slides or overhead transparencies

Section 1

Anatomy and Physiology

Objectives
(Slide 10-1)

At the conclusion of the chapter the student will be able to:

1. **Write a list of the major bones of the body.**
2. **Define the following:**

Ligaments	**Tendons**
Cartilage	**Appendicular vs axial skeleton**

3. **List the 3 types of muscle and describe their functions.**
4. **Write a list of major muscles of the upper and lower extremities and their functions.**
5. **List 3 types of joints and explain their range of motion.**

Instructor Preparation

Reading preparation for the lesson:

EMT Prehospital Care, Chapter 10, pages 429-444

Optional reading:

Guyton, A.C.: Textbook of Medical Physiology. 8th Edition, W.B. Saunders. Philadelphia, PA 1990

Solomon, E.P., Phillips G.A.: Understanding Human Anatomy and Physiology. W.B. Saunders. Philadelphia, PA 1987

Suggested Learning Activities

Using a lecture format with the aid of slides, overhead transparencies or charts, provide an overview of anatomy and physiology of the musculoskeletal system.

Display different types of splints for students during lecture.

Use skeleton to show various bones and ranges of motion.

When possible, have students palpate structures or monitor activities.

Content

I. Introduction **(Slide 10-2)**
- A. Fractures and injuries to ligaments, tendons and muscles account for a large percentage of all injuries
- B. Motor vehicle accidents, falls, and sports-related injuries are common causes
- C. Bones are strong structures that give mobility and support to the body
- D. Significant force is needed to cause fractures and often results in injury to surrounding soft tissue
- E. Complications include injury to nerves, blood vessels and adjacent organs
- F. Knowledge of anatomy and physiology and the common mechanisms of injury is essential to assessment and treatment
- G. Often there are associated fractures to search for based upon identifying specific types of injury
- H. The EMT and paramedic should not be distracted by gross deformities and overlook more serious injuries

II. Anatomy and Physiology
- A. Skeletal system **(Slide 10-3)**
  - 1. The skeletal system provides protection and support
  - 2. Muscles are attached to permit movement
  - 3. Types and functions of bones vary greatly throughout the body, e.g., bones of middle ear vs femur
  - 4. Bones
    - a) 206 bones throughout the axial and appendicular skeleton
    - b) The axial skeleton: the skull, the spine and the ribs primarily provide protection to the vital organs and permit motion in the spine and chest
    - c) The appendicular skeleton consists of the upper and lower extremities, shoulder and pelvic girdle and provides erect position, mobility and protection of the pelvic organs
  - 5. Cartilage **(Slide 10-4)**
    - a) Cartilage is the softer precursor of bone
    - b) Present throughout the body
    - c) Cartilage persists at sites of bone growth, at the anterior margins of the ribs, and at articulations to provide a smooth, friction-free surface
    - d) Cartilage also exists in the ears, trachea and other airways and in the nose
  - 6. Ligaments
    - a) Connective bands that attach bone to bone
    - b) Maintain the stability of joints
    - c) May become stretched or torn [sprain]
  - 7. Tendons
    - a) Connect muscle to bone and pull or move bones as muscles contract
    - b) Can be overstretched or torn during violent injury

Content

8. Anatomy of bone **(Slide 10-5)**
   a) Bones must withstand the forces of weight bearing, gravity and muscular movement and also be lightweight
   b) There are two basic types of bone tissue: compact and spongy bone
   c) Compact bone is dense and provides the greatest strength
   d) Spongy bone is latticework structure for lightweight and good support against compression forces
   e) The shaft of a bone is known as the diaphysis
      (1) Diaphysis consists primarily of compact bone
   f) The end of the diaphysis is known as the metaphysis and is recently developed bone in growing children
   g) The end of a bone is the epiphysis
      (1) Epiphysis consists primarily of spongy bone covered by a thin layer of compact bone
      (2) The joint surface is covered by an articular cartilage to provide a friction-free cushion and interface
   h) The epiphysis and metaphysis are separated by a growth plate of cartilage
   i) Types of bones **(Slide 10-6)**
      (1) Long bones consist of spongy ends and compact shaft; e.g., the femur, tibia, fibula, humerus, metacarpals, etc.
      (2) Short bones are primarily spongy bone, i.e., carpal bones, tarsal bones, etc.
      (3) Flat bones, i.e., ribs and sternum, consist of spongy bone between two layers of compact bone
      (4) Irregular bones, i.e., scapula, vertebrae, spongy bone with compact bone around it, amount of spongy vs compact bone varies
   j) Marrow is contained within the shafts of long bones and the meshwork of spongy bone
      (1) Red marrow is primarily in spongy bone; is responsible for red blood cell production
      (2) Yellow marrow is contained within the shaft of long bones; consists of fat and scattered blood cells
   k) Periosteum is a fibrous membrane that covers bone except at the articular surfaces
      (1) It provides an attachment point for muscles and tendons
      (2) Contains blood vessels to provide nutrition for bone
      (3) Some bones have a nutrient artery, which provides the major blood supply
9. Bone growth **(Slide 10-7)**
   a) Skeleton of a fetus is initially cartilage; becomes ossified at about 7 weeks [sites of cartilage change to bone]
   b) Long bones contain epiphyseal plates, which are growth centers
      (1) These plates are a weak point in children and are often the site of injury
      (2) Injuries to epiphyseal plates may affect future growth

Content

10. Bone remodeling
    a) There are two different types of bone cells: one lays down new bone while the other breaks down existing bone for repair and remodeling
    b) During growth, there is more bone formation than breakdown
    c) During middle age, growth and breakdown are relatively evenly matched
    d) During old age, breakdown exceeds remodeling, resulting in weaker bones [osteoporosis]
11. Bone healing
    a) Following a fracture, bleeding occurs at the fracture site and cells die
    b) Cells capable of laying down new bone accumulate
    c) These cells break down and reabsorb old bone for remodeling
    d) Healing is influenced by age, condition of the patient, alignment, and complications, i.e., infections and impaired blood supply
    e) Early proper handling is important to healing and reducing soft tissue damage [immobilization]

B. Muscular system **(Slide 10-8)**
1. Muscles are tissues capable of contraction and relaxation
2. Contraction results in movement
3. There are three types of muscle
    a) Voluntary muscle results in movement of the skeleton and is under conscious control
        (1) Attached to muscles via tendons to allow movement of one bone to another
    b) Smooth muscle controls autonomic muscles, i.e., peristalsis, blood vessels and airways
        (1) Involuntary or smooth muscle is not under conscious control
    c) Cardiac muscle is similar in structure to skeletal or voluntary muscle and functions automatically via its own pacemaker to pump blood
        (1) Cardiac muscle is not under conscious control and is directed by the autonomic nervous system

C. Specific bones, muscles, joints
1. Upper extremities **(Slide 10-9)**
    a) Shoulder and humerus
        (1) Shoulder is formed by three bones, the humerus, scapula and clavicle
        (2) The scapula is an irregular, shaped bone, which lies between the second and seventh ribs posteriorly on the thorax
            (a) The acromion process can be felt at the lateral edge of the shoulder
            (b) The glenoid fossa articulates with the humerus
            (c) The coracoid process lies on the lateral side where muscles attach

Content

(d) The triangular body of the scapula lies over the posterior ribs and is covered by thick muscles
(e) The medial border is readily seen and palpated
(3) The clavicle is located on the anterior-superior portion of the thorax and can be palpated
(a) Serves as an attachment of the upper extremity to the axial skeleton
(b) The clavicle is fractured from direct force or when forces are transmitted from the arm or shoulder
(4) The humerus is a long bone in the upper arm extending from the glenoid fossa of the scapula to the olecranon fossa of the elbow **(Slide 10-10)**
(a) Forms a ball-and-socket joint at the shoulder and permits a wide range of motion
(b) Shaft widens near the elbow and shoulder to form articulations
(c) The medial and lateral epicondyles are palpable at the elbow and are attachments for muscles

(5) Major muscles of the shoulder include deltoid, pectoralis major, trapezius and latissimus dorsi
(a) Deltoid inserts in medial aspect of humerus and abducts shoulder and aids in flexion and extension of arm
(b) Pectoralis major adducts and rotates arm medially
(c) Trapezius raises the clavicle
(d) Latissimus dorsi adducts, extends and rotates arm medially
b) Elbow and forearm **(Slide 10-11)**
(1) Elbow is made up of articulation of lower humerus and proximal ends of radius and ulna
(2) Proximal end consists of olecranon, which articulates with humerus
(3) Radius is parallel to the ulna on the lateral aspect of the arm
(4) They are joined by ligaments
(5) The elbow is a hinge joint
(6) Major muscles that operate the forearm are the triceps and the biceps (both located on the upper arm)
(7) Medial rotation is referred to as pronation; lateral rotation is supination
c) Wrist and hand **(Slide 10-12)**
(1) Wrist is composed of eight small carpal bones
(2) Carpal bones articulate with radius and ulna, which allows flexion, extension, abduction, adduction and circumduction

Content

(3) Metacarpals consist of five long bones, which extend from the wrist to the fingers (phalanges)
(4) There are three phalanges in each finger except for the thumb, which contains two

2. Lower extremities
   a) Pelvis and femur **(Slide 10-13)**
      (1) Pelvis is a ringlike structure consisting of the sacrum and coccyx posteriorly and two innominate bones on either side, which meet anteriorly at the symphysis pubis
         (a) Innominate bones consist of three fused bones: the ilium, the ischium and the pubis
            i) These three bones form the acetabulum or hip socket joint
            ii) The ischial tuberosity bears weight in the sitting position
            iii) The pubis is comprised of a body and superior and inferior pubic rami
         (b) Pelvis protects internal organs and supports the weight of the body
      (2) The femur is the largest and strongest bone in the body **(Slide 10-14)**
         (a) The head of the femur articulates with the acetabulum to form the hip joint
         (b) The femoral neck extends about two inches and attaches to the shaft at the greater and lesser trochanters
         (c) The shaft of the femur widens distally at its posterior end where the medial and lateral condyles are easily palpable
   b) Knee and lower leg **(Slide 10-15)**
      (1) The tibia is the major weightbearing bone of the lower leg
         (a) It widens distally and proximally to form the ankle and knee joints
         (b) The tibia runs anteriorly and superficially and is easily palpable
         (c) Proximally, the medial and lateral condyles form an articular surface with femoral condyles
         (d) Strong ligaments hold joint together
      (2) The patella is a small flat bone contained within the tendon of the quadriceps muscle **(Slide 10-16)**
         (a) Has cartilage surface and articulates with femoral condyles
      (3) The knee joint is a hinge joint and permits some rotation
      (4) The fibula is a smaller long bone running parallel, lateral and posterior to the tibia
         (a) It articulates with tibia and is palpable just below the knee [posterior]
         (b) Not a weight-bearing bone; serves as a point for muscle attachment of ankle joint

Content

c) Ankle and foot **(Slide 10-17)**
(1) Bones of the foot include several tarsal bones, five metatarsals and fourteen phalanges
(2) The ankle is formed by articulation of the tibia, fibula and talus bones
(3) Talus bone rests upon calcaneus, or heel bone
(4) Ligaments attach to lateral and medial malleoli, which are palpable
(5) Primary movement is flexion and extension with other complex motion

d) Major muscles of the lower extremities **(Slide 10-18)**
(1) Gluteus maximus extends and rotates thigh laterally
(2) Hamstrings flex leg and extend and rotate thigh
(3) Tibialis anterior allows dorsiflexion of the foot
(4) Gastrocnemius plantar flexes the foot

Section 2

Musculoskeletal Injuries

Objectives
(Slide 10-19)

At the conclusion of the chapter the student will be able to:

1. **List four forces that cause musculoskeletal injury.**
2. **List four types of fractures and a related mechanism of injury for each.**
3. **List three common complications of fractures and dislocations.**
4. **Describe the assessment needed to identify nerve or blood vessel complications in the upper and lower extremities.**
5. **List the mechanisms of injury, types of fractures, associated injuries, and treatment for fractures and dislocations to the following bones and joints:**

Scapula	**Humerus**	**Ulna**	**Radius**
Shoulder	**Clavicle**	**Carpals**	**Phalanges**
Pelvis	**Hip**	**Femur**	**Patella**
Tibia	**Fibula**	**Tarsals**	

6. **List the steps of application for the following devices:**
   - **Rigid splint for the forearm**
   - **Sling and swathe**
   - **Elbow splint in angulated and straightened positions**
   - **Wrist and hand splint**
   - **Finger splint**
   - **Rigid splint for the lower extremity**
   - **Pillow splint**
   - **Sager traction splint**
   - **Hare traction splint**
   - **Air splint**

Instructor Preparation

Reading preparation for the lesson:

EMT Prehospital Care, Chapter 10, pages 445-485

Optional reading:

Prehospital Trauma Life Support Committee of The National Association of

EMTs: Pre-Hospital Trauma Life Support. 2nd Edition, Emergency Training. Akron, Ohio 1990

Suggested Learning Activities
Using a lecture format with the aid of slides, overhead transparencies, or charts, provide a presentation of musculoskeletal trauma. **Demonstrate splinting techniques and principles.** **Provide case histories that illustrate different types of muscular skeletal trauma.**

Content

III. Musculoskeletal System Injuries **(Slide 10-20)**
  A. Injuries to the musculoskeletal system include:
    1. Fractures
      a) Break in the continuity of bone
      b) Complete, incomplete, or hairline crack
    2. Dislocations
      a) Displacement of bones in a joint from their normal anatomic position
      b) Due to stretching or tearing of ligaments
      c) May be associated with fractures, sprains and strains
      d) Signs and symptoms similar to fractures
    3. Sprains
      a) Injuries to ligaments
      b) Resulting from stretching forces
    4. Strains
      a) Injuries to muscles or tendons
      b) Overstretching or violent contractions
      c) Severity
        (1) Minor--overstretching of some of the fibers
        (2) Major- complete disruption of ligament or tendon
  B. Mechanism of injury **(Slide 10-21)**
    1. Predicts the location and type of fracture
    2. First assessment of the trauma victim
    3. Forces may be direct or indirect
      a) a)Direct forces may cause fracture at point of impact
        (1) A car bumper striking the tibia
        (2) A gunshot wound shattering a bone
        (3) Falling person landing on feet and breaking heel bones
      b) Indirect forces result in injury at a location other than the point of impact
        (1) Fall on an outstretched hand with a dislocated shoulder
        (2) Twisting force, i.e., an ice skater catches blade while doing a spin and fractures tibia
    4. Pathologic fractures result when bone diseases have destroyed and weakened bone **(Slide 10-22)**
      a) Minimal stress may lead to fracture
      b) Bone cancer, congenital diseases, and osteoporosis are examples
      c) Ordinary activities, e.g., stepping off a curb, may result in fracture
    5. Stress fractures are fractures that result from overuse or continuous activity **(Slide 10-23)**
      a) Cumulative effect of repetitive stress, e.g., jogging
      b) Can occur in athletes, joggers, or military recruits usually in lower extremities

Content

C. Types of fractures **(Slide 10-24)**
1. Closed fracture
a) A simple fracture has no break in the skin over the fracture site
b) Fracture does not communicate with the external environment
2. Open or compound fracture
a) Communicates with the external environment because the skin above the site has been broken
b) Risk of infection increased and should be covered with a sterile dressing
c) Results from penetrating wounds, lacerations, crush injuries, sharp bone fragments
3. Other Classifications **(Slide 10-25)**
a) Transverse - fractures usually produced by a direct force applied perpendicular to a bone **(Slide 10-26)**
b) Spiral fractures - long, sharp, and pointed bone ends, and are produced by twisting forces **(Slide 10-27)**
c) Oblique - produced by a twisting force with an upward thrust, fractured ends at oblique angle **(Slide 10-28)**
d) Greenstick - fractures in long bones of children under the age of ten, bone remains intact **(Slide 10-29)**
e) Comminuted - multiple (always more than two) fragments and are caused by severe violence **(Slide 10-30)**
f) Impacted - forces that drive bone fragments firmly together, may have function of extremity **(Slide 10-31)**
g) Compression - Spongy bones collapse from transmitted forces, bones are driven together
h) Avulsion - Forceful contraction of muscle against resistance, tearing a fragment of bone **(Slide 10-32)**

D. Signs and symptoms of fractures **(Slide 10-33)**
1. Pain and tenderness
a) Most common symptom of a fracture
b) Point tenderness at the fracture site
c) Referred pain distal or proximal to injury
2. Deformity **(Slide 10-34)**
a) Angulation of long bones
b) Protuberance of the bone end against soft tissues
c) Overriding or separation of bone fragments by opposing muscles
3. Swelling and discoloration **(Slide 10-35)**
a) Fluid or blood loss at the site of injury
b) Early sign, or it may occur some time after injury
c) Compare extremities to differences
4. Loss of use
a) Pain on movement
b) Disruption of bones, ligaments, or tendons
c) Neurovascular compromise
5. Crepitus
a) Grating sensation or sound
b) Bone fragments rubbing against one another
c) Should not deliberately attempt to elicit

Content

6. Exposed bone **(Slide 10-36)**
    a) Bone ends protruding through the skin
    b) Obvious sign of an open fracture
    c) Increased risk of infection

E. Signs and symptoms of a dislocation **(Slide 10-37)**
1. Result from both direct and indirect violence
2. Some patients have recurrent dislocations due to previous injuries
3. Signs and symptoms of fractures may be present
4. Signs that are more specific or common for dislocation
    a) Loss of movement
    b) Deformity at a joint
    c) Joint locked in a deformed position
    d) Pain and swelling over the joint
    e) Signs of neurovascular compromise
5. Common sites **(Slide 10-38)**
    a) Shoulder
    b) Elbow
    c) Fingers
    d) Hip
    e) Knee
    f) Ankle

F. Signs and symptoms of sprains **(Slide 10-39)**
1. Pain
2. Swelling
3. Disability
4. Instability/dislocation of the joint
5. Most common site of sprain is the ankle joint

G. Complications of Fractures **(Slide 10-40)**
1. Bleeding
    a) Can be life-threatening especially if there are multiple fractures or open fractures
    b) Fractures of the pelvis and femur are particularly serious
    c) Signs of blood loss
        (1) Swelling
        (2) Discoloration
        (3) Signs of shock
2. Vascular injuries **(Slide 10-41)**
    a) Mechanisms of vascular injury
        (1) Vessels can be pinched or torn by bone
        (2) Penetrating injuries
        (3) Spasm
        (4) Compressed by soft tissue swelling
        (5) Occluded by thrombosis
    b) Common sites of vascular injury
        (1) Shoulder
        (2) Elbow
        (3) Knee
        (4) Foot

Content

c) Signs and symptoms **(Slide 10-42)**
(1) Distal pulses absent
(2) Skin color
(3) Temperature
(4) Capillary return
(5) Pain
(6) Numbness, tingling, prickling
(7) Sensory loss
(8) Paralysis distal to the injury
(9) Five P's: pain, pulselessness, pallor, paresthesias (numbness or tingling, prickling), and paralysis
d) Always check for vascular compromise before and after applying splinting
3. Peripheral nerve injury **(Slide 10-43)**
a) Mechanisms of nerve injury
(1) Range from contusion to complete disruption
(2) Torn bone ends can tear or pinch the nerve
(3) Displaced joints can stretch or compress a nerve
(4) Violent forces, e.g., gunshot wounds, can cause direct damage
b) Common sites of nerve injury **(Slide 10-44)**
(1) Clavicle
(2) Shoulder
(3) Humerus
(4) Elbow
(5) Wrist
(6) Hip and femur
(7) Knee
(8) Spinal cord
c) Signs and Symptoms of Nerve Injury **(Slide 10-45)**
(1) Numbness
(2) Pain
(3) Abnormal sensation
(4) Loss of motor ability.
4. Injuries to the viscera **(Slide 10-50)**
a) Fractured pelvis--bladder, urethra, rectum and lower intestine, and reproductive organs
b) Thoracic injuries--hemothorax, pneumothorax and rupture of the spleen and liver
5. Fat embolism **(Slide 10-51)**
a) Fat can enter the bloodstream and become lodged in pulmonary arteries
b) Fractures of the long bones and pelvis have been noted to cause fat embolism
c) Usually within one to three days following injury; can occur earlier

Content

H. History and physical assessment **(Slide 10-52)**
   1. Scene survey--determine mechanism of injury
   2. Primary survey
      a) Assume spine injuries during assessment and treatment
      b) Airway, breathing, circulation first
      c) Open chest wounds, shock take priority over fractures
      d) Do not become distracted by a grotesquely angulated fracture
   3. Secondary survey **(Slide 10-53)**
      a) Position of a passenger in a car
      b) Seat belts were worn?
      c) Speed at impact?
      d) Height of a fall?
      e) Position of the body at impact?
      f) History **(Slide 10-54)**
         (1) Events immediately before an accident
         (2) Did a patient trip and fall?
         (3) Did patient become dizzy, loose consciousness, and then fall?
      g) Head-to-toe survey **(Slide 10-55)**
         (1) Expose and inspect for abrasions, bruises, or deformities
         (2) Patterns of skin wounds
         (3) Examination of the bony pelvis **(Slide 10-56)**
            (a) Instability requires a break in two places
            (b) May be associated with significant blood loss
            (c) Compress the iliac crests posteriorly and medially **(Slides 10-57 and 10-58)**
            (d) Palpate symphysis pubis gently to check for tenderness **(Slide 10-59)**
         (4) Extremities **(Slide 10-60)**
            (a) Note open wounds, deformity, swelling, discoloration, other signs of fracture
            (b) Note tenderness, creptius, palpable deformity
            (c) Compare one extremity to other to note subtle differences in size
            (d) Be systematic, move from proximal to distal
            (e) Neurovascular assessment
               i) Distal pulses
               ii) Capillary return and color
               iii) Motor check of feet and hands
               iv) Sensory check of feet and hands **(Slide 10-61)**
               v) Hypovolemic shock can also cause pallor and weak or absent distal pulses

I. Management **(Slide 10-62)**
   1. Goals of management
      a) Reduce pain
      b) Prevent further injury by immobilization
         (1) Prevents motion of bone fragments or dislocated joints

Content

(2) Minimizes pain and further damage to surrounding soft tissues
(3) May reduce blood loss
c) Minimizing complications will speed healing
2. Principles of splinting **(Slide 10-63)**
a) Treat the patient as a whole, lifesaving measures come first
b) Assume a fracture until proven otherwise
c) Minimize movement of injured part
d) Pad splints
e) Splint fracture site and adjacent joints
f) Check and recheck neurovascular function
g) Straighten grossly angulated fractures to permit proper immobilization and transport
(1) With resistance or pain, splint in the position found
(2) May restore blood flow
(3) Never forcefully straighten a locked extremity
h) Cover open wounds
3. Types of splints **(Slides 10-64 and 10-65)**
a) Rigid
(1) Cardboard, wood, metal, or plastic, which should be well padded
(2) Come in lengths of a few inches for fingers to five feet for the lower extremities
b) Air splints
(1) Soft plastic splints, filled with air to provide circumferential support
(2) Various lengths and configurations for use on distal upper and lower extremity
(3) PASG can serve as an air splint for patients with lower extremity or pelvic fractures
(4) Air pressure must be reevaluated with changes in environmental temperature
c) Wire ladder
(1) Constructed of thin metal rods
(2) Can be shaped and molded to conform to a fractured extremity
(3) Should be well padded before application
d) Pillow
(1) Splint for an ankle or as an adjunct for dislocations
(2) Attached with safety pins, bandages, or cravats
e) Sling and swathe
(1) Used in the treatment of upper extremity injuries
(2) Bought commercially or improvised
f) Traction
(1) Consists of a metal frame and a pulley system to apply traction to the lower extremity
(a) Thomas' splint
i) Simple metal frame used in conjunction with bandage materials

Content

(b) Hare, Kippel, or Sager
i) Splints with preattached velcro fasteners and mechanical pulleys
(2) Used to immobilize fractures of femur, hip, or upper tibia and fibula
g) Improvised
(1) Blankets
(2) Magazines
(3) Cardboard
(4) Other materials that accomplish immobilization
(5) Device less important than the principles of treatment
4. Methods of splintings
a) Rigid splint to the humerus **(Slides 10-66 to 10-67)**
b) Rigid splint to forearm **(Slides 10-68 to 10-69)**
c) Splint to arm in straightened position **(Slides 10-70 to 10-72)**
d) Splint to elbow in angulated position **(Slides 10-73 to 10-75)**
e) Splint to wrist **(Slides 10-76 to 10-80)**
f) Finger splint **(Slide 10-81)**
g) Air splint to upper extremity **(Slides 10-82 to 10-84)**
h) Spine board immobilization **(Slide 10-85)**
i) Hare traction splint **(Slides 10-86 to 10-98)**
j) Other traction splints **(Slides 10-99 to 10-100)**
k) Sager traction splint **(Slides 10-101 to 10-108)**
l) Rigid splint to leg **(Slides 10-109 to 10-113)**
m) Pillow splint **(Slide 10-114)**

IV. Upper extremity injuries
A. Clavicle **(Slide 10-115)**
1. Mechanism of injury
a) Direct blow to the anterior upper chest or a fall on shoulder
b) Side hit in auto collision
c) Falls on the outstretched hand, force transmitted to clavicle
2. Types of fractures
a) Direct blows cause fractures along clavicle
b) Indirect forces--fracture at junction of middle and lateral thirds
c) Fracture to middle third often results in deformity
d) Fracture to lateral third of the bone is seldom displaced
e) Dislocated at sternum or the scapula
f) Dislocations of sternoclavicular joint are usually anterior and are palpable
g) Occasionally dislocated posteriorly at sternum, where it may compress vessels
3. Signs and symptoms
a) Pain in the shoulder and at fracture site
b) Arm held against chest with hand supporting elbow
c) Shoulder may drop and be rotated inward
d) Visible and palpable deformity

Content

4. Associated injuries
    a) Rib cage
    b) Underlying vessels (subclavian) and nerves
    c) Lungs and the pleura
5. Treatment
    a) Sling and swathe
    b) Position of comfort

B. Scapula **(Slide 10-116)**
1. Mechanisms of injury
    a) Requires violent blow to fracture
    b) Indicates great force sustained
    c) Raise concern about damage to thorax
2. Types of fractures
    a) Spine, body, or other processes
    b) May be associated with dislocations
3. Signs and symptoms
    a) May be some palpable irregularity, swelling, pain, and ecchymosis
    b) Patient may hold the arm against the chest (adduction) and resist abduction
4. Associated injuries
    a) Ribs, spine, and lungs
    b) Violent forces necessary to fracture
5. Treatment
    a) Sling and swathe
    b) Position of comfort

C. Dislocation of the acromioclavicular joint **(Slide 10-117)**
1. Acromion process is attached to lateral aspect of clavicle
2. Ligaments can be sprained resulting in dislocation
3. Mechanism of injury
    a) Direct forces striking downward on the lateral aspect of the shoulder
    b) Falls on the outstretched arm
4. Signs and symptoms
    a) Acromioclavicular joint pain aggravated by movement
    b) Visible or palpable deformity **(Slide 10-118)**
5. Treatment
    a) Sling and swathe
    b) Position of comfort

D. Dislocations of the shoulder **(Slide 10-119)**
1. Displacement of head of the humerus from glenoid
2. Mechanisms of injury
    a) Usually displaced anteriorly
    b) Fall with arm abducted and externally rotated
    c) Fall on outstretched hand
    d) Posterior dislocation results from forceful blow anteriorly

Content

3. Types of dislocations/fractures
    a) Humeral head anterior to scapula
    b) Posterior (5% of shoulder dislocations)
    c) Associated with fractures of proximal humerus
4. Signs and symptoms
    a) Loss of rounded contour of the shoulder **(Slide 10-120)**
    b) Humerus may be palpable anteriorly and medially
    c) Patient resists adduction and internal rotation
    d) Posterior dislocation--arm stiffly at side with internal rotation
5. Associated injuries
    a) Fractures to the shoulders
    b) Nerve and vessel injury
6. Treatment
    a) Sling and swathe
    b) Pillow or blanket between the chest and arm for additional support
    c) Position of comfort

E. Proximal humerus **(Slide 10-121)**
1. Mechanism of injury
    a) Direct violence to lateral shoulder
    b) Fall on outstretched arm with the elbow extended **(Slide 10-122)**
    c) Twisting forces
2. Types of fractures
    a) Displaced or impacted
    b) Impacted fractures may permit motion and use
3. Signs and symptoms
    a) Obvious deformity
    b) Impacted fractures present with less pain, ecchymosis and ability to use the arm
    c) Ecchymosis may gravitate downward after a day or two **(Slide 10-123)**
4. Associated injuries
    a) Nerves of the upper arm
    b) Bleeding
5. Treatment
    a) Sling and swathe
    b) Supine position, can be bound to the side with swathes

F. Shaft of the humerus **(Slide 10-124)**
1. Mechanism of injury
    a) Direct blows
    b) Indirect twisting forces
    c) Fall on the elbow or outstretched hand
    d) Common site for pathologic fractures **(Slide 10-125)**
2. Types of fractures
    a) Same as other long bone fractures
    b) Deformities caused by opposing muscles

Content

3. Signs and symptoms
    a) Obvious deformity possible
    b) Angulation or shortening
4. Associated injuries
    a) Radial nerve causing wrist drop
    b) Inability to dorsiflex the wrist and hand
    c) May be obvious on neurovascular evaluation
5. Treatment
    a) 9-inch padded splint to the humerus
    b) Sling and swathe
    c) Supine position, bound to the side with swathes

G. Distal humerus **(Slide 10-126)**
1. Mechanism of injury
    a) Commonly seen in children and older adults
    b) Direct blows over the olecranon
    c) Fall on outstretched arm in flexion
    d) Twisting forces generated on an extended arm
2. Types of fractures
    a) Severe displacement can result in open fractures
    b) Associated with elbow dislocations
3. Signs and symptoms
    a) Deformity may be obvious with shortening
    b) Ecchymosis and swelling from bleeding
4. Associated injuries
    a) Nerve and vascular injury
    b) Volkmann's ischemic contracture
    c) Progressive and increasing pain due to ischemia
    d) Fingers and wrist flexed
    e) Passive extension of the fingers is painful
    f) Other signs of vascular compromise
5. Treatment
    a) If pulse is present splinting in the position found
    b) Rigid armboard with a sling and swathe
    c) If no distal pulse, attempt to straighten
    d) Distal pulse should be rechecked after splinting

H. Elbow **(Slide 10-127)**
1. Mechanism of Injury
    a) Direct blows can fracture the elbow
    b) Fall on the outstretched hand with elbow flexed
    c) Hyperextension of the elbow joint and falls cause dislocations
2. Types of Fractures/Dislocations
    a) Dislocations usually posteriorly displaced
    b) Associated with fractures
    c) Children between one and four years are susceptible to slippage of the radial head
        (1) Ligaments stretched after sudden traction on an outstretched arm
        (2) Nursemaid's elbow

Content

3. Signs and Symptoms
    a) Deformity with posterior protrusion **(Slide 10-128)**
    b) Apparent shortening of the forearm
    c) Pain, swelling and inability to move the joint
4. Associated Injuries
    a) Dislocations of elbow
    b) Nerve and vascular damage
    c) Volkmann's contracture
5. Treatment
    a) If pulse present, splint in the position found
    b) Bridged splint from humerus to forearm
    c) Sling applied around wrist to support arm
    d) Signs of vascular compromise, attempt to restore circulation by gentle straightening

I. Forearm -- radius and ulna **(Slide 10-129)**
1. Mechanism of Injury
    a) Direct blows when arm assumes defensive posture
    b) Fall on the outstretched hand **(Slide 10-130)**
    c) Site of fracture depends on position of arm during fall
2. Types of Fractures
    a) Displacement fracture from force of the trauma
    b) Deformity from opposing muscles
3. Signs and Symptoms
    a) Deformity obvious on inspection
    b) Other signs of fracture
4. Associated injuries
    a) Displaced fractures associated with nerve damage
    b) Dislocation of elbow
5. Treatment
    a) Armboard extending from the hand to the elbow
    b) Sling and swathe
    c) Long armboard or air splint can be used to immobilize the forearm in the extended position

J. Wrist **(Slide 10-131)**
1. Mechanism of injury
    a) Fall on the hand
    b) Position of the hand will determine fracture
    c) Punches with a flexed fist
2. Types of fractures
    a) Colles's fracture **(Slide 10-132)**
        (1) Distal radius
        (2) Dorsal angulation
    b) Displaced anteriorly
        (1) Less common
        (2) Fall on hand with the wrist flexed
    c) Either occurs with or without fracture of distal ulna
    d) Nondisplaced fractures also occur

Content

3. Signs and symptoms
    a) Pain and tenderness
    b) Colles's fractures have a "dinner fork" deformity
4. Associated injuries
    a) Nerve injuries
    b) Affecting sensation and movement
5. Treatment
    a) Rigid splint or an air splint
    b) Bulky dressing in the hand
    c) Elevated and supported with a sling

K. Hands and fingers **(Slide 10-133)**
1. Mechanism of injury
    a) Direct blows
    b) Crushing injuries in the home and the work place
    c) Closing doors or industrial presses
    d) Punching causes head of metacarpal or boxer's fracture
    e) Jamming of fingers as ball strikes the tips of extended fingers
2. Types of fractures
    a) Shaft fractures can result in deformity
    b) Dislocation causes obvious deformity with locking in a deformed position
3. Signs and symptoms
    a) Pain, swelling, loss of motion
    b) Angulation of the fingers
4. Associated injuries
    a) Nerves, tendons and vessels
    b) Early care is important to minimize complications
5. Treatment
    a) Hand
        (1) Splinted in the position of function
        (2) Board splint
    b) Fingers
        (1) Padded tongue blade
        (2) Commercial finger splints
        (3) Taped to next finger with padding between the fingers

V. Lower extremity fractures

A. Pelvis **(Slide 10-134)**
1. Mechanism of injury
    a) Direct compression forces
        (1) Side to side
        (2) Anterior-posterior
        (3) Inferior straddle injuries
    b) Indirectly by forces transmitted from the femur
    c) Usually indicates major violence
2. Types of fractures
    a) Fractures anywhere along pelvic ring **(Slide 10-135)**
    b) Two or more fractures will result in instability

Content

c) Fractures of the pubic bone
d) Fractures of the acetabulum from femoral head
3. Signs and symptoms
a) Pain in the pelvis
b) Violent mechanism of injury
c) Bruising or deformity
d) Tenderness, deformity, crepitus, or instability
e) Gently compress the iliac crests medially and posteriorly
f) Gently press the pubic bone
4. Associated injuries
a) Because of violent forces, multiple trauma is commonly associated
b) Hypovolemic shock due to blood loss
(1) Half the patients who suffer open fractures die from bleeding or infection
(2) Each fracture may cause approximately 500 ml blood loss
c) Death rate exceeds 10%
d) Rupture to the internal viscera
5. Treatment
a) Immobilization on a long spine board
b) PASG with signs of shock

B. Hip joint dislocations **(Slide 10-136)**
1. Mechanism of injury and types of fractures
a) Posterior dislocations
(1) Most common, usually resulting from dashboard injuries
(2) More apt to result when the hip is flexed, adducted and internally rotated
(3) Femoral head slips posteriorly out of the acetabulum
(4) Thigh can be locked in an abnormal position
b) Central dislocation
(1) Fall may force the head of the femur directly through acetabulum
(2) Lateral force from side hit in car
(3) Femoral head may protrude into the pelvis
(4) May be stable appearance to leg
c) Anterior dislocation
(1) Much less common
(2) Occurs when the thigh is abducted, flexed, and externally rotated
(3) Force is applied to the back of the thigh as in a fall
(4) Femoral head is then forced forward out of the socket
(5) Joint locks in an abnormal position
2. Signs and symptoms **(Slide 10-137)**
a) Locking of the hip joint in an abnormal position
(1) Posterior--thigh and knee are flexed and internally rotated
(2) Anterior--hip is flexed with the thigh widely abducted and externally rotated
(3) Central--shortening of the leg and limitation of motion

Content

3. Associated injuries
    a) Associated knee injuries
    b) Nerve injuries
        (1) Cause footdrop (inability to dorsiflex the foot)
        (2) Sensory deficits of the foot
4. Treatment
    a) Limb should be supported in the position found with rolled blankets
    b) When possible, attach one leg to the other
    c) Secure to the long backboard

C. Hip fracture **(Slide 10-138)**

1. Mechanism of injury
    a) Common in the elderly
    b) Usually occurs after falls
    c) Violent force is required to cause fractures in younger people
2. Types of fractures **(Slide 10-139)**
    a) Femoral head and neck
    b) Intertrochanteric
3. Signs and symptoms
    a) External rotation and shortening of the leg
    b) Deformities do not always occur
    c) Pain or tenderness may be only sign
4. Treatment options
    a) Traction splint
    b) Tie the legs together after placing blankets or pillows between the legs
    c) PASG when there are signs of hypovolemia

D. Femur **(Slide 10-140)**

1. Mechanism of injury
    a) High-impact motor vehicle accidents
    b) Falls from heights
    c) Gunshot wounds
    d) May occur in younger population
    e) Elderly with osteoporosis fracture distal femur after a fall on a flexed knee
2. Types of fractures
    a) Femoral shaft
        (1) Area below the lesser trochanter to the junction of middle and lower thirds
        (2) Can be angulated
    b) Distal femur
        (1) May involve the knee joint
        (2) Risk of injury to the femoral or popliteal artery and vein
3. Signs and symptoms **(Slide 10-141)**
    a) Marked swelling and/or deformity
    b) Angulated or rotated
    c) Evidence of open fractures

Content

4. Associated injuries
    a) Blood loss can be significant
    b) May impair circulation of the foot
    c) Fat embolism (pulmonary)
        (1) Usually occurs after one to three days
        (2) May be a cause of unexplained dyspnea
    d) May also be significant trauma to other body organs and fractures in hip and knee
5. Treatment
    a) Traction splint
    b) Angulated fractures should be gently straightened
    c) PASG for patients in shock

E. Patella **(Slide 10-142)**
1. Mechanism of injury
    a) Direct blows, dashboard of a car
    b) Violent contraction of the quadriceps muscle
    c) Dislocations can occur following blows to the edge of the patella
2. Types of fractures
    a) Direct blows
    b) Nondisplaced fractures
    c) Dislocation laterally
3. Signs and symptoms
    a) Fracture fragments might be palpable
    b) Swelling and bruising
    c) Dislocated patella is palpable lateral from its normal position
    d) History of chronic dislocations
4. Associated injuries
    a) Associated fractures of joint
    b) Hip dislocations
    c) Femur fractures
5. Treatment
    a) Splint the knee in extension
    b) If unable to straighten, splint in position found

F. Knee joint **(Slide 10-143)**
1. Mechanism of injury
    a) Hyperextension injuries **(Slide 10-144)**
    b) Rotation injuries about a planted foot
    c) Direct trauma from a car bumper
2. Types of injuries
    a) Overstretching of the ligaments
    b) Complete disruption of ligaments
    c) Associated fractures
3. Signs and symptoms
    a) Instability or abnormal position of the knee
    b) Limitation of movement
    c) Laxity or abnormal movement
    d) Pain and swelling
    e) Patient may have heard a pop

Content

4. Treatment
    a) Gently straighten
    b) Rigid splint

G. Dislocations of the knee **(Slide 10-145)**

1. Mechanism and types of injury
    a) Extended beyond normal range of motion
    b) Tearing of the ligaments
    c) Complete dislocation of the knee
    d) Dislocated in any direction
2. Signs and Symptoms
    a) Grotesque deformity
    b) Associated nerve and vascular damage
3. Associated Injuries
    a) Injuries to the vessels (particularly the popliteal artery)
    b) Nerve injury
4. Treatment
    a) Gently straighten by applying manual traction
    b) Immobilized with a traction splint <u>without traction</u>
    c) Rigid splint or long-leg air splint
    d) Reassess distal neurovascular function

H. Tibia and fibula **(Slide 10-146)**

1. Mechanism of injury
    a) Direct forces, i.e., pedestrian struck by a car bumper **(Slide 10-147)**
    b) Twisting forces
    c) Fatigue fractures
2. Types of fractures
    a) Transverse, oblique
    b) With greater forces, comminuted and angulated
    c) Open fractures are relatively common
3. Signs and symptoms
    a) Tibia (superficial) lends itself to examination
    b) Small deformities may be palpated
4. Associated injuries
    a) Compromised distal circulation
    b) Compartment syndrome with pain and signs of poor distal circulation
5. Treatment
    a) Long-leg rigid splints
    b) Full-leg air splints
    c) PASG for signs of hypovolemic shock

I. Ankle **(Slide 10-148)**

1. Mechanism of injury
    a) Rotational injuries
    b) Difficult to differentiate sprains and fractures
2. Types of fractures
    a) Distal fibula and tibia usually occur from torsional forces
    b) Sprains on the lateral and medial sides of the ankle
    c) Sprains result in pain, swelling and possible instability

Content

3. Signs and symptoms **(Slide 10-149)**
    a) Pain and swelling are common
    b) Severe injuries present with grotesque deformity
4. Associated injuries
    a) Dislocations
    b) Neurovascular compromise
5. Treatment
    a) Gently straighten deformities
    b) Pillow splint, air splint or rigid splint

J. Foot

1. Mechanism of injury and types of fractures
    a) Falls on the heel can cause fractures of the calcaneus **(Slide 10-150)**
    b) Twisting injuries can fracture the other bones. Dropping a heavy object onto the foot is common
2. Signs and symptoms
    a) Bones are palpable
    b) Palpate calcaneus in a patient who has fallen and landed on the feet
3. Associated injuries
    a) Calcaneus fractures are associated with injuries to vertebrae
    b) Other bones of the lower extremities
    c) Wrist fracture
4. Treatment
    a) Air splint or pillow splint
    b) Rigid splints applied posteriorly
    c) Isolated fractures of toes can be taped to the neighboring toe

Chapter 10

MUSCULOSKELETAL INJURIES

Examination

1. The appendicular skeleton consists of the:

   a. skull, spine, ribs, sternum
   b. pelvis, spine, skull, lower extremities
   c. upper extremities, lower extremities, skull, chest
   d. upper extremities, lower extremities, shoulder, pelvis

Match the term in column B with the description in column A.

Column A		Column B	
2.	a softer precursor of bone that is present throughout the body and persists at sites of bone growth and at joints to provide a smooth, friction-free surface	a.	ligaments
3.	connective bands of tissue that attach bone to bone and maintain the stability of joints	b.	tendons
4.	thin bands of tissue that attach muscle to bone and initiate movement of joints	c.	cartilage
5.	the injury present when tendons are overstretched or torn following trauma or forceful muscular contraction	d.	sprains
6.	the injury present when ligaments are torn or stretched resulting in instability of the joint	e.	strains

Match the bones in column B to the appropriate type of bone in column A.

Column A		Column B	
7.	short bone	a.	tibia
8.	irregular bone	b.	scapula
9.	long bone	c.	carpal bone
10.	flat bone	d.	sternum

11. The epiphyseal plate is the:

    a. fibrous membrane that covers bone except at the articular surfaces
    b. portion of bone responsible for the production of red blood cells
    c. site of active bone growth for the long bones
    d. relatively strong point in the young child's bone

12. The marrow of the bone is the:

    a. fibrous membrane that covers bone except at the articular surfaces
    b. portion of bone responsible for the production of red blood cells
    c. site of active bone growth for the long bones
    d. relatively strong point in the young child's bone

13. The periosteum is the:

    a. fibrous membrane that covers bone except at the articular surfaces
    b. portion of bone responsible for the production of red blood cells
    c. site of active bone growth for the long bones
    d. relatively strong point in the young child's bone

Match the structures or location of muscles in column B to the appropriate type of muscle in column A.

Column A		Column B	
14.	smooth muscle	a.	digestive system
15.	cardiac muscle	b.	triceps
16.	skeletal muscle	c.	heart

Match the name of the bone in column B to the appropriate location in the body in column A.

Column A		Column B	
17.	upper arm	a.	femur
18.	lower arm	b.	fibula
19.	thorax	c.	humerus
20.	pelvis	d.	metatarsals
21.	upper leg	e.	ulna
22.	lower leg	f.	metacarpals
23.	hand	g.	sacrum
24.	foot	h.	sternum

25. The hip is an example of a __________ joint.

    a. hinged
    b. ball-and-socket
    c. fused
    d. gliding

26. Displacement of bones in a joint from their normal anatomical position is called a:

    a. compression injury
    b. dislocation
    c. sprain
    d. strain

27. During old age there may be more bone breakdown than formation, resulting in weaker bones. This process is called:

    a. a stress fracture
    b. osteoporosis
    c. bone deficiency syndrome
    d. bone remodeling

Match the description in column B with the type of fracture in column A.

Column A	Column B
28. compression	a. produced by a twisting force
29. oblique	b. fracture associated with no break in the skin
30. transverse	c. fragment of bone due to a forceful muscle contraction
31. avulsion	d. result when spongy bones collapse from transmitted forces that drive bones together
32. open	e. multiple fragments of bone at the fracture site
33. impacted	f. fracture associated with a break in the skin
34. greenstick	g. produced by a twisting force with an upward thrust
35. comminuted	h. fracture perpendicular to bone produced by direct force
36. spiral	i. incomplete fracture common in children
37. closed	j. fracture resulting in bone driven into bone

38. The most common symptom of a fracture is:

    a. deformity
    b. discoloration
    c. crepitus
    d. pain

39. A grating sensation or sound indication of bone fragments rubbing against one another is called:

    a. friction rub
    b. Homan's sign
    c. rhonchi
    d. crepitus

40. All of the following may indicate vascular or nerve injury in a fractured extremity:

    a. paralysis, pallor, and pain
    b. purple skin, paresthesia, and paralysis
    c. palpitations, pain, and pallor
    d. palpitations, paresthesia, and pallor

Match the type of force in column B to the appropriate mechanism of injury in column A (one item in column B can be used twice).

Column A	Column B
41. a gunshot wound shattering a bone	a. twisting force
42. a skater fracturing the tibia after the blade is trapped in a ridge in the ice	b. indirect force
43. a cervical spine fracture after falling and landing on the heels	c. direct force
44. a car bumper stikes the tibia	

45. Of the following, absence of capillary refill in a single extremity is most suggestive of:

    a. hypovolemic shock and vasoconstriction
    b. vascular compromise due to a fracture or dislocation
    c. spinal shock causing vasoconstriction to one side of the body
    d. cardiac tamponade causing poor cardiac output

46. A primary rule of fracture management is to splint the fracture site and the:

    a. surrounding tissues
    b. distal extremity
    c. adjacent joints
    d. proximal extremity

Match the average amount of blood loss due to a closed fracture in column B with the fracture site in column A.

Column A		Column B	
47.	radius and ulna	a.	1000 ml
48.	humerus	b.	500 ml
49.	pelvis	c.	150-250 ml
50.	femur	d.	1500-3000 ml
51.	tibia and fibula	e.	250 ml

Match the type of splint in column B with the description in column A.

Column A		Column B
52.	made of padded cardboard, wood, metal, or plastic	a. traction splint
		b. pillow splint
53.	environmental temperature can impair function	c. rigid splint
54.	can be shaped and molded to conform to an extremity	d. sling and swathe
		e. wire ladder splint
55.	best ankle splint	f. air splint
56.	made from triangular bandages	
57.	best splint for femur fracture	

Match the splinting method in column B with the injury in column A.

Column A		Column B
58.	fractured scapula	a. rigid three foot and five foot splint
59.	fractured wrist	b. sling and swathe
60.	fractured tibia	c. flexible aluminum splint
61.	fractured finger	
62.	fractured pelvis	d. rigid nine inch splint
		e. long spine board

63. When applying the traction splint the splint is adjusted so that the end of the splint is approximately:

   a. even with the length of the injured leg
   b. even with the length of the uninjured leg
   c. 6 inches below the patient's foot
   d. 12 inches below the patient's foot

64. A patient presents with a closed fracture to the medial tibia-fibula. The fracture site is grossly angulated. You should:

   a. gently straighten the leg and then splint
   b. splint the leg in the position you find it
   c. straighten the leg even if resistance is encountered
   d. apply a Hare traction splint to properly protect the leg from further injury

65. Which of the following fractures (in and of itself) is highly suggestive of a severe mechanism of injury and a likelihood of underlying chest trauma?

   a. clavicle
   b. humerus
   c. scapula
   d. shoulder

66. A fall with the arm adducted to the side, or a force striking downward on the lateral aspect of the shoulder may result in a dislocation to the:

   a. elbow
   b. shoulder
   c. acromioclavicular joint
   d. hand

67. Fractures of the wrist that have a classic "dinner fork" deformity are called ___________ fractures.

   a. Volkmann's
   b. Homan's
   c. Colles'
   d. Brown's

68. When splinting the hand it is important to place the hand in the position of:

   a. extension
   b. rotation
   c. function
   d. articulation

69. Instability of the pelvis suggests a minimum of ___ fractures of the pelvic ring.

    a. two
    b. three
    c. four
    d. five

70. The stability of the pelvis is evaluated by gentle compression of the iliac bones:

    a. medially and anteriorly
    b. anteriorly and laterally
    c. medially and posteriorly
    d. superiorly and posteriorly

Match the mechanism of injury in column B with the type of hip dislocation in column A.

Column A	Column B
71. anterior	a. car dashboard against knee
72. posterior	b. fall onto the side of the hip
73. central	c. thigh is abducted, flexed, and externally rotated and a force is applied to the back of the thigh

74. A 75-year-old male complains of pain to the left hip after a fall. He is able to stand and bear weight with pain. You suspect:

    a. an anterior dislocation of the hip
    b. a central dislocation of the hip
    c. a posterior dislocation of the hip
    d. a fracture of the hip

75. The classic presentation resulting from a hip fracture is:

    a. internal rotation and shortening
    b. internal rotation and thigh flexion
    c. external rotation and shortening
    d. external rotation and thigh flexion

Skill Performance Sheet

Applying a Sling and Swathe

Student's Name_______________________ Date_________

Performance Standard	**Performed**	**Failed**
Supports extremity during procedure		
Exposes and examines extremity		
Check distal pulse and function		
Places sling with long end over opposite shoulder and apex toward injured side		
Ties sling at side of neck to avoid pressure		
Secures end of sling with knot or twist		
Attaches swathes		
Check distal pulse and function		
Leaves fingernails exposed		

Comments____

____

____

____

Instructor _______________ Circle one: Pass Fail

Skill Performance Sheet

Rigid Splint for Humerus Fracture

Student's Name______________________________ Date__________

Performance Standard	**Performed**	**Failed**
Check distal pulse		
Apply 9" splint to medial arm		
Apply sling		
Attach swathe		
Check distal pulse and function		
Leave fingernails exposed		

Comments____

____

____

____

Instructor ___________________ Circle one: Pass Fail

Chapter 10

Skill Performance Sheet

Splint Arm in the Straightened Position

Student's Name________________________ Date________

Performance Standard	Performed	Failed
Maintain immobilization distal and proximal to injury		
Check distal pulse		
Place splints medial and lateral		
Attach splints with cravats or bandage		
Attach arm to body with cravats		
Check distal pulse and function		

Comments____

____

____

____

Instructor ______________ Circle one: Pass Fail

Skill Performance Sheet

Applying Splint to Elbow in Angulated Position

Student's Name__________________________ Date_________

Performance Standard	**Performed**	**Failed**
Check distal pulse		
Bridge splint from upper arm to forearm		
Attach with cravats or bandage		
Place sling without direct pressure on elbow		
Check distal pulse and function		

Comments____

____

____

____

Instructor ________________ Circle one: Pass Fail

Chapter 10

Skill Performance Sheet

Applying Splint to Wrist

Student's Name________________________________ Date__________

Performance Standard	Performed	Failed
Check capillary refill		
Maintain distal and proximal immobilization and position splint medially		
Place hand in position of function with rolled bandage or gauze		
Attach splint with cravats or bandage		
Apply sling and swathe (optional) and elevate hand		
Check distal circulation and function		

Comments____

____

____

____

Instructor ____________________ Circle one: Pass Fail

Skill Performance Sheet

Applying Finger Splint

Student's Name________________________ Date________

Performance Standard	**Performed**	**Failed**
Check capillary refill		
Position finger splint or tongue blade from fingertip to heel of hand		
Tape splint in place		
Apply sling and elevate hand		
Check distal circulation and function		

Comments____

____

____

____

Instructor ________________ Circle one: Pass Fail

Chapter 10

Skill Performance Sheet

Applying an Air Splint

Student's Name______________________________ Date__________

Performance Standard	**Performed**	**Failed**
Check distal pulse		
EMT #1 maintains distal and proximal immobilization		
EMT #2 wraps splint on his/her arm		
Splint is slid onto patient's arm		
Splint is inflated		
Check for correct pressure by pressing small dent in splint		
Check distal pulse and function		

Comments____

____

____

____

Instructor ____________________ Circle one: Pass Fail

Skill Performance Sheet

Applying a Hare Traction Splint

Student's Name______________________________ Date__________

Performance Standard	Performed	Failed
EMT #1 checks distal pulse while EMT #2 maintains immobilization at the knee		
Cuts pants away		
Inspects injured area		
Attaches ankle hitch and maintains traction with ankle hitch		
Measures and adjusts length of splint		
Places splint with ischial bar at base of buttocks		
Applies traction with crank until patient feels comfort or length of injured leg matches good leg		
Attaches straps above and below knee		
Checks distal pulse and function		

Comments____

____

____

____

Instructor ___________________ Circle one: Pass Fail

Skill Performance Sheet

Applying a Sager Traction Splint

Student's Name____________________________ Date__________

Performance Standard	**Performed**	**Failed**
Check distal pulse		
EMT #1 maintains immobilization at knee		
Positions splint and attaches ischial strap		
Attaches the ankle hitch		
Applies traction with ankle hitch by pulling bar		
Applies supports over upper and lower leg		
Checks distal pulse and function		

Comments____

____

____

____

Instructor __________________ Circle one: Pass Fail

Skill Performance Sheet

Applying a Rigid Leg Splint

Student's Name____________________________ Date_________

Performance Standard	**Performed**	**Failed**
EMT #1 maintains immobilization		
EMT #2 cuts away pants and checks a distal pulse		
Aligns splints on medial and lateral sides of the legs		
Attaches splints with cravats or bandages		
Elevates the leg		
Check distal pulse and function		

Comments____

____

____

____

Instructor __________________ Circle one: Pass Fail

Chapter 10

Skill Performance Sheet

Applying a Pillow Splint to an Ankle

Student's Name____________________________ Date_________

Performance Standard	**Performed**	**Failed**
Check distal pulse		
Wraps pillow around heel and ankle		
Attaches with cravats or bandages		
Check distal circulation and function		

Comments____

____

____

____

Instructor __________________ Circle one: Pass Fail

Chapter 11

ENVIRONMENTAL INJURIES

Materials and Equipment for Lesson

1. Anatomy slides, overhead transparencies, drawings or flipcharts
2. Handouts
   - Heat and cold emergencies
   - Burn emergencies
   - Radiation emergencies
   - Diving emergencies
   - Hazmat emergencies
3. Slide projector, overhead projector, flipchart and/or blackboard

Section 1

Heat and Cold Emergencies

Objectives
(Slide 11-1)

At the conclusion of the chapter the student will be able to:

1. **List two ways heat can normally be produced in the body.**
2. **List five ways that the body normally loses heat.**
3. **List four predisposing factors to heat-related illness.**
4. **List the mechanisms, signs and symptoms, and treatment of the following heat-related disorders:**
   - **Heat cramps**
   - **Heat exhaustion**
   - **Heat stroke**
5. **Define hypothermia.**
6. **Describe the differences between the following types of hypothermia emergencies.**
   - **Acute immersion**
   - **Subacute exposure**
   - **Chronic exposure**
7. **List four predisposing factors to hypothermia.**

8. List the signs and symptoms associated with the following degrees of hypothermia:
- **Mild Hypothermia -- 32 - 35 C**
- **Moderate Hypothermia -- 26 - 32 C**
- **Severe Hypothermia -- < 26 C**

9. List the management steps for hypothermia.

10. List the signs and symptoms and management steps for the following types of local cold injuries:
- **Frostnip**
- **Superficial frostbite**
- **Deep frostbite**
- **Trenchfoot or immersion foot**
- **Chilblains**

Instructor Preparation

Reading preparation for the lesson:

EMT Prehospital Care, Chapter 11, pages 488-499

Optional reading:

Auerbach P.S., Gheehr E.C. (eds): Management of Wilderness and Environmental Emergencies. New York, Macmillan, 1983

Suggested Learning Activities

Using a lecture format with the aid of slides, overhead transparencies or charts, provide a presentation on heat and cold emergencies.

Provide case history examples of heat and cold emergencies.

Content

I. Overview **(Slide 11-2)**
  A. Body maintains a relatively constant temperature at 98.6°F or 37 degrees Celcius
  B. Normal deviation 35.8 to 37.7°C (96.4 - 99.8°F)
  C. Hard exercise causes core temperature to rise to 40°C
  D. During sleep temperature may drop to 35.8°C (96.8°F)
  E. Greater variances are not tolerated
  F. If body temperature is too low or too high the body can lose ability to regulate
  G. Environment dramatically fluctuates
    1. Heat must be produced through metabolic activity
    2. Lost through circulatory system

II. Heat regulation **(Slide 11-3)**
  A. Core temperature
    1. References to body temperature refer to core temperature
    2. Core temperature is maintained within narrow limits
    3. Greater variances in temperature occur on body shell
    4. Gradual fall from core temperature to shell (muscle, subcutaneous tissue, skin) **(Slide 11-4)**
    5. Regions also vary, example of skin: **(Slide 11-5)**
      a) Arms and legs - 31-32°C
      b) Forehead 34°C
      c) Toes 27°C
      d) Core 37.1°C
    6. Core temperature is measured rectally and orally
      a) Rectal is generally one degree F greater
      b) Axillary temperature is generally one degree F lower than the oral
  B. Heat production **(Slide 11-6)**
    1. Metabolic processes within the body generate heat
    2. Metabolism at rest is called the basal metabolism
      a) Provides a constant supply of heat
      b) In comfortable environments generates more than enough
      c) Can be increased by hormones under influence of CNS
      d) Muscular activity can increase heat production
        (1) Shivering--involuntary muscular activity
        (2) Metabolism and muscular activity could cause the core temperature to rise to dangerous levels
        (3) Excess heat is released to the environment through the skin
    3. Heat is gained when outside temperature exceeds body temperature
  C. Heat loss **(Slide 11-7)**
    1. Radiation
      a) Transfer of heat from a warmer to a cooler environment; not in contact with the body
      b) In proportion to difference between body and environment
      c) At 70°F room temperature, the body radiates heat
      d) When environment exceeds body temp., heat is gained

Content

2. Conduction
   a) Transfer of heat to objects in direct contact
   b) Influenced by properties of the materials
      (1) Water conducts heat faster than air
         (a) Wet clothing (5x)
         (b) Immersion in cold water (25x)
   c) Air surrounding body is heated by conduction
   d) Air is poor conductor
   e) Heat surrounding body serves to insulate unless there is convection
3. Convection
   a) Heat carried away by air currents
   b) Removing warmed air and replacing with cooler air
   c) Wind velocity influences heat loss
      (1) Wind chill factor
      (2) At 50°F, a 20-mile-per-hour wind makes it feel like 32°F.
4. Evaporation
   a) Loss of heat when moisture vaporizes on the body surface
   b) Rate depends on temperature, movement of air, and humidity
   c) Air can hold more water vapor as temperature rises
   d) When humidity is high, less evaporates
   e) When sweat runs off body, less cooling occurs
   f) When environmental temperature exceeds body temperature, evaporation becomes major mechanism for heat loss
5. Respiration
   a) Inhaled air is heated or cooled to body temperature
   b) Body loses heat when inhaled air is cooler than body
   c) Body gains heat when the inhaled air is warmer than body
   d) Minimal factor in humans, under normal conditions: **(Slide 11-8)**
      (1) Radiation, 60%
      (2) Evaporation, 22%
      (3) Conduction and convection, 15%
      (4) Smaller amounts through respiration, urine, and feces
6. Environmental conditions have great influence on heat loss

D. Mechanisms of control
1. Brain **(Slide 11-9)**
   a) Hypothalamus sets the body's thermostat
      (1) Regulates temperature by influencing:
         (a) Metabolic rate
         (b) Cardiovascular system
         (c) Skin circulation
      (2) When high temperatures are noted, skin vessels are directed to vasodilate
      (3) When cold is noted, metabolic rate will increase
      (4) Other receptors in the skin and spinal cord
         (a) Cause shivering (increased heat production)
         (b) Inhibit sweating
         (c) Induce vasoconstriction

Content

2. Cardiovascular system **(Slide 11-10)**
    a) Brings heated blood from core to skin
    b) Vasodilation vs constriction of vessels regulates blood flow to skin
    c) During heat stress widespread vasodilation occurs and this contributes to heat exhaustion
3. Skin **(Slide 11-11)**
    a) Skin is interface between external and internal environments
    b) Primary role in heat regulation
        (1) Insulates and regulates heat loss through changes in blood flow to skin
        (2) Evaporation of sweat

III. Heat emergencies **(Slide 11-12)**
  A. Three general types
    1. Heat cramps--muscular cramps
    2. Heat exhaustion--cardiovascular overload
    3. Heat stroke--complete failure
  B. Predisposing factors **(Slide 11-13)**
    1. Climate
        a) Temperature, humidity, and wind play large role
        b) Temperature will determine heat loss and gain by radiation and conduction
        c) High humidity will decrease the rate of evaporation
        d) Mortality increases threefold during heat waves
    2. Exercise and training
        a) Muscular activity greatly increases heat production
        b) Temperatures may rise to 40°C on hot humid days with exercise
        c) Athletes are high-risk group
        d) As one trains
            (1) Sweating begins earlier
            (2) More sweating occurs
            (3) Sweat can increase from 1 to 3 liters per hour
        e) Water is essential on hot days
            (1) Hypovolemia
            (2) Salt loss
        f) Salt and water replacement is essential
    3. Age
        a) Very old and very young are at increased risk
        b) Tendency to wrap infants in hot places increases risk
        c) Neonate is at greater risk because of poor thermoregulatory mechanisms
        d) Lack of mobility in infant and elderly, e.g., bedridden without air conditioning
    4. Preexisting illness
        a) Heart disease and dehydration compromise response to heat
        b) Obesity increases insulating effect
        c) Febrile illness
        d) Parkinson's due to constant muscle tremors
        e) Debilitated or retarded have less ability to care for self

Content

5. Alcohol and drugs
   a) Alcohol causes vasodilation
   b) Amphetamines and cocaine increase heat production
   c) Tranquilizers and antihistamines can affect the hypothalamus and inhibit sweating
   d) Diuretics can result in dehydration
   e) Drugs affecting judgment can prevent people from taking appropriate precautions

C. Heat cramps **(Slide 11-14)**
1. Mechanism
   a) Painful muscular contractions of heavily exercised muscles
   b) Caused by loss of sodium due to sweating and replacement with fluids without salt
   c) During exercise or hard work
2. Signs and symptoms **(Slide 11-15)**
   a) History of muscle cramping
   b) Immediately following exertion
   c) Excessive sweating
3. Treatment **(Slide 11-16)**
   a) Move patient to cooler environment
   b) Replace fluid and salt
      (1) Dilute salt solution
      (2) Gatorade or similar drinks
      (3) 1/2 teaspoon or less of salt in a quart of water
      (4) Stretch cramped muscles

D. Heat exhaustion **(Slide 11-17)**
1. Mechanisms
   a) Inability of the cardiovascular system to respond to the added demands
   b) Vasodilation of skin vessels
   c) Period of sweating and volume loss
   d) Mildly hypovolemic
   e) Previously dehydrated patient will be more prone
2. Signs and symptoms **(Slide 11-18)**
   a) Hot environment
   b) May have had a period of exertion
   c) Skin moist
   d) Core body temperature may be elevated (to 102°F)
   e) Weakness or exhaustion
   f) Inadequate flow to organs can result in dizziness, feeling faint, nausea, and headache
   g) Skin can appear gray or cold sometimes pink
   h) BP may be normal or orthostatic hypotension
   i) Tachycardia
3. Treatment **(Slide 11-19)**
   a) Move to cooler environment
   b) Given modest amount of fluids (one to two liters), same as heat cramps

Content

c) Fan to speed the cooling
d) Supine with legs elevated
e) Gatorade or a half-teaspoon of salt in a liter of water is a suitable replacement fluid.

E. Heat stroke **(Slide 11-20)**
1. Life-threatening emergency
2. High mortality rate
3. Primary measure is to lower body temperature
4. Mechanisms **(Slide 11-21)**
a) Can occur in any aged individual
b) Failure of the heat regulation mechanism
c) Temperature may rise quickly
d) When core temperature rises to 107°F
(1) Direct damage to cells occurs
(2) Particularly brain and blood vessels
e) Risk factors same as above (age, drugs, etc.)
f) Mortality can run as high as 80% if untreated
5. Signs and symptoms **(Slide 11-22)**
a) Altered mental status ranging from confusion to coma
b) High body temperatures (above 104°F)
c) Hot, dry skin (may be moist, particularly in younger individuals)
d) May be pink or flushed or ashen
e) Tachycardia
f) Increased respiratory rate
g) May be hypotensive
h) Seizures are not uncommon
6. Treatment **(Slide 11-23)**
a) Lower body temperature
(1) Fanning
(2) Move to cooler temperature
(3) Remove clothing
(4) Ice packs in neck, armpits, and groin
(5) Sheets or towels moistened with cool water
(6) Never use isopropyl alcohol
(7) High concentration of oxygen
b) Transport as medical emergency to hospital

IV. Cold emergencies **(Slide 11-24)**
A. Local injuries such as frostnip and frost-bite
B. Hypothermia
C. Time and temperature are major factors
1. Below freezing--short time
2. Above freezing--longer time
D. Frostbite involves freezing of the water between and within body cells
E. Results in ice crystal formation
F. Trenchfoot is localized cold injury without ice crystal formation
G. Hypothermia is core temperature below 35°C **(Slide 11-25)**
1. Body's ability to produce and regulate heat is unable to cope with environment

Content

2. Severe stresses such as icy water immersion can overwhelm mechanisms and result in death
3. Compromised ability to generate heat or prevent heat loss, may become hypothermic at room temperature

H. Rewarming done best in the hospital **(Slide 11-26)**

I. Prehospital care is directed toward
1. Preventing further heat loss
2. Protecting the injured parts
3. Transport

J. Physiologic response to cold **(Slide 11-27)**
1. Body normally produces more than sufficient heat
2. In temperate climates more than 90% of heat generated must be lost
3. Mechanisms described above
4. Man deals with extremes by creating environments that insulate and warm **(Slide 11-28)**
    a) Clothing
    b) Buildings
    c) Heating systems
5. When faced with cold **(Slide 11-29)**
    a) Increase in the metabolic rate
    b) Vasoconstriction
    c) Shivering
6. Shivering **(Slide 11-30)**
    a) Begins around 35°C (95°F)
    b) May continue for a few hours
    c) Malnourished or insulin shock patients may deplete energy stores in a shorter period
    d) Abolished by physical activity
    e) Certain drugs may suppress shivering response
    f) Usually stops below 31°C (87.8°F)
    g) Muscle rigidity is noted
    h) Once it stops temperature may drop precipitously
7. Central nervous system signs **(Slide 11-31)**
    a) May appear as early as 34°C (92°F) and will progress with drop in temperature
        (1) Amnesia and slurred speech
        (2) Irrational behavior
        (3) Stupor and coma as the temperature drops further
    b) Judgment may be disturbed
    c) Movement becomes impeded
    d) Hypothermic process will become more rapid
8. Other factors **(Slide 11-32)**
    a) Metabolism decreases 6% for every degree centigrade drop in body temperature
    b) Decrease in oxygen requirements increases the time from clinical to biological death
    c) Patients may have recovery even with long period in cardiac arrest

Content

K. Hypothermia **(Slide 11-33)**

1. Depends on several factors
   a) Type of exposure (water vs air)
   b) Time in environment
   c) Temperature
2. Acute immersion hypothermia **(Slide 11-34)**
   a) Immersion in icy waters
   b) Can result in death within 15 minutes
   c) Rarely does one survive for more than an hour
   d) At water temperatures of 15.5°C exposure of 6 hours is the upper limit
3. Subacute exposure **(Slide 11-35)**
   a) Exposure to air will result in longer survival times than submersion
   b) If clothing becomes soaked time is reduced
   c) Wind velocity plays a significant role
4. Chronic exposure **(Slide 11-36)**
   a) Over a period of hours or days
   b) Usually in compromised individuals
   c) Disease, drug intoxication make individual susceptible
   d) Shock states can compromise heat production and compensatory actions

Case Example **(Slide 11-37)**

> EMTs responded to an "unconscious" call in an apartment building. On arrival they discovered a 55 year old man who was found by his neighbor, unresponsive, with a large scalp laceration and a pool of blood on the floor. The laceration was not actively bleeding. The man was unresponsive to verbal and painful stimuli, had a BP of 80/60, R 12, and P 80, and a smell of alcohol on the breath. The skin was pale, cool and dry. A diagnosis of hypovolemic shock was made and PASG was applied resulting in an improvement in BP to 100/80 -- with no change in pulse or mental status. Further assessment and treatment in the hospital confirmed the diagnosis of hypovolemic shock from a scalp laceration and revealed a core temperature of 31°C. The paramedics noted that the apartment in which the patient was found was of normal temperature. A significant alcohol level was noted on blood analysis.

   e) Illustrates that extreme environmental temperatures are not necessary
   f) Factors
      (1) Alcohol resulting in vasodilation and unconscious
      (2) Shock
      (3) Radiation and conduction loss exceeded heat production
5. Predisposing factors (same as above)
   a) Climate **(Slide 11-38)**
      (1) Temperature, humidity, and wind play large role
      (2) Temperature will determine heat loss and gain by radiation and conduction

Content

(3) High humidity will decrease the rate of evaporation
(4) Mortality increases threefold during heat waves

b) Exercise and training
(1) Muscular activity greatly increases heat production
(2) Temperatures may rise to 40°C on hot humid days with exercise
(3) Athletes are high-risk group
(4) As one trains
(a) Sweating begins earlier
(b) More sweating occurs
(c) Sweat can increase from 1 to 3 liters per hour
(5) Water is essential on hot days
(a) Hypovolemia
(b) Salt loss
(6) Salt and water replacement is essential

c) Age
(1) Very old and very young are at increased risk
(2) Tendency to wrap infants in hot places increases risk
(3) Neonate is at greater risk because of poor thermoregulatory mechanisms
(4) Lack of mobility in infant and elderly, e.g., bedridden without air conditioning

d) Preexisting illness
(1) Heart disease and dehydration compromise response to heat
(2) Obesity increases insulating effect
(3) Febrile illness
(4) Parkinson's due to constant muscle tremors
(5) Debilitated or retarded have less ability to care for self

e) Alcohol and drugs
(1) Alcohol causes vasodilation
(2) Amphetamines and cocaine increase heat production
(3) Tranquilizers and antihistamines can affect the hypothalamus and inhibit sweating
(4) Diuretics can result in dehydration
(5) Drugs affecting judgment can prevent people from taking appropriate precautions

6. Signs and symptoms

a) Mild hypothermia -- 32-35°C **(Slide 11-39)**
(1) Cool skin
(2) Shivering
(3) Difficulty in speech and movement
(4) Amnesia
(5) Vital signs may be normal

b) Moderate hypothermia -- 26-32°C. **(Slide 11-40)**
(1) Shivering stops and is replaced with muscular rigidity
(2) Pulse and respirations may be depressed
(3) Pupils may dilate

Content

(4) Pulse may become irregular
(5) As temperature approaches 28°C ventricular fibrillation may develop

c) Severe hypothermia -- < 26°C **(Slide 11-41)**
(1) Unresponsive to pain
(2) Ventricular fibrillation and cardiac arrest are likely

7. Treatment **(Slide 11-42)**
a) Determined by time to transport and the degree of hypothermia
b) Reduce further heat loss
(1) Replace wet clothes with dry clothes or blankets
(2) Sleeping bags
(3) Warm environment
c) Resuscitation techniques **(Slide 11-43)**
(1) Supplemental oxygen approximately 50%
(2) Ventilate
(a) Do not hyperventilate
(b) Causes arrythmias
(3) Carefully insert airway devices to avoid gag reflex
(4) Careful assessment of pulses before initiating cardiac compressions
(a) Peripheral pulses may be difficult to palpate
(b) Unnecessary cardiac compressions may precipitate VF
d) Active rewarming **(Slide 11-44)**
(1) Application of heat internally or externally
(2) Most techniques are not recommended in the field
(3) Internal techniques as applicable in a hospital
(a) Instillation of warmed IV fluids
(b) Peritoneal dialysis (with heated fluids)
(c) Hemodialysis (heated fluids)
(d) Warmed humidified oxygen
(e) Guided by core temperature
(4) In the field monitoring is not possible and active rewarming is limited to **(Slide 11-45)**
(a) Warm humidified oxygen
(b) Application of local heat to large superficial vessels
(c) Warm fluids with sugar to conscious patient with gag reflex
(5) In restricted circumstances **(Slide 11-46)**
(a) Immersion in a tub of hot water (105°F)
(b) Application of warmed blankets or hot water bottles to shell
(c) Not recommended for all patients because of "rewarming shock"
i) Sudden dilatation of peripheral vessels
ii) Increase in the size of the circulatory system
(d) When far from medical facility active rewarming may be necessary

Content

- e) Transport
    - (1) Should be undertaken as soon as possible
    - (2) Avoid rough rides
- 8. Prevention of hypothermia **(Slide 11-47)**
    - a) Clothing must give adequate insulation
        - (1) Protection from wind and moisture
        - (2) Layering
        - (3) Wet clothing should be removed
        - (4) Cover body and head
    - b) Avoid contact with good conductors such as metal, snow, and water
    - c) Alcohol should be avoided
    - d) Smoking should be avoided
    - e) Carbohydrates and movement are necessary to sustain heat production
    - f) Know physical abilities and limitations
    - g) Seek shelter

L. Local injuries **(Slide 11-48)**

- 1. Tend to occur to extremities, exposed ears, nose, chin, cheeks
- 2. Vasoconstriction in response to cold leaves less heat to warm the superficial parts
- 3. Water in the superficial tissues freezes
- 4. Entire area may become frozen
- 5. Ice crystals form and cause damage to cellular structure
- 6. Recovery is possible with proper rewarming
- 7. Upon rewarming **(Slide 11-49)**
    - a) Marked vasodilation
    - b) Swelling from capillary leakage
    - c) Thrombosis in small vessels can affect circulation
        - (1) Stagnation of blood flow
        - (2) Mottled appearance
        - (3) Obstructed venous flow may appear bluish or purplish
- 8. Frostnip **(Slide 11-50)**
    - a) Completely reversible injury
    - b) Intense vasoconstriction to cold exposure
    - c) May appear as a sudden blanching of the skin
    - d) Loss of feeling and sensation
    - e) Victim unaware of process
    - f) Skin will not be hardened
    - g) Can be warmed
        - (1) Other warm body part
        - (2) Blowing warm breath on the area
    - h) Rewarmed area may be red and tingling
- 9. Superficial frostbite **(Slide 11-51)**
    - a) Freezing within upper layers of skin
    - b) White and waxy
    - c) Firm to the touch
    - d) Tissues beneath will be soft and resilient

e) After thawing the skin may appear flushed or mottled
f) There may be edema and blisters after 1-24 hours
g) Area is usually painful

10. Deep frostbite **(Slide 11-52)**
    a) Freezing extends throughout the dermis
    b) May involve subcutaneous tissues, muscle, tendons, neurovascular structures, and even bone
    c) Skin becomes white and feels frozen
    d) Resists depression
    e) Difficult to gauge the extent of deep frostbite
    f) Rethawed area may appear mottled
    g) Demarcation separating injured from healthy tissue
    h) Treatment **(Slide 11-53)**
        (1) Should not be undertaken in the field
        (2) Time consuming and can delay assessment of hypothermia and evacuation
        (3) Complications are best handled in the hospital
        (4) Insulate area with clothing or blanket
        (5) Remove wet clothing
        (6) If thawed, do not break blisters
        (7) Cover with sterile dressings
        (8) Separate fingers and toes
        (9) Handle with care
        (10) Patient should avoid walking on frostbitten extremity; expecially if thawed or partially thawed
        (11) Oxygen
        (12) Where transport may be significantly delayed t **(Slide 11-54)**
            (a) Immerse part into a basin of water large enough to not touch walls
            (b) Preheat and maintain water temperature at about 40.6^{o}C -- 105 F
            (c) Keep it between 37.8 and 43.3^{o}C
            (d) Too warm a temperature may harm the part
            (e) Lesser temperatures are not effective
            (f) Keep the water circulating
            (g) Patient will feel pain on rethawing
            (h) Complete when the part is soft and color and sensation are present
            (i) Sterile dressings
            (j) Dressings between toes and fingers
            (k) Can take from 20 to 40 minutes

11. Trenchfoot or immersion foot **(Slide 11-55)**
    a) Exposure (10 -12 hours) to above-freezing temperatures (below 10°C, 50°F) and dampness
    b) Common in wartime when soldiers stood for long periods of time in cold wet trenches
    c) Causes damage to the small vessels and nerves and occurs in stages

Content

d) In response to the cold **(Slide 11-56)**
(1) Vessels vasoconstrict
(2) Paleness or blueness, diminished pulses
(3) Edema
(4) Decreased or absent sensation
(5) Diminished pulses

e) This phase is followed by **(Slide 11-57)**
(1) Increase in circulation to the area
(2) Foot may appear hot and red and dry
(3) Pulses may be bounding
(4) Extreme painful
(5) Skin can atrophy
(6) Ulcers and gangrene can follow

f) Treatment **(Slide 11-58)**
(1) Keep warm and dry
(2) Protect from weight bearing and further injury

12. Chilblains **(Slide 11-59)**
a) Abnormal vascular response to mild cold
b) Itching, redness, and swelling on the dorsal surfaces of hands and feet
c) Following exposure to above-freezing temperatures
d) Most often affect women, children, and patients with vascular and collagen diseases

Section 2

Burns

Objectives
(Slide 11-60)

At the conclusion of the chapter the student will be able to:

1. **List three types of burns.**
2. **List the three classifications of burn depth and describe the appearance of each.**
3. **List the percentage of body surface area for the head, chest, abdomen, groin, and upper and lower extremities for the adult and child using the "Rule of Nines."**
4. **List four regions of the body that when burned are considered critical.**
5. **List four complicating historical or physical factors that are considered when determining the severity of burns.**
6. **Describe burns as minor, moderate, or severe based upon percentage of body surface area of second- and third-degree burns.**
7. **List three signs of inhalation injury.**
8. **Describe the management of thermal burns.**
9. **Describe the basic management of chemical burns.**
10. **Describe the special management considerations for the following types of chemical burns:**
    - **Dried Chemicals [Lime]**
    - **Phosphorus**
    - **Sodium and Potassium**
    - **Hydrofluoric Acid**
    - **Phenols**
11. **Describe the basic management of electrical burns.**

Chapter 11

Instructor Preparation

Reading preparation for the lesson:

EMT Prehospital Care, Chapter 11, pages 499-509

Optional reading:

Auerbach PS, Gheehr EC (eds):Management of Wilderness and Environmental Emergencies. New York, Macmillan, 1983

Suggested Learning Activities
Using a lecture format with the aid of slides, overhead transparencies, or charts, provide a presentation on burns. **Provide case history examples of burn emergencies.**

Content

V. Burns **(Slide 11-61)**
- A. Caused by thermal [heat], chemicals, or electrical injury
- B. Affect about two million persons per year
- C. About 3 to 5% are life-threatening
- D. Most thermal burns occur in home
- E. Result of flames or scalding water
- F. Under three years of age hot liquids are the most common source of burns
- G. Ages 3 to 14 clothing fire is the most common source
- H. Over age 60 blackouts or general debilitation may contribute
- I. Smoke can contain a number of toxins **(Slide 11-62)**
    - 1. Most common carbon monoxide
    - 2. Colorless, tasteless, odorless gas
    - 3. Impairs oxygen transport
    - 4. Contributes to over half the deaths

VI. Thermal burns **(Slide 11-63)**
- A. Overview
    - 1. Skin
        - a) Barrier to infection, water loss
        - b) Major thermoregulatory organ
        - c) Sensory organ
        - d) Epidermis is relatively impermeable to water and bacteria
        - e) Dermis contains several structures
            - (1) Blood vessels, nerves
            - (2) Hair follicles, sweat ducts
            - (3) Sebaceous glands
        - f) Subcutaneous tissue serves protective and insulating role
    - 2. Problems that follow burns include **(Slide 11-64)**:
        - a) Loss of temperature control
        - b) Loss of body fluids and water
        - c) Infection
    - 3. Prehospital care **(Slide 11-65)**
        - a) Stop the burning process
        - b) Remove patient from smoky environment
        - c) Give supplemental oxygen
        - d) Prevent infection
        - e) Transport
        - f) Treat airway obstruction and associated injuries
        - g) Maintain body temperature
        - h) Minimize pain
- B. Limits of heat tolerance **(Slide 11-66)**
    - 1. Degree of heat and the length of exposure are critical
    - 2. Above 60°C will cause cell death
    - 3. Below 45°C -- no cell damage occurs
    - 4. Above 45°C -- variable damage depending on the duration

Content

5. Effects of chemical burns depend on the type, concentration, and duration of exposure
6. Effects of electrical burns depend on voltage, resistance, and the length of contact

C. Classification and assessment **(Slide 11-67)**
1. First degree
    a) Involve the epidermis only
    b) Sunburn is a common example
    c) Skin appears reddened, dry, and warm to touch
    d) Painful
    e) Pain may not be present for several hours
    f) Slight edema
    g) Slightly elevated temperature
    h) Heal spontaneously after peeling
2. Second degree **(Slide 11-68)**
    a) Involve epidermis and upper dermis
    b) Partial-thickness burns
    c) Commonly caused by flash injuries or spills, scalds
    d) Different appearances depending on the extent of dermal injury
        (1) Edema and blisters
        (2) Surface may be moist or weeping
    e) Blisters should be left intact
    f) Color may vary
        (1) Pink or red and blotchy
        (2) Deeper -- may be darker or pale and colorless
    g) Vary in their sensitivity
        (1) Can be extremely painful
        (2) Deeper will be normal or decreased sensation
        (3) Very deep may have no sensation
    h) Difficult to distinguish from third degree
3. Third degree **(Slide 11-69)**
    a) Involve full thickness of the epidermis and dermis
    b) Caused by extreme heat or prolonged exposure
    c) Skin
        (1) Charred, yellow-brown, dark red, or white and translucent
        (2) Thrombosed veins are visible
        (3) No pain or sensation
        (4) Texture is leathery
        (5) Loss of resilience
        (6) Can restrict movement and expansion of underlying structures
        (7) Especially over large surface or circumferential
            (a) Can constrict blood flow
            (b) Restrict chest expansion
            (c) Can progress over time
            (d) In the hospital incisions are made to allow chest wall expansion or blood flow through limbs

Content

(8) Lose ability to generate tissue
(9) Require skin grafting

4. Fourth degree **(Slide 11-70)**
   a) Involve skin and subcutaneous tissue, muscle, and even bone
   b) Electrical burns can cause damage as current travels through the body
5. Extent of burns **(Slide 11-71)**
   a) Body is approximated into 9% and 18% to estimate burns
      (1) Head and neck -- 9%
      (2) Each arm -- 9%
      (3) Front of the torso -- 18%
      (4) Back of the torso -- 18%
      (5) Each leg -- 18%
      (6) Genitalia -- 1%
   b) Summation accounts for 100%
   c) Palm represents about 1%; might be used to estimate and describe smaller areas
   d) Infant estimate changes due to head and leg differences
      (1) Head and neck - 18%
      (2) Each arm - 9%
      (3) Front of the torso - 18%
      (4) Back of the torso - 18%
      (5) Each leg - 14% (or 13.5%)
      (6) Genitalia - 1%
6. Location **(Slide 11-72)**
   a) Critical areas due to tendency for infection, loss of function, or respiratory involvement
   b) Face, perineum and genitalia, and the feet and hands
   c) Circumferential burns can obsruct blood flow through extremities and restrict breathing
7. Complicating factors **(Slide 11-73)**
   a) Old age
   b) Inhalation injuries
   c) Associated injuries or medical conditions
   d) Preexisting conditions
8. Burn severity classification **(Slide 11-74)**
   a) Burns are classified by severity for patient triage and transport decision
   b) Local protocols will use burn severity to determine facility selection
   c) National criteria may be adjusted to reflect local resources
   d) American College of Surgeons Criteria
      (1) Minor
         (a) Second degree less than 15% in adult
         (b) Second degree less than 10% in child
         (c) Third degree less than 2%

Content

(2) Moderate
(a) Second degree less than 15 to 25% in adult
(b) Second degree less than 10 to 20% in child
(c) Third degree 2 to 10%
(3) Major
(a) Second degree more than 25% in adult
(b) Second degree more than 20% in child
(c) Third degree more than 10%
(d) Significant burns to hand, face, feet, and perineum
(e) Inhalation injury
(f) Fractures or mechanical trauma
(g) Significant diseases, e.g., diabetes
(h) Ages less than 5, more than 60

D. Treatment of thermal burns **(Slide 11-75)**
1. Stop the burning process
2. Remove from the burning or smoky environment
3. Cool water by facecloth or immersion may help reduce severity of burn when applied shortly after the accident
4. Cool compresses (not more than 20% of the body) for pain
5. Assess for airway compromise **(Slide 11-76)**
a) Respiratory distress
b) Stridor, hoarseness
c) Use of accessory muscles
d) Cyanosis
e) Other signs of respiratory distress
f) Signs of inhalation injury
g) Administer high-concentration oxygen, humidified if possible
6. Treat for shock
7. Obtain history **(Slide 11-77)**
a) Circumstances surrounding the burn
b) Source and duration of the thermal injury
c) Smoke inhalation?
d) Was the patient in a closed space or did he suffer unconsciousness?
e) Preexisting medical conditions
8. Sterile or clean dressings or sheets **(Slide 11-78)**
9. Remove rings or bracelets
10. Never apply ointments or any other substance
11. Leave blisters intact
12. In cool environments maintain body temperature
13. Transport according to local protocols

E. Smoke inhalation **(Slide 11-79)**
1. Most common cause of death in fires
2. Hot air containing noxious gases and small particles
3. Death from smoke, four general ways **(Slide 11-80)**:
a) Consumes oxygen in environment
b) Carbon monoxide
(1) Binds with hemoglobin
(2) Interferes with oxygen transport

Content

(3) Small concentrations can result in death
(4) 200x greater affinity for hemoglobin than does oxygen
(5) All smoke inhalation victims should be considered to have inhaled carbon monoxide
(6) Treat with oxygen

c) Cyanide impairs tissues ability to use oxygen
(1) Cyanide poisons the tissues and interferes with oxygen metabolism
(2) Sources of cyanide in fires include polyurethane, polyacrylonitrile, wool, and silk

d) Direct injury to the airways from heat and irritant gases
(1) Leads to swelling of the airway
(2) Bronchospasm, and damage to the delicate alveoli
(3) Moist heat common cause
(4) Irritant gases can damage capillaries and cause edema

4. History **(Slide 11-81)**
a) Duration of exposure
b) Type of burning materials
c) Was the victim exposed to steam?
d) Trapped in a closed space?
e) If rescuers overcome, were they wearing self-contained breathing apparatus?
f) Note the time the victim was removed

5. Symptoms of smoke inhalation **(Slide 11-82)**
a) Burning of the eyes, nose, and throat
b) Tearing, coughing, tightness in the chest
c) Shortness of breath with moderate exertion

6. Physical examination **(Slide 11-83)**
a) Burns of the face
b) Singed nasal hairs
c) Hoarseness, stridor
d) Erythema and particles in the oropharynx
e) Carbonaceous (black particles) sputum
f) Wheezes and rales
g) Cyanosis, tachypnea, and tachycardia
h) Cherry-red color noted (occasionally) to occur with carbon monoxide poisoning

7. Treatment **(Slide 11-84)**
a) Removal from environment
b) High-concentration humidified oxygen
c) Transport rapidly if signs of airway obstruction

VII. Chemical burns **(Slide 11-85)**

A. General principles
1. Cause burns similar to thermal
2. Concentration and the duration of exposure are important
3. Chemicals continue to burn until they are removed
4. Immediate and thorough irrigation essential treatment **(Slide 11-86)**
a) Large amounts of water for 20 to 30 minutes
b) Splashes should be avoided

Content

c) Garden hoses or showers are ideal
d) Pressure should be adjusted to avoid traumatic injury to burned tissues
5. Acids and alkali are the most common
6. Alkalis tend to take longer to remove
7. In general one should not use a neutralizing agent
a) Wastes time finding one
b) Chemical reaction may produce heat
B. Dried chemicals (Lime) **(Slide 11-87)**
1. Powdered or dried chemicals should be brushed off
2. Water may activate burning reaction
3. Contaminated clothing and shoes removed before irrigation. Chemicals may collect in pants cuffs and shoes
5. Irrigate with large amounts of water
C. Special considerations
1. Phosphorus **(Slide 11-88)**
a) Yellow or white phosphorus
b) Chemicals used in munitions, insecticide, and fertilizer industries
c) Combusts when exposed to air
d) Affected parts should be submerged in water or covered with soaked dressings
2. Sodium and potassium **(Slide 11-89)**
a) Ignite spontaneously in air
b) Also react with water to form more caustic forms
c) Smoldering fragments embedded in the skin should be:
(1) Extinguished with a fire extinguisher
(2) Smothered with sand
(3) Or covered with petroleum jelly
3. Hydrofluoric acid **(Slide 11-90)**
a) Caustic to the skin and penetrates into the dermis
b) Continues to cause injury until deactivated
c) Water is used for irrigation as with other acid burns
d) Deactivation of penetrated particles requires calcium chloride or calcium gluconate or magnesium oxide paste
e) Advanced EMT units carry calcium salt solutions
4. Phenols **(Slide 11-91)**
a) Phenols and cresol can penetrate skin and be absorbed systemically
b) Treatment with polyethylene glycol (PE) and methylated spirits in a 2:1 mixture
c) If available should be applied prior to water irrigation
d) May be available on site of industrial accident
VIII. Electrical burns **(Slide 11-92)**
A. Definition of electricity
1. Fundamental entity of nature
2. Consisting of negative and positive kinds

Content

3. Composed respectively of electrons and protons, or possibly of electrons and positrons
4. In natural phenomena (as lightning or the aurora borealis)
5. Utilized in the form of electric currents

B. General principles **(Slide 11-93)**

1. 1000 deaths per year, high-risk groups
    - a) Children from infancy to 4 years who chew through wires or play with electrical outlets
    - b) Men working in industrial settings
2. Types of electrical injuries **(Slide 11-94)**
    - a) Lightning
    - b) Downed power lines
    - c) Malfunction of home appliances
    - d) Contact with TV antennas to high-tension power line
    - e) High tension power lines (adolescent boys)
3. Electricity burns tissues when entering body **(Slide 11-95)**
4. High-voltage arcs can hit people a distance away
5. Death can occur when vital organs are struck
6. Rescuers must take due precautions to protect self and victim from further injury
7. What is electricity? **(Slide 11-96)**
    - a) Movement of electrons from a point of higher to lower concentration
    - b) Amperage -- number or volume of electrons
    - c) Voltage -- force with which movement occurs
    - d) Resistance -- degree of hindrance to electron flow
    - e) Amperage = voltage/resistance
8. Exposure to low voltage is less serious than to high voltage **(Slide 11-97)**
    - a) Fatalities have occurred with voltage as low as 45 to 60 cycles/second
    - b) Human muscle response is in the range from 40 to 150 cycles/second
    - c) Household current can easily initiate tetanic contractions
    - d) Steady tonic contraction of the muscle can prevent release of the electrified object
9. Amperage is usually more pertinent to the extent of injury **(Slide 11-98)**
    - a) Amperage and resistance are seldom known
    - b) As the amperage increases, different consequences are possible:
        - (1) Tingling of the skin
        - (2) Tetanic contractions
        - (3) Respiratory arrest
        - (4) Cardiac arrest

Content

10. Resistance is a measure of the hindrance to electron flow through a given material **(Slide 11-99)**
    - a) Copper wires offer relatively low resistance
    - b) Rubber has a very high resistance
    - c) Wood has high resistance and burns
    - d) Ground **(Slide 11-100)**
        - (1) Webster: "large conducting body, as the earth, used as a common return for an electrical circuit and an arbitrary zero of potential"
        - (2) Cars are insulated from the ground because of rubber tires
    - e) Downed power line in contact with a car may leave the occupants unharmed **(Slide 11-101)**
        - (1) As long as they themselves avoid contact with the ground
        - (2) If they step out of car (while touching the car) they will be part of the circuit
    - f) When electricity penetrates skin, current will follow path of least resistance **(Slide 11-102)**
        - (1) Skin and bone -- high resistance
        - (2) Muscle offers less
        - (3) Vessels and nerves -- least resistance
        - (4) Significant internal injury can occur, which cannot be judged externally
    - g) Wet skin offers much less resistance
    - h) Household current can result in ventricular fibrillation

C. Burns to skin **(Slide 11-103)**
- 1. Burns can extend from first-degree to fourth-degree burns
- 2. Third and fourth degree can vary in appearance from gray-white areas to charred
- 3. Arcs can cause burns
- 4. The longer the contact the greater the burn

D. Arc burns **(Slide 11-104)**
- 1. Current can travel through air
- 2. Heat radiating from the core of the arc is called the flash
- 3. Intense heat can cause thermal injury
- 4. Clothing can catch on fire

E. Assessment and treatment **(Slide 11-105)**
- 1. Assess whether hazards continue to exist
    - a) If there are fallen wires summon the power company or rescue personnel
    - b) Downed wire should be considered as charged until authorities confirm that power is off
    - c) When encountering victims entrapped in a vehicle in contact with a downed wire **(Slide 11-106)**
        - (1) Have them stay in the vehicle
        - (2) Do not touch the vehicle
        - (3) If there is a fire in the car, victims should jump out or throw small children without completing a circuit between the car and the ground

Content

(4) Assess ABC's
(5) The cervical spine precautions
(6) Look closely for any fractures and splint appropriately
(7) Cover wounds with sterile dressings
(8) Transport to the hospital

Chapter 11

Section 3

Radiation Injuries

Objectives
(Slide 11-107)

At the conclusion of the chapter the student will be able to:
1. Define ionizing radiation.
2. Describe the purpose of a dosimeter and a survey instrument.
3. Describe the difference between irradiation and contamination.
4. Define external contamination, internal contamination, and incorporation.
5. Describe the penetrating ability and relative hazards of the four kinds of ionizing radiation.
6. List the factors affecting the severity of radiation injury.
7. Describe the role of the radiologic monitor or radiation safety officer.
8. List the four radiation protection principles and explain their use in reducing radiation exposure.
9. Describe the role of prehospital personnel in patient management and decontamination of radiation victims at the scene and at the hospital.
10. Discuss the maximum allowable exposures for rescue personnel performing lifesaving actions and in less urgent emergencies.

Instructor Preparation

Reading preparation for the lesson:

EMT Prehospital Care, Chapter 11, pages 509-525

Optional reading:

Auerbach PS, Gheehr EC (eds):Management of Wilderness and Environmental Emergencies. New York, Macmillan, 1983

Suggested Learning Activities

Using a lecture format with the aid of slides, overhead transparencies, or charts, provide a presentation on heat and cold emergencies.

Provide case history examples of radiation emergencies.

Display radiation monitoring devices.

Content

IX. Definitions **(Slide 11-108)**

A. Radiation

1. The process of emitting radiant energy [energy traveling as wave motions];
2. Specifically the energy of electromagnetic waves in the form of waves or particles
3. Process by which energy is propagated through space or matter not affected by it

B. Ionizing radiation

1. Any radiation displacing electrons from atoms or molecules
2. Thereby producing ions
3. Alterations in molecules within cells can disrupt normal function

C. Radioactive

1. The ability of a substance to emit rays or particles from its nucleus.

D. Radioactivity

1. The property possessed by some elements [as uranium] of spontaneously emitting alpha and beta particles and gamma rays by the disintegration of the nuclei of its atoms

E. Isotope

1. One of two or more atoms with the same atomic number [the same chemical element] but with different atomic weights
2. The nuclei of isotopes have the same number of protons but different numbers of neutrons.
3. Isotopes of an element have very nearly the same chemical properties but somewhat different physical properties
4. "Unstable" isotopes break down spontaneously to smaller atoms and in the process they emit radioactive energy as particles or waves

F. Irradiated **(Slide 11-109)**

1. A person or substance exposed to ionizing radiation
2. For example, someone who has been x-rayed is said to have been irradiated and represents no threat to persons who come in contact with them

G. Contamination

1. Radioactive material is physically present on a person or object
2. It can be spread to others

H. Decontamination

1. The process by which radioactive material is removed from a person or object

I. Roentgen

1. Special unit of exposure to radiation
2. Measured from ionizing effect of radiation on air molecules within a chamber

J. Rad

1. Special unit of absorbed dose of radiation
2. When ionizing radiation passes through matter, some of its energy is imparted to the matter
3. The amount absorbed per mass of material is called the absorbed dose

Content

K. Rem
   1. Special unit of dose equivalent
   2. Equivalent to absorbed dose in rads multiplied by the quality factor, the distribution factor, and other modifying factors
L. Physical half-life **(Slide 11-110)**
   1. The time required for a radioactive substance to lose 50% of its activity by decay
M. Radiation injuries **(Slide 11-111)**
   1. Radiation is a form of energy transmission
   2. Effects of ionizing radiation
   3. Radiation with the potential to alter the function of the body's cells by altering or ionizing
   4. Can cause biochemical changes in the cells
      a) Immediate
      b) Future
   5. High doses of radiation sustained over a short time can lead to an <u>acute radiation syndrome</u>
   6. Smaller doses may:
      a) Increase risk of cancer
      b) Result in cataracts
      c) Affect growth and life span
   7. There are set limits of occupational exposure **(Slide 11-112)**
   8. Small amounts of radiation are not harmful, radiation exposure occurs normally
      a) Sun
      b) Earth
      c) Manmade objects
   9. Radiation cannot be perceived by our senses
      a) Injuries may not be felt
      b) Workers wear instruments to monitor the exposure
   10. Radiation injuries were not common (after WWII and prior to Chernobyl)
      a) Fewer than 1000 persons involved in serious radiation accidents
      b) About 450 receiving medically serious dose
      c) Fewer than 21 fatalities
      d) Health workers were not injured giving treatment
   11. Most accidents occurred in the workplace
      a) Experts usually available
      b) Provisions for decontamination usually available
   12. Transportation accidents
      a) Radioactive wastes along highways
      b) EMTs at traffic accident
         (1) Know how to summon help
         (2) Understanding of the basic principles

(3) Initiate lifesaving interventions
(4) Prevent unnecessary exposure to themselves, the public, and the accident victims

X. Basic Biophysics **(Slide 11-113)**
- A. Atom consists of protons, neutrons, and electrons
  - 1. Most atoms are stable
  - 2. Some elements exist in more than one form
    - a) Same number of protons
    - b) Different numbers of neutrons
    - c) Called <u>isotopes</u>
      - (1) Some are "unstable"
      - (2) Break down spontaneously to smaller atoms. Emit energetic rays or particles
      - (3) Isotopes have specific names such as U 238 or 238 Uranium.
    - d) Common units of measurement
      - (1) Roentgen
      - (2) Rad
      - (3) Rem
      - (4) Curie
    - e) Can result in an electronically measurable charge in the air
- B. Types of radiation **(Slide 11-114)**
  - 1. The average annual exposure from natural sources ranges from 100 to 400 mrem/year in United States
  - 2. Alpha
    - a) Positively charged particle consisting of two protons, two neutrons
    - b) Identical to a helium nucleus with a 2+ charge
    - c) Least penetrating form
      - (1) Travels only a few centimeters in air
      - (2) Stopped by a sheet of paper, clothing, and the epidermis
      - (3) Only dangerous if ingested, inhaled, or absorbed through broken skin
    - d) Transuranic isotopes most common source
  - 3. Beta **(Slide 11-115)**
    - a) Charged particles that have the mass of an electron
    - b) Neither a negative nor a positive charge [called positrons]
    - c) Can travel less than 1 foot to several feet. Travel somewhat deeper than alpha into the dermal layer where they are stopped
    - d) Can cause burns similar to thermal burns
    - e) Can be stopped by protective clothing
    - f) Usually are only dangerous if they result in internal contamination
    - g) Alpha and beta particles can cling to the skin or clothing or contaminate a person
  - 4. Gamma rays **(Slide 11-116)**
    - a) High-energy electromagnetic radiation similar to x-rays but more energetic

Content

b) Can penetrate the body and cause damage
c) Biochemical transformation
(1) Instant
(2) Long term
d) Do not cause contamination of the victim
e) No risk to others
f) Victim exposed is irradiated
g) Can travel long distances and penetrate most materials with ease
(1) Dense materials such as lead are the best shielding
5. Neutrons **(Slide 11-117)**
a) Uncharged particles found in the nucleus of an atom
b) Emissions occur in nuclear reactors
c) Much more penetrating than alpha and beta particles
d) Can "activate" the body and materials in the path such as rings, belt buckles, coins
e) They are not common
C. Contamination vs irradiation
1. Contamination **(Slide 11-118)**
a) Contamination may be external and/or internal
(1) External contamination--radioactive materials limited to skin and clothing. Internal contamination--materials enter into the body
(a) Ingestion
(b) Inhalation
(c) Break in the skin
(2) Materials can be incorporated as part of the body's structure (internal)
(3) External contamination itself is rarely a medical emergency
(a) Primary concern is unnecessary spread of radioactive materials to the patient, the rescuer, and others
(4) Primary concern is with internal contamination
(a) Prompt institution of medical care
(b) Eliminate
(c) Dilute
(d) Bind up
(e) Block the effects
b) Contamination should not interfere with medical care
2. Irradiation **(Slide 11-119)**
a) Gamma rays pass through or penetrate a person but do not remain as radioactive
b) Victim is said to have been irradiated
c) Presents no greater risk to another person
d) Risk to rescuers is only from source
3. Types of Patients **(Slide 11-120)**
a) Irradiated with no contamination
b) External contamination

Content

c) Internal contamination via inhalation, ingestion, or break in the skin
d) Simple trauma
e) Combination of any of the above conditions

XI. Patients with Radiation Injuries **(Slide 11-121)**
A. Irradiated patients
1. Result from overexposure to unshielded radioactive sources
a) Industries that use sealed radioisotope sources
b) Injuries at weapons research or reprocessing facilities
2. No threat to bystanders
B. External contamination **(Slide 11-122)**
1. Radioactive dust particles, or solid, liquid, or gas materials on the skin or clothing
2. May emit alpha, beta, or gamma radiation
3. External contamination can occur
a) Hospitals
b) Universities
c) Many industries
d) Explosions
e) Fires
f) Apparatus breakage
g) Container ruptures
h) Transportation accidents
C. Internal contamination **(Slide 11-123)**
1. Inhalation
a) Dust, gaseous substances, or particles following fires or explosions
b) Obtain nasal swabs if possible
(1) May be done by personnel at the site
(2) Recommended before contamination efforts commence
(3) Moistened cotton-tipped applicators are used to swab each nostril
(4) Placed in a sealed container for laboratory analysis
(5) Labeled with the subject's name, time, and date
2. Ingestion **(Slide 11-124)**
a) Causes
(1) Ingestion of contaminated foods or liquids, touching lips with contaminated hands
(2) Other accidental or suicidal ingestions of isotopes
(3) Can occur with inhaled radioactive materials through the pharynx
b) Internal contamination rarely constitutes a significant threat to the rescuer
(1) Vomitus should be treated as external contamination
(2) There should be no smoking, eating, or drinking in a contaminated area

Content

3. Absorption **(Slide 11-125)**
    a) Can enter the body through an open wound or burn and be absorbed
    b) In explosion, solid particles or fragments may be embedded in the skin
    c) Some isotopes, tritium, radioactive iodine may pass through intact skin
    d) Ascertain the properties of the contaminant

XII. Measuring instruments **(Slide 11-126)**
  A. Dosimeters or personnel monitoring devices
    1. Radiation-measuring instruments used to monitor the total accumulation of radiation
    2. Worn by individuals who work with radioactive particles or by rescue personnel
    3. Worn on the torso
    4. Measure similar to the total whole body radiation
    5. The unit of measurement
      a) Roentgen [R]
      b) Milliroentgen [mR] [1/1000 of a roentgen]
    6. Basic types
      a) Film badges or photographic film
      b) The pocket dosimeter
        (1) Charged or zeroed prior to use
        (2) Eliminates need to subtract background
  B. Survey instruments **(Slide 11-127)**
    1. Measure the <u>rate of exposure</u> in terms of roentgens per hour or milliroentgens per hour
    2. The Geiger-Mueller counter
    3. Can be calibrated in roentgens per hour [R/hr] or milliroentgens per hour [mR/hr]
    4. Civil defense survey meters are designed to measure gamma radiation, and some detect beta radiation
    5. Special instruments for alpha radiation detection are also available
    6. Purpose
      a) Rescuers can determine risk
      b) Can predict exposure over time
      c) To determine if a victim or rescuer has been contaminated
  C. Radiation safety officers or radiologic monitors should have expertise to use and interpret results
  D. EMTs should follow advice of officer

XIII. Acute Radiation Syndrome and Factors Affecting Severity **(Slide 11-128)**
  A. Severity of a radiation exposure is affected by **(Slide 11-129)**:
    1. Strength of source
    2. Type of radiation
    3. Duration of exposure
    4. Area of the body exposed

Content

5. Distance from source
6. Shielding
7. Age and condition of a patient

B. Acute radiation syndrome **(Slide 11-130)**

1. High dose over short time
   a) Results from damage to the bone marrow, GI tract, nervous and cardiovascular systems
      (1) 50 rem--may have no visible effects but a small percentage may show depression of WBCs (white blood cells)
      (2) 100 rem--nausea and vomiting occur in a small percentage of exposed persons
      (3) 200 rem--most will show signs of nausea and vomiting, depression of the bone marrow
      (4) 400 rem--about 50% of the exposed individuals will die within weeks
      (5) 600 rem--near 100% lethality without medical intervention
      (6) 1000 rem--GI complications begin to appear at immediate onset
      (7) 3000 rem--hypotension, central nervous syndrome with rapid onset of drowsiness, uncoordination, and convulsion
2. Smaller doses (genetic effects) **(Slide 11-131)**
   a) 5--25 rem--detectable by chromosome analysis
      (1) Sperm count is reduced
      (2) Procreation should be avoided for a period of time following exposure
      (3) Pregnant women should avoid any exposure at site of radiation accidents

Natural and Medical Radioactive Sources
(Slide 11-132)

SOURCE	DOSE
Cosmic	42 mrem/year
Terrestrial	44 mrem/year
Chest x-ray	66 mrem/year
Lumbar spine x-ray [4 views]	10,000 mrem/year

Content

C. Strength of the radioactive source **(Slide 11-134)**
   1. The stronger the radioactive source, the greater the dose received at a fixed distance

D. Type of radiation.
   1. Gamma radiation and neutrons are the most penetrating
   2. Alpha and beta particles are nonpenetrating through intact skin and damage is limited with careful decontamination
   3. Internal contamination with alpha and beta requires elimination of isotope to block toxic effects

E. Duration of exposure
   1. Doses fatal if absorbed over a short interval may be tolerated if absorbed over a longer time period
   2. Rescuers can gauge the amount of time
      a) if source emits 100R/hr, 15 minutes in the area may result in absorption of 25R
      b) Rescue workers can reduce individual exposure by sharing time spent in the danger zone
      c) The shorter the time spent in a radiation field, the less radiation will be absorbed by the body

F. Area of the body exposed **(Slide 11-135)**
   1. Different parts of the body can tolerate different amounts of radiation
   2. Permissible occupational standards for hands are several times those for the gonads or the whole body
   3. Shielding parts of the body during medical or dental x-rays is an example of limiting body exposure

G. Distance from the source
   1. Greater the distance less absorbed radiation
   2. Double the distance decreases radiation exposure by factor of 4

H. Shielding
   1. Lead aprons
   2. Dense materials
   3. Protective clothing should be utilized

Content

XIV. Emergency Care **(Slide 11-136)**

A. EMTs may be called to administer emergency care at a radiation accident

B. If monitoring or rescue expected of EMT, then specialized training should be provided in use of:

1. Survey instruments
2. Protective clothing
3. Decontamination procedures

C. Protection and containment

1. First priority is to protect self and others
2. A safety zone should be established
3. Protective gear should be utilized
4. Protection principles must be followed

D. Identification of source

1. Is there a risk?
2. Type of isotope[s] involved identified through:
    a) On-site personnel
    b) Patients
    c) Labels on containers
    d) Shipping papers
    e) The DOT guidebook
    f) Sample of internal contamination (nose swab)
    g) Sample of vomitus or other body secretions

Placard Information
(Slide 11-137)

Label	Dose Rate At Surface [mR/hr]	Dose Rate At 3 feet [mR/hr]
Radioactive White I	< 0.5 mrem/hr	---
Radioactive Yellow II	0.5-50	<1
Radioactive Yellow III	50-200	1-10

E. Notification **(Slide 11-138)**

1. Know the responsible state and/or local agency
2. Department of Energy Regional Coordinating Office for Radiological Assistance
3. Radiation Emergency Assistance Center/Training Site [REAC/TS]
    a) Provides a 24-hour consultation
    b) [615] 576-3131 Monday through Friday [8:00 am to 4:30 pm]
    c) [615] 482-2441 beeper 241, a 24-hr telephone at Oak Ridge Hospital
    d) Writing REAC/TS, Box 117, Oak Ridge, Tennessee 37830

Content

4. Chemtrex is another source of information [800] 424-9300.
5. Notify receiving hospital
    a) A radiation accident has occurred
    b) Number of victims who are contaminated and not contaminated
    c) Extent of the injuries
    d) Type of isotope[s]
    e) Update as necessary

F. Protection principles **(Slide 11-139)**
1. Limit exposure to the smallest portion of the body
2. Limit time of exposure
3. Maintain the greatest possible distance
4. Use suitable shielding
5. Limit exposures in lifesaving situations
6. Planned Occupational Exposures (emergency conditions)
    a) Risk benefit concept
    b) Doses cannot be specified but must be held to lowest limit
    c) Lifesaving actions: search and removal
        (1) Volunteers and/or professional rescue personnel
        (2) Should be broadly familiar with the consequences
        (3) Women capable of reproduction should not take part
        (4) Volunteers above the age of 45 should be selected
        (5) Planned dose to the whole body should not exceed 100 rem
        (6) Hands and forearms may receive additional dose of up to 200 rem
        (7) Internal exposure should be minimized by protective gear
        (8) Limited to once in a lifetime
        (9) Persons receiving exposures should avoid procreation for a period up to a few months
    d) Actions in less urgent circumstances
        (1) Volunteers should be broadly familiar with exposure consequences
        (2) Women capable of reproduction shall not take part
        (3) Planned whole body dose shall not exceed 25 rem
        (4) Planned dose of hands and forearms shall not exceed 100 rem
        (5) Internal exposure shall be minimized by protective gear
        (6) Actions should be limited to once in a lifetime (From NCRP Report No.39, pp 99-101)
7. Safety zone **(Slide 11-140)**
    a) A safety zone should be maintained
    b) Keep onlookers 150 ft away
    c) Contain area
8. Use of protective gear
    a) For greatest safety to the rescuers, protective clothing should be utilized (at minimum)
        (1) Gloves
        (2) Masks

Content

(3) Surgical gowns
(4) Shoe covers (or paper bags)
(5) Film badge with the name
(6) Large-size surgical trousers
(7) Pullover shirts
(8) Waterproof shoe covers
(a) Attached to the cuffs of trousers with tape
(b) Surgical gown is put on with a pair of surgical gloves, which can be taped to the sleeves
(9) A surgical hood and mask
(10) Second pair of surgical gloves
(11) Second dosimeter should be attached to the neck of the gown

b) Full protective clothing may be required depending on chemical nature of contaminants

9. Assessment
a) Exposure at life-threatening levels--rapid removal from the danger zone
b) ABC's should commence
c) Determine the relative safety
d) If contamination is the main hazard
(1) lifesaving care should be rendered to the victim after donning gear
(2) Avoid internal contamination from mouth-to-mouth ventilation
(3) Use other appropriate positive-pressure ventilation devices
e) Removing the victim's clothing will generally remove 80 to 90% of contamination
(1) Seal it in a plastic bag and label it
(2) Leave it in the contaminated zone
f) Rarely is the contaminated victim a threat to the rescuers
g) If the patient is contaminated
(1) Areas around wounds should be assessed and cleansed to prevent internal absorption
(2) Nares should be assayed with a cotton swab
h) If internal contamination, the time factor until medications are administered becomes important

10. Assaying for contamination **(Slide 11-141)**
a) External
(1) The radiologic monitor will assay for beta and gamma survey meter
(2) Record results along with the areas of distribution on a body diagram
(3) Survey directly over the wound or from samples of the wound secretions
(4) Wipes from the wounds may be saved as samples

Content

- b) Internal
    - (1) Nasal swabs and samples should be saved in tightly lidded and labeled containers
    - (2) Label all urine, vomitus, and feces
    - (3) This may be done at hospital depending on protocols

11. Treatment **(Slide 11-142)**
    - a) Decontamination
        - (1) Prevent or minimize transfer of contaminants to an internal site
        - (2) Reduce the amount of radiation dosage from the contaminant
        - (3) Prevent the spread of contamination to other persons and areas
    - b) Establishment of priorities **(Slide 11-143)**
        - (1) Care for contaminated wounds and body orifices first
        - (2) Then focus on areas with the highest levels of radioactivity
        - (3) Consider chemical properties
            - (a) Corrosive
            - (b) Toxic
            - (c) Soluble vs insoluble
            - (d) Do the guidelines for removal vary?
            - (e) Information may be available from consulting guides
        - (4) Remove the clothes and cover the patient with a blanket
        - (5) Contaminated clothing may be left at the site in labeled plastic bags
    - c) Removal from the intact skin **(Slide 11-144)**
        - (1) Limit mechanical, thermal, or chemical irritation to the skin
            - (a) Soft brush and gentle soaps should be used to avoid skin irritation
            - (b) Tepid water should be used
            - (c) Scrub the area gently for 3 to 4 minutes, rinse for 2 to 3 minutes
            - (d) Blot the area dry and remonitor
            - (e) Repeated scrubs may be necessary
            - (f) If contamination persists after 2 to 3 washes
                - i) Lava soap or;
                - ii) Half Tide detergent and half cornmeal can be used
            - (g) If still more decontamination, use Clorox full strength for small areas. Dilute solution for large areas if contamination persists
            - (h) Decontamination stops when radioactivity can not be reduced to a lower level
            - (i) Do not shave hair

Content

(j) Ambulatory patients can shower or a sink or basin can be used
(k) Use a clean towel following each shower. Avoid getting wash water into body orifices
(l) Water should be saved if feasible

d) Wounds and body orifices **(Slide 11-145)**
(1) Wounds
(a) Drape the area around the wound
(b) Irrigate repeatedly with saline, water, or 3% hydrogen peroxide
(c) Drapes and dressings should be removed as they become contaminated
(d) Use forceps to remove contaminated particles
(e) Embedded fragments may have to be removed surgically
(f) Monitor the irrigation fluid
(g) Remonitor the wound
(h) After decontaminated, cover with sterile waterproof dressing
(i) Decontaminate the area around the wound. Contaminated burns are treated as any other burn
(2) Body orifices
(a) Decontaminate by irrigation
(b) Alert patient may rinse, brush teeth, and spit out the fluid, avoiding swallowing
(c) Nasogastric tube may be passed to remove contaminated stomach contents
(d) With eyes, use a gentle stream diverted away nasal area

e) Internal contamination
(1) Treat as a medical emergency and obtain expert advice
(2) Special medications are needed to eliminate effects

f) Arrival at the hospital **(Slide 11-146)**
(1) Special entrance
(2) Notification
(3) Floor coverings
(4) Dirty areas
(5) The emergency physician and the radiation safety officer will meet the ambulance
(6) Physician will assess for life-threatening injuries
(7) Radiation safety officer determines whether the victim is contaminated
(8) The ambulance stretcher is placed on the covered floor
(9) Patient can then be transferred to a clean stretcher

(10) EMTs may be asked to remain in the ambulance until they are decontaminated
(a) Remove outer gloves first, turning them inside out as they are pulled off
(b) Give dosimeter to radiation safety officer
(c) Remove all tape at trouser cuffs and sleeves
(d) Remove outer surgical gown, turning it inside out; avoid shaking
(e) Remove surgical shirt
(f) Remove head cover
(g) Pull surgical trousers over shoe covers
(h) Remove shoe cover from foot
(i) Monitor shoe
(j) Step over the line, remove other shoe cover, and have other shoe monitored
(k) Remove inner gloves
(l) Feet and hands monitored for final time
(m) Shower

12. The transportation accident **(Slide 11-147)**
a) Perform lifesaving functions
b) If a pair of gloves and coveralls are present, put them on
c) Place the patient directly on a stretcher
d) Blanket may be placed over the patient
e) Move patient at least 20 yards from the accident vehicle if not moved immediately
f) Other people who are potentially contaminated
(1) Stay 20 yards away from vehicle
(2) Do not leave scene
g) Place a blanket under the stretcher and over patient
h) Notify the hospital
i) Notify the state police
j) Unwrap patient in dirty area
k) Lift the patient onto a clean hospital stretcher
l) EMT should remove outer clothing and place it in a plastic bag
m) Do not shake clothes or blanket
n) EMT should wash and shower
o) Should exit through same area
p) Multiple patients, return and proceed as described previously

Chapter 11

Section 4

Diving Accidents

Objectives
(Slide 11-148)

At the conclusion of the chapter the student will be able to:

1. **Define air embolism [from diving] and list the signs and symptoms.**
2. **Define decompression sickness and list the signs and symptoms.**
3. **List the general steps of management for a diving accident.**
4. **Explain the function of a hyperbaric chamber.**
5. **Describe the mechanism of barotrauma.**

Instructor Preparation

Reading preparation for the lesson:

EMT Prehospital Care, Chapter 11, pages 525-528

Optional reading:

Auerbach PS, Gheehr EC (eds):Management of Wilderness and Environmental Emergencies. New York, Macmillan, 1983

Suggested Learning Activities

Using a lecture format with the aid of slides, overhead transparencies, or charts, provide a presentation on diving accidents.

Provide case history examples of diving emergencies.

Content

XV. Diving accidents **(Slide 11-149)**

A. In 1984 there were approximately 2.8 mil SCUBA divers in the United States of America

B. Accident rate of 5/100,000

1. All types of injuries
2. Majority involve decompression sickness and air embolism

C. Physics and gases **(Slide 11-150)**

1. Definitions

a) Pressure

(1) Force applied per unit atmospheric area;

(2) Amount of pressure or force exerted by the earth's atmosphere varies with elevation

b) Gauge pressure

(1) Pressure being measured above atmospheric pressure

(2) In diving due to the pressure of water

(3) Atmospheric pressure not taken into account

c) Absolute pressure is gauge pressure plus atmospheric pressure

d) Ambient pressure--absolute pressure surrounding an object or diver

e) Hydrostatic pressure-pressure of a column of water above, and acting on a body immersed in the fluid

D. Pressure and the diver's body **(Slide 11-151)**

1. Exposed to atmosphere on surface of earth
2. Pressure becomes greater as we descend in water

a) One atmosphere = 14.7 lbs psi at sea level

b) Each additional 33 ft of water = one additional atmosphere of pressure

c) Gases in body can be compressed under pressure

d) Solid and liquid are not compressed

e) During descent nitrogen molecules dissolve in tissues

f) Breathing scuba tank, more nitrogen is loaded into the tissues

g) During gradual ascent nitrogen load reverses itself **(Slide 11-152)**

(1) Molecules move from the tissues to the blood and out with exhaled air

(2) Ordinarily occurs without complications

h) If diver surfaces rapidly (greater than 60 ft per minute)

(1) Gas within body will expand faster than it can be eliminated

(2) "Bubbler" of nitrogen will form in the tissues and within bloodstream

(3) Causes symptoms known as the "bends"

i) Hyperbaric chamber (recompression therapy) speeds up gas elimination process

Content

E. Decompression sickness **(Slide 11-153)**
   1. Bends or caissons disease
   2. Bubbles are carried by the bloodstream
      a) Brain, spinal cord
      b) Joints and muscles
      c) Inner ear
      d) Cause circulation blockage
   3. Over 50% of cases develop symptoms within one hour of the dive
   4. 90% within 6 hours
   5. Mild symptoms **(Slide 11-154)**
      a) Fatigue and weakness
      b) Skin rash
   6. Severe symptoms
      a) Pain
         (1) Localized
         (2) Deep burning pain in joints
         (3) Increases with time
      b) Paralysis or weakness
      c) Unstable walking
      d) Respiratory difficulties [chokes]
      e) Unconsciousness upon surfacing
      f) Spinal bends
         (1) Sharp back pain
         (2) Radiates to the front
         (3) Paresthesias of the extremities
         (4) Progress to unstable gait, then paralysis
   7. Risk factors **(Slide 11-155)**
      a) Older people with poor circulation
      b) Overweight people
      c) Scar tissue from past injuries
      d) Poor physical condition
      e) Fatigue
      f) Diving with a hangover
      g) Hard work at depth
      h) Cold water
      i) Multiple dives per day over a period of 7 to 10 days

F. Air embolism **(Slide 11-156)**
   1. Symptoms
      a) Bloody froth at the mouth
      b) Dizziness
      c) Visual blurring
      d) Disorientation
      e) Numbness or paralysis in extremities
      f) Convulsions
      g) Respiratory arrest

G. History **(Slide 11-157)**
   1. Did the victim breathe compressed air under water?
   2. How many dives have been made?
   3. What was the depth and bottom time of each dive?

Content

4. What was the surface interval between dives?
5. Type of equipment used?
6. Dive activity and environmental factors?
7. Type of entry into the water?
8. Presence of a buddy?
9. Kind of breathing gas used?

H. Emergency care **(Slide 11-158)**

1. Place victim on left side with head and chest inclined downward
2. Maintain open airway and prevent aspiration
3. Administer oxygen
4. Maintain body temperature
5. Give the conscious victim nonalcoholic liquids
6. IV fluids for unconscious victims
    a) Ringer's lactate
    b) Normal saline
7. Contact diving physician for consultation (National Divers Alert Network 919 684-8111)
8. In water, recompression should never be attempted

I. Barotrauma **(Slide 11-159)**

1. Diver is unable to equalize the pressure in the body's air-filled cavities during descent
2. Results in barotrauma or squeeze
3. Most commonly affected areas are ears
4. Can occur in sinuses, face, lungs, or total body in a dry diving suit
5. Caused by changing environmental pressures (flying or diving)
6. Middle ear maintains equal pressure via air movement through the eustachian tubes
7. Changes in pressure before equalization cause distortion and rupture of eardrum
    a) Normally pressure on inside of tympanic membrane matches that on outside
    b) If diver cannot equalize pressure due to blockage of the eustachian tube, rupture of the eardrum can result
    c) Patients with barotrauma of ear present with pain and/or hearing loss
    d) Upper respiratory infections may predispose patients to barotrauma
8. No prehospital treatment

Chapter 11

Section 5

Hazardous Materials

Objectives
(Slide 11-160)

At the conclusion of the chapter the student will be able to:

1. **Describe the genral protection principles used at a hazmat incident.**
2. **Describe the significance and uses of placards, labels and bills of lading in hazardous material accidents.**

Instructor Preparation

Reading preparation for the lesson:

EMT Prehospital Care, Chapter 11, pages 528-534

Optional reading:

United Sates Department of Transportation:Hazardous materials Guidebook:Guidebook for Hazardous Materials Incident. Washington, DC, Department of Transportation, 1984

Suggested Learning Activities

Using a lecture format with the aid of slides, overhead transparencies, or charts, provide a presentation on hazardous materials.

Provide case history examples of hazmat incidents.

Content

XVI. Hazardous materials
- A. Overview **(Slide 11-161)**
  1. First rule of a hazmat incident - do no harm
  2. Hazmat incident may not be obvious to bystanders and EMS personnel
     - a) Both may be in great danger
     - b) Danger may not be evident immediately
     - c) Signs and symptoms may be delayed
  3. EMT must utilize other resources i.e. police, fire, federal agencies to be effective
- B. Safety rules **(Slide 11-162)**
  1. Responding EMTs should wear full turn-out gear
     - a) Helmet
     - b) Coat
     - c) Gloves
     - d) Self-contained-breathing-apparatus (when appropriate)
       - (1) Personnel must be trained in its use
       - (2) Gear can be hazardous when used improperly
  2. Primary responsibility of EMT is to provide emergency care
     - a) Hazmat incident control is usually the function of rescue or fire personnel
     - b) EMT may assume a safety role prior to arrival of hazmat team
     - c) After hazmat team arrival EMT should focus on medical care

  3. The scene **(Slide 11-163)**
     - a) One's senses provide information when arriving on hazmat scene
       - (1) Look at scene from distance whenever possible
       - (2) Use binoculars if available
       - (3) Remain upwind
       - (4) Observe for smoke indicating ignition of material
       - (5) Listen for noises suggesting explosions of leaks of material
       - (6) If strange odor is noted retreat to safer location
       - (7) If scene is safe initiate rescue efforts
       - (8) If you suspect dangers contact support personnel
     - b) Staging area **(Slide 11-164)**
       - (1) Area where assessment and care is provided prior to transport
       - (2) Identify early in the call
       - (3) Factors in selecting a staging area
         - (a) Is it far enough from scene of incident to be safe?
         - (b) Is it upwind and/or uphill to avoid gas or run off from scene?
         - (c) Can decontamination be done in this area safely?
         - (d) Will it allow easy flow of vehicles to and from the scene?

Content

c) Identification of hazardous materials **(Slide 11-165)**
(1) Overview
(a) Very important early in the response
(b) Special precautions and equipment may be needed
(c) The need for decontamination must be identified early
(d) Unique actions may be required based on type of material
(2) Methods for identification
(a) Placards **(Slide 11-166)**
i) Signs that identify material
ii) Specific by color, symbols, category name, and numbers
iii) Located on vehicles
iv) Time is a crucial factor
v) Vehicle may not be appropriately marked
(b) Bill of lading **(Slide 11-160)**
i) Usually stored on vehicle
ii) Identifies material and special information
(c) Hazmat guidebook **(Slide 11-167)**
i) Number of books available on hazmat i.e.
i) United Sates Department of Transportation: Emergency response guidebook to initial response to hazardous materials incident. Published by Department of Transportation
ii) Provide information on various materials
iii) Should be carried in all vehicles
ii) Uses placard and other identification systems to identify product
iii) Provides important safety information
(d) Chemical transport emergency center (Chemtrec) **(Slide 11-168)**
i) Agency provides advice on hazmat incidents
ii) Available 24 hrs/day, 7 days a week
iii) Telephone number 1-800-424-9300
iv) Communication usually occurs through coordinating agency
v) You should have the following information when calling
i) Identification number of product
ii) Name of product
iii) Name of manufacture
iv) Name of shipper
v) Type of vehicle or container involved
vi) Location of incident
vii) Weather conditions
viii) Particulars of the site
ix) Name and number of contact person

Content

(e) Other resources are available
i) Consult local protocols
ii) Follow local guidelines

C. Communications **(Slide 11-169)**
1. One of the most important elements of hazmat response
2. Whenever possible, all pertinent Information should be retrieved from the dispatcher
3. Upon arriving at the scene the following should be relayed to the dispatcher
a) Concise overview of situation
b) Estimated number of victims
c) Identification of hazardous material
d) Immediate dangers i.e. gas, explosion, fire, etc.
e) Type of assistance needed
f) Status of scene
(1) Safety of public
(2) Traffic
(3) Weather
(4) Wind direction
g) Information described above for chemtrec
4. Dispatch frequency must be controlled for important communications
5. Interagency communication on scene **(Slide 11-170)**
a) Appropriate frequency allocation for incidents must be planned in advance
b) Coordination of resources is an essential aspect of a hazmat scene
c) Codes must also be determined to reduce inappropriate radio time
d) Where radio communication is impaired "runners" may be used for on-scene communication

D. Incident command and triage **(Slide 11-171)**
1. Command
a) Same principles as disaster management
b) Person ultimately in charge of the disaster response
c) Fire or police chief, EMS chief, mayor or county executive
d) May vary with type of incident or political structure
2. Triage
a) Safety is most important factor during triage
b) Same principles as disaster
c) Triage may be conducted on scene or staging area depending on incident
d) Equipment should be readily available to treat and transport victims

E. Decontamination **(Slide 11-172)**
1. Take victim to safe area where clothing can be removed and initial washdown can take place
a) Should not be the staging area
b) Should be warm enough to permit irrigation of patient
c) Run off from wash down should be carefully controlled

Content

2. Washdown of exposed areas must be done for a minimum of 10-15 minutes
    a) Some material may not be washed away with water
    b) Consultation with experts should be done first
    c) Make sure that run off does not endanger other persons
    d) Protective clothing for rescue personnel is essential
    e) SCUBA may be needed in some instances
3. Move patient to another area for second wash down and patient care
4. Decontaminate vehicle prior to secondary response
5. Place or clothing or other contaminated material in appropriate container

XVII. Patient care **(Slide 11-173)**

A. Principles for patient care are no different for hazmat incident
1. A,B,Cs
2. Spinal immobilization considerations when appropriate
3. Self protection is essential

B. Example protocol (Adapted from New York City Emergency Medical Services. Basic Life Support Treatment Protocols, New York, New York, 1990)
1. Always do 10 second survey
2. Never underestimate size of the spill or incident
3. Establish and maintain communications with borough or citywide dispatcher
4. Stay upwind and upgrade at all times
5. Monitor weather and wind changes
6. Do not breathe any smoke, fumes, or vapors
7. Do not touch or walk through any spilled materials
8. Do not eat, drink or smoke at incident scene
9. Do not touch your face, mouth, or eyes
10. Eliminate all sources of ignition, such as, flares, flames, sparks, smoking, flashes, flashlights, gas and diesel engines, and portable radios
11. Do not drive through spilled materials
12. Identify substance if possible using DOT emergency response guidebook
13. Inform dispatcher of your findings
14. Observe all safety precautions and directions as set forth by incident commander, police, fire department, EPA, DEP
15. All orders should be taken face to face
16. Remain clear of all restricted ares until declared safe by incident commander

Chapter 11

ENVIRONMENTAL EMERGENCIES

Examination

1. Heat is distributed throughout the body by the:

   a. respiratory system
   b. nervous system
   c. digestive system
   d. cardiovascular system

2. The metabolism necessary to maintain cellular function at rest is called the __________ metabolism:

   a. central
   b. basal
   c. autonomic
   d. vascular

3. Heat can be lost from the body through:

   a. radiation, conduction, respiration, shivering
   b. respiration, convection, shivering, radiation
   c. radiation, evaporation, respiration, convection
   d. evaporation, shivering, convection, conduction

4. Radiation is the:

   a. transfer of heat from a warmer environment to a cooler environment that is not in direct contact with the body
   b. transfer of heat to objects in direct contact with the body
   c. loss of heat that occurs when moisture vaporizes on the body's surface
   d. movement of warm air around the body by air currents and the replacement of this warm air with cooler air

5. Convection is the:

   a. transfer of heat from a warmer environment to a cooler environment that is not in direct contact with the body
   b. transfer of heat to objects in direct contact with the body
   c. loss of heat that occurs when moisture vaporizes on the body's surface
   d. movement of warm air around the body by air currents and the replacement of this warm air with cooler air

6. When the environmental temperature approaches or exceeds body temperature, _________ is the only mechanism of heat loss:

   a. convection
   b. evaporation
   c. radiation
   d. respiration

7. Under normal conditions, most heat loss occurs via

   a. evaporation
   b. conduction
   c. convection
   d. radiation

8. The body's "thermostat," which regulates temperature by influencing the metabolic rate, the cardiovascular system, and the skin, is located on the:

   a. cerebellum
   b. brainstem
   c. hypothalamus
   d. pituitary

9. Under heat stress, when the skin vessels are dilated, the blood flow to the skin can increase to _____ ml per minute:

   a. 1000
   b. 2000
   c. 3000
   d. 4000

10. The three general types of heat emergencies are:

   a. heat cramps, heat exhaustion, heat prostration
   b. heat cramps, heat stroke, febrile seizures
   c. heat cramps, heat exhaustion, heat stroke
   d. heat stroke, heat hyperdiaphoresis, heat prostration

11. The group of individuals who are at increased risk of heat emergencies includes:

   a. teenagers
   b. men between 30 and 50
   c. women between 30 and 50
   d. the very young and the very old

Match the explanations in column B to the predisposing factors of heat-related emergencies in column A.

Column A		Column B	
12.	heart disease	a.	compromised cardiovascular response
13.	obesity	b.	increased insulation results in less heat loss
14.	febrile illness	c.	increased heat production
15.	Parkinson's disease	d.	muscle tremors produce heat
16.	mental retardation	e.	inability to care for themselves

17. Alcohol causes ________________ and can cause a gain in heat when the environmental temperature is above body temperature.

    a. vasoconstriction
    b. vasodilation
    c. increased pulse
    d. high blood pressure

18. The treatment for heat cramps includes:

    a. moving the patient to a cooler environment
    b. covering the patient with a blanket to prevent hypothermia
    c. placing ice under the armpits to rapidly cool the patient
    d. administering IV fluids rapidly that have been cooled in a refrigerator

Match the signs and symptoms in column B with the heat-related condition in column A.

Column A		Column B	
19.	Heat cramps	a.	very high temperature, dry skin, altered mental state
20.	Heat stroke	b.	muscular cramps following exercise
21.	Heat exhaustion	c.	weakness, cool sweaty skin, rapid pulse, and elevated core temperature

22. The treatment of heat stroke includes:

    a. cooling with an alcohol sponge bath, rapid transport and oxygen, fanning with wet sheets on the body
    b. cooling with an alcohol sponge bath, rapid cooling with ice at arterial points, rapid transport and oxygen
    c. rapid transport and oxygen, cooling with ice at arterial points, fanning with wet sheets on the body
    d. covering the patient with blankets to prevent hypothermia, rapid transport and oxygen, fanning with wet sheets on the body

23. A core body temperature less than 35°*C*, best defines:

    a. frostbite
    b. chilblains
    c. hypothermia
    d. frostnip

24. The involuntary contraction of small groups of muscles that can generate great amounts of heat is called:

    a. vasoconstriction
    b. shivering
    c. peristalsis
    d. muscle flexion

25. The first signs that the central nervous system is affected owing to hypothermia include:

    a. coma and delayed capillary refill
    b. amnesia and slurred speech
    c. stupor and hypotension
    d. coma and bradycardia

26. Acute immersion hypothermia is a very severe form of cold injury because:

    a. water is a very good conductor of heat
    b. water vapors freeze your nasal mucosa
    c. inhalation of water causes bronchoconstriction
    d. cold water causes vasodilation and shock

Categorize the items in column A as either mild, moderate, or severe signs or symptoms of hypothermia.

Column A		Column B	
27.	unresponsive to pain	a.	mild
28.	significant hypotension	b.	moderate
29.	difficulty in speech	c.	severe
30.	shivering		
31.	muscular rigidity		
32.	ventricular fibrillation		
33.	slowing of pulse and respirations		

34. The goals of the prehospital treatment of hypothermia are to:

    a. completely rewarm the patient in the field
    b. reduce further heat loss and transport rapidly
    c. administer 100% oxygen and hyperventilate the patient
    d. hyperventilate the patient if respiratory assistance is needed

35. Which of the active rewarming techniques are recommended for field use:

    a. gastric lavage with warm fluids through a nasogastric tube
    b. warm IV fluids and peritoneal lavage
    c. warmed humidified oxygen and warm packs at arterial points, e.g., armpits
    d. applying battery-operated heated electric blankets

36. To combat hypoperfusion CPR should be started on hypothermic patients when:

    a. the pulse drops below 50
    b. the pulse drops below 40
    c. the pulse drops below 30
    d. pulselessness is absolutely certain

37. A completely reversible cold injury secondary to intense vasoconstriction to cold exposure is called:

    a. frostnip
    b. chilblains
    c. deep frostbite
    d. superficial frostbite

38. The cold injury that may involve the freezing of subcutaneous tissues, muscle, and tendons is called:

    a. frostnip
    b. chilblains
    c. deep frostbite
    d. superficial frostbite

39. If a frostbitten foot should thaw prior to arrival at the hospital, you should:

    a. break blisters to relieve pressure
    b. cover with sterile dressings
    c. encourage the person to walk to improve circulation
    d. rub the foot with snow to prevent total rewarming

40. In a wilderness situation where transport is not possible, rewarming of a localized cold injury should be performed at water temperatures of:

    a. 100°F
    b. 102°F
    c. 105°F
    d. 110°F

41. A patient has been burned by hot water. This type of injury is called a(n) __________ injury:

    a. electrical
    b. thermal
    c. chemical
    d. aqueous

42. The most common toxin in smoke that is produced by burning material is:

    a. carbon dioxide
    b. carbon tetrachloride
    c. carbon monoxide
    d. carbon chloride

43. The organ most commonly injured by thermal burns is the:

    a. skin
    b. lungs
    c. arterial system
    d. heart

44. The two most critical variables in thermal burn injuries are:

    a. degree of heat and length of exposure
    b. type of heat and thickness of skin
    c. distance from patient and pigment of skin
    d. age of patient and pigment of skin

45. Skin that is reddened and is dry and warm to the touch best describes a ___ degree burn:

    a. first
    b. second
    c. third
    d. fourth

46. Which layer(s) are injured in a second degree burn?

    a. the dermis
    b. the subcutaneous
    c. the fatty tissue
    d. the fascia

47. Which of the following burn areas are likely to be most painful:

    a. first degree
    b. second degree
    c. third degree
    d. forth degree

48. A burn injury that extends completely around a body part such as an arm is called a __________ burn:

    a. complete
    b. circular
    c. conclusive
    d. circumferential

Match the burned body parts in column A to the correct percentage in column B.

Column A		Column B	
49.	a baby's entire head	a.	46%
50.	both legs of an adult	b.	27%
51.	both arms and the entire torso	c.	18%
52.	an adult's entire head	d.	9%
53.	both legs, the genitalia, and one arm of an adult	e.	36%
54.	The anterior surface of the torso and the entire head in the adult	f.	54%

55. Calculation of the extent of burns is made according to:

    a. the rules of nine
    b. 20% for each extremity and 20% for the torso
    c. the burn degree scale
    d. the type of burn injury

56. Which of the following body areas are considered "critical" when evaluating a burn patient:

    a. armpits, perineum, face
    b. face, genitalia, chest
    c. perineum, face, genitalia
    d. face, back, hands

Indicate which of the following burn management steps are correct prehospital care by TRUE (T) or FALSE (F):

57. ______ apply sterile dressing

58. ______ stop the burning process

59. ______ cover burns with ointments

60. ______ apply cool compress if burn is greater than 20%

61. ______ maintain body temperature

62. The most common cause of death from fires is:

    a. severe burns
    b. infection
    c. airway obstruction
    d. smoke inhalation

63. A toxic gas that has an affinity for hemoglobin 200 times greater than does oxygen is:

    a. nitrogen
    b. carbon dioxide
    c. carbon monoxide
    d. helium

64. The cherry-red color that occurs with carbon monoxide poisoning comes from:

    a. the color of carboxyhemoglobin
    b. inadequate tissue perfusion
    c. increased carbon dioxide in the blood
    d. decreased oxygen in the blood

65. You should initiate immediate and thorough irrigation of the injured area for patients suffering from:

    a. electrical burns
    b. first-degree burns
    c. chemical burns
    d. thermal burns

Match the <u>specific</u> treatments that are needed (either in the emergency department or in the industrial setting) in column B to the agent in column A.

Column A		Column B	
66.	dried calcium oxide	a.	submerge in water
67.	phosphorus	b.	application of calcium gluconate dressing
68.	sodium and potassium metals	c.	cover with petroleum jelly
69.	hydrofluoric acid	d.	brush off before irrigation
70.	phenols	e.	irrigat with 2:1 mixture of polyethylene glycol and mentholated spirits

71. Electricity is often described in terms of the following three variables:

    a. amperage, capacity, wattage
    b. wattage, voltage, resilience
    c. wattage, amperage, capacity
    d. amperage, voltage, resistance

72. When electric current passes through the body it:

    a. stays on the skin's surface
    b. follows an internal path of least resistance
    c. dissipates quickly once it encounters the bone
    d. causes minor damage internally and extensive damage externally

73. Which of the following materials provides the <u>greatest</u> degree of resistance to electrical flow:

a. water
b. rubber
c. copper
d. steel

74. High-voltage traveling through air that generates intense heat that can cause thermal burns is called an:

a. air burn
b. jump burn
c. light burn
d. arc burn

75. The property possessed by some elements of spontaneously emitting alpha and beta particles and gamma rays by the disintegration of nuclei of its atoms best defines:

a. radiation
b. ionizing radiation
c. isotope
d. radioactivity

76. The term used to describe a person or substance exposed to ionizing radiation is called:

a. contamination
b. irradiated
c. roentgen
d. radioactive

77. The time required for a radioactive substance to lose 50% of its activity by decay is called:

a. radioactive loss equation
b. contamination safety time zone
c. physical half-life
d. isotope frequency rate

Match the type of radiation in column B to the description in column A.

Column A		Column B	
78.	The least penetrating form of radiation, which travels only a few centimeters in the air	a.	alpha
		b.	gamma
79.	High-energy electromagnetic radiation similar to x-rays. Can penetrate and cause severe damage to tissues, but cannot contaminate others in contact with the patient	c.	beta
80.	Can travel one foot to several and can penetrate into the dermal layer of the skin. Also can contaminate the patient and make him a danger to others		

81. A dosimeter is used to measure the:

a. radiation emitted over 1 minute's time
b. total accumulation of radiation
c. rate of exposure in roentgens per hour
d. type of radiation present

82. A Geiger counter is used to measure the:

a. radiation emitted over 1 minute's time
b. total accumulation of radiation
c. rate of exposure in roentgens per hour
d. type of radiation present

83. All of the following are factors that affect the severity of a radiation exposure <u>except</u>:

a. type of radiation
b. the temperature in the area
c. area of the body exposed
d. distance from the source

84. A national organization that can be consulted in the event of a radiation injury for information on how to proceed goes by which of the following initials:

a. AHA
b. REACTS
c. NACOT
d. RADS

85. A syndrome that may occur when high doses of radiation are absorbed over a short period of time, and results from damage to the bone marrow is called:

    a. radiation toxicity
    b. radiation necrosis
    c. hyperradiation syndrome
    d. acute radiation syndrome

86. The DOT emergency response guidebook recommends a safety zone at a radiation accident should be at least ________ feet upwind from the accident.

    a. 50
    b. 100
    c. 150
    d. 500

87. Prior to bringing a contaminated patient into the emergency department you should:

    a. identify the correct designated "dirty" path and room to bring the patient to
    b. remove all blankets from the patient and carry them into the emergency department
    c. remove your protective clothing and bring the patient to the room
    d. hand-carry all contaminated material in before you bring the patient into the emergency room

Match the definition in column B to the term in column A that is connected with diving and its effects on the human body.

Column A	Column B
88. hydrostatic pressure	a. amount of force exerted by earth's atmosphere, which varies with elevation
89. atmospheric pressure	b. gauge pressure plus atmospheric pressure
90. absolute pressure	c. pressure of a column of water above and acting on a body immersed in it

91. When a diver ascends too rapidly (faster than 60 feet/minute) nitrogen "bubbles" can form in tissues and the bloodstream, resulting in a condition called decompression sickness, Caisson disease, or:

    a. barotrauma
    b. altitude sickness
    c. hydroencephalopathy
    d. the bends

92. A form of decompression sickness that is caused by nitrogen bubbles forming in the spinal cord is called:

    a. central neurogenic bends
    b. posterior bends
    c. spinal bends
    d. cord parathesia

93. The most dangerous problem a diver can develop is:

    a. an air embolism
    b. central neurogenic hyperventilation
    c. pleurisy
    d. blurred vision

94. The deep and burning pain of decompression sickness is most often felt in the ______________ since this area can least tolerate the expansion of tissues.

    a. mid thigh
    b. joints
    c. head
    d. chest

95. Decompression in a hyperbaric chamber is:

    a. a treatment for decompression sickness utilized at least one week after the injury
    b. useful only if initiated within 1 hour of the injury
    c. the definitive treatment for decompression sickness
    d. not as useful as recompression in the water

96. When the diver is unable to equalize the pressure differential in the body's air-filled cavities during descent, the result can be:

    a. barotrauma
    b. altitude sickness
    c. hydroencephalopathy
    d. the bends

97. The primary responsibility of an EMT at a hazardous material incident is:

    a. containment
    b. decontamination
    c. emergency medical care
    d. removal

98. When reacting to a documented HAZMAT incident it is important to establish a treatment and transport location for the patient, called a:

    a. command center
    b. staging area
    c. communications area
    d. transport area

99. Signs that identify hazardous materials by color, symbols, category names, and numbers are called:

    a. the bill of lading
    b. computerized HAZMAT identification system
    c. material data safety sheets
    d. placards

100. A 24-hour-a-day resource service available to provide advice on how to handle chemical emergencies is the:

    a. chemical transport emergency center (CHEMTREC)
    b. computerized hazmat identification system (CHIS)
    c. United States Department of Transportation emergency response guide (USDOT-ERG)
    d. medical decontamination task force advisory board (MDTFAB)

Chapter 12

MEDICAL EMERGENCIES

Materials and Equipment for Lesson

1. Anatomy slides, overhead transparencies, drawings or flipcharts
2. Handouts
   - Diabetic emergencies
   - Anaphylaxis
   - Poisons and overdose
   - Communicable diseases
3. Slide projector, overhead projector, flipchart and/or blackboard

Section 1

Diabetic Emergencies

Objectives
(Slide 12-1)

At the conclusion of the chapter the students will be able to:	
1.	Define diabetes.
2.	Describe the purpose and function of insulin.
3.	List 4 signs or symptoms of diabetic coma.
4.	List 4 signs or symptoms of insulin shock (hypoglycemia).
5.	Describe the predisposing causes of insulin shock.
6.	Describe the predisposing causes of diabetic coma.

Instructor Preparation

Reading preparation for the lesson:

EMT Prehospital Care, Chapter 12, pages 538-545

Suggested Learning Activities
Using a lecture format with the aid of slides, overhead transparencies or charts, provide a presentation on diabetic emergencies. **Provide case history examples of diabetic emergencies.**

Content

I. Diabetes overview **(Slide 12-2)**
   A. A disease that results from inadequate secretion of insulin
   B. Insulin helps regulate utilization and storage of glucose
   C. Glucose is a sugar molecule used by the cells for energy
      1. Absorbed after eating into the bloodstream
      2. Glucose rises, insulin is secreted and moves glucose into cells
      3. Used for energy or stored for future use
   D. Body depends on glucose for basic energy needs
   E. Most cells also use other sources of fuel
   F. Brain depends almost exclusively on glucose
      1. When deprived, brain function is altered
      2. Unconsciousness, seizures and cell death can occur
   G. Complications of diabetes
      1. Related to too high or low a blood sugar
      2. From the abnormal metabolism due to lack of insulin
      3. Two major life threatening conditions
         a) Diabetic ketoacidosis (diabetic coma)
         b) Hypoglycemia (low blood sugar or insulin shock)

II. Regulation of glucose metabolism **(Slide 12-3)**
   A. Actions of insulin **(Slide 12-4)**
      1. Produced in specialized cells in pancreas, called the islets of langerhans
      2. Glucose rises in the blood after a meal
      3. Body secretes insulins
      4. Causes movement of glucose and other food products into cell
         a) Immediate utilization as fuel
         b) Storage for future needs
         c) Stored in liver and muscle as glycogen
         d) Converted into adipose tissue
         e) After transfer, blood glucose falls
         f) Insulin secretion is reduced
      5. Body uses glucose and fats for fuel
      6. Between meals, fats are utilized
      7. Brain must have adequate supply of glucose
      8. Brain cannot burn fats for its energy needs
   B. Actions of glucagon **(Slide 12-5)**
      1. Causes stored glucose to be released and to be synthesized from other molecules
      2. Secreted in different cells in pancreas than insulin
      3. Secreted when blood sugar falls
      4. Glycogen converts to glucose molecules, which enter blood
      5. Cells make glucose from other molecules
      6. Actions of insulin and glucagon maintain constant glucose levels after eating and between meals
      7. Also released during exercise or stress or reduced periods of intake
      8. Glucagon can be injected to treat hypoglycemia

Content

C. Actions of epinephrine **(Slide 12-6)**
1. Released during stress or exercise
2. Has a glucagon like effect
3. In hypoglycemia causes release of glucose from liver
4. During stress increases supply of glucose and fat
5. Signs of epinephrine release may be noted with hypoglycemia
    a) Pale, cool skin
    b) Tachycardia
    c) Sweating
    d) Normal or slightly elevated blood pressure

III. Diabetes **(Slide 12-7)**

A. Relative or absolute lack of insulin

B. Untreated patient would have high blood glucose with loss in the urine and abnormal metabolism

C. Type I - insulin dependent diabetics **(Slide 12-8)**
1. Severe or absolute lack of insulin
2. Juvenile diabetes
3. Require treatment with insulin
4. Must be injected intramuscularly on daily basis
5. Careful attention to their diet
6. Different types of insulin: pork, beef, human DNA
7. Different formulations which vary in time of onset, peak effect and duration
    a) Can be mixed or taken at different times
    b) To manage predictable peaks of glucose
    c) Adjusted to lifestyle and metabolism
8. Must balance food intake with medication
    a) Insulin intake and no food = hypoglycemia
    b) Overeat and no insulin = diabetic ketoacidosis
9. Other factors affecting balance
    a) Infections and fever may increase insulin need; exercise increases the glucose requirements
    b) Diabetics learn to adjust food intake and insulin
    c) Test urine or blood for glucose

D. Type II - non-insulin-dependent diabetics **(Slide 12-9)**
1. Develop diabetes later in life
2. May not require insulin injections
3. Maturity onset diabetes
4. Some can control by diet alone
5. Others require oral medications
6. Some require insulin

E. Complications of diabetes **(Slide 12-10)**
1. Accelerated atherosclerosis
2. Narrowing of vessels
    a) Coronary artery disease
    b) Cerebrovascular disease
    c) Kidney disease
    d) Blindness
    e) Ulcers on distal lower extremities

Content

3. Nerve damage **(Slide 12-11)**
    a) Symmetrical (bilateral) loss of sensation
    b) Numbness, pain
    c) Combination of impaired circulation and nerve damage cause "diabetic foot"
        (1) Repeated traumas to foot due to loss of sensation
        (2) Failure to heal due to poor circulation
        (3) Gangrene or necrosis of the toes results
4. Protein depletion, weight loss, and weakness
5. Prone to infections
6. Infections can cause diabetic ketoacidosis

IV. Diabetic emergencies **(Slide 12-12)**
  A. Diabetic ketoacidosis (DKA)
    1. Relatively prolonged insulin deficiency
    2. Blood glucose rises
    3. Fatty acids are produced in blood
    4. Can be life threatening
    5. Types of patients **(Slide 12-13)**
        a) Known diabetic who fails to balance insulin and diet
        b) Diabetics stressed by illness, infections, and fever
        c) Diabetics with severe disease
        d) First presentation of diabetes
    6. Onset is gradual, may take days to two weeks
    7. Signs and symptoms of DKA **(Slide 12-14)**
        a) Signs of dehydration
            (1) Glucose rises in blood
            (2) Excess is excreted in the urine and pulls water along; signs of dehydration:
                (a) Urinate frequently (polyuria)
                (b) Increased thirst (polydipsia)
                (c) Increased appetite (polyphagia)
                (d) Vomiting worsens fluid loss and prevents replacement
            (3) Abdominal pain is frequent in children
            (4) If uncorrected, hypovolemic shock develops
        b) Signs of acidosis **(Slide 12-15)**
            (1) Body shifts to fat metabolism
            (2) By-products include fatty acids (ketoacids)
            (3) Blood becomes acidotic
            (4) Some acids converted to acetone
            (5) Acetone vaporizes and causes fruity breath odor
            (6) Body breathes faster and harder to blow off carbon dioxide (carbonic acid)
            (7) Deep and rapid breathing is called Kussmaul's
            (8) Acidosis alters consciousness and coma occurs
        c) Dehydration leads to vascular collapse and death
        d) Correction of dehydration and acidosis, and insulin is needed
        e) Hyperosmolar coma **(Slide 12-16)**
            (1) Signs similar to DKA

Content

(2) Elevated glucose, dehydration
(3) No acidosis
(4) Altered mental status
(5) No ketone breath and hyperventilation
f) Alcoholics **(Slide 12-17)**
(1) Can develop ketoacidosis without hyperglycemia
(2) Due to fasting and breakdown of alcohol by the liver
(3) May even be hypoglycemic
(4) Have ketone odors and hyperventilation
g) Distinctions in field not important **(Slide 12-18)**

B. Hypoglycemia **(Slide 12-19)**
1. Abnormally low blood sugar
2. Most common and treatable diabetic problem
3. Types of patients
a) Failure to balance food intake with insulin administration
(1) Took insulin
(2) Missed meals
(3) Insulin action peaks and glucose falls
b) Insulin-secreting tumors
c) Prolonged fasting
d) Administration of hypoglycemic drugs
e) Liver failure
f) Alcohol consumption and fasting
g) Excessive insulin secretion
4. Signs and symptoms **(Slide 12-20)**
a) Altered mental status, extremely variable
(1) Combativeness, hostility and bizarre behavior (mistaken for psychosis)
(2) Sleepy or lethargic
(3) Confusion
(4) Seizures or coma
(5) If untreated, leads to brain death
b) Early signs **(Slide 12-21)**
(1) Hunger
(2) Nausea
(3) Uneasiness, weakness
(4) Increased salivation
c) Later signs (adrenaline release) **(Slide 12-22)**
(1) Tachycardia
(2) Cold, pale, clammy skin
(3) Dilated pupils
(4) Increased nervousness and trembling
(5) Excitability
d) Signs and symptoms vary from patient to patient
e) Some ambulances test glucose level with blood sticks

V. Assessment of diabetic patient **(Slide 12-23)**
A. Patients or family may offer diabetic history as part of chief complaint
B. Altered mental status, bizarre behavior, seizures, or coma
C. Shortness of breath or abdominal pain (DKA)

Content

D. History of present illness **(Slide 12-24)**
  1. Patient has taken insulin and not eaten?
  2. Patient has not taken insulin?
  3. Frequent urination, thirst and hunger?
  4. When did you last take your medications?
  5. When did you last eat?
  6. When did you measure blood or urine?
  7. What were the results? **(Slide 12-25)**
  8. Do you test your urine for acetone?
  9. When and what were the results?
  10. Recent infection or stress?
  11. Have you taken sugar or glucagon?
  12. Have you had similar episodes in the past?
  13. If so, what was the problem?

E. Past medical history **(Slide 12-26)**
  1. Diabetes
  2. Heart disease
  3. High blood pressure
  4. COPD

F. Physical exam **(Slide 12-27)**
  1. Kussmaul's respiration?
  2. Breath odor
  3. Signs of dehydration
  4. Evidence of adrenaline release?

VI. Treatment of diabetic patients **(Slide 12-28)**

A. Primary treatments
  1. Administration of oral or intravenous glucose
  2. Administration of intramuscular glucagon
  3. Either can rapidly reverse a hypoglycemia

B. Conscious patients
  1. Oral glucose solutions are preferred
  2. Soda, juices, mix sugar in water
  3. Other glucose-rich solutions

C. Unconscious patients
  1. Cannot be given oral fluids
  2. Some systems allow EMTs to administer IV glucose or IM glucagon
  3. Test for gag reflex (tongue blade on back of throat)
  4. No gag reflex or patient is lethargic **(Slide 12-29)**
    a) IV glucose
      (1) Intravenous 50 ml of a 50% solution of glucose can be administered
      (2) Pre-treatment blood sample drawn to test for glucose at the hospital
    b) Intramuscular glucagon **(Slide 12-30)**
      (1) Can increase blood sugar in 8 - 10 minutes
      (2) Usually responds in 5 -20 minutes
      (3) May not work in some patients
        (a) Very young children
        (b) Alcoholics

Content

(c) Malnourished individuals
(4) Give 1 mg. intramuscularly
c) Intramuscular injection (glucagon)
(1) Assemble equipment **(Slide 12-31)**
(2) Check medication **(Slide 12-32)**
(3) Wipe top of diluting solution **(Slide 12-33)**
(4) Inject air and draw solution **(Slide 12-34)**
(5) Wipe top of medication **(Slide 12-35)**
(6) Injected solution **(Slide 12-36)**
(7) Shake vial to mix **(Slide 12-37)**
(8) Withdraw solution
(9) Select site (mid deltoid) **(Slide 12-38)**
(10) Prep site **(Slide 12-39)**
(11) Inject at 90° angle **(Slide 12-40, 12-41)**
(12) Check for blood **(Slide 12-42)**
(13) Inject medication **(Slide 12-43)**
(14) Remove needle **(Slide 12-44)**
(15) Massage area
(16) Properly dispose of needle and syringe

D. Supportive care **(Slide 12-45)**
1. Airway management
2. Supplemental oxygen
3. Maintenance of body temperature
4. Proper positioning appropriate for shock or coma
5. Rapid transport

Section 2

Anaphylaxis

Objectives
(Slide 12-46)

At the conclusion of the chapter the students will be able to:
1. List 2 signs and symptoms of anaphylaxis for each of the following body systems: **Skin and general signs** **Cardiovascular System** **Respiratory System**
2. List 3 common agents which cause anaphylaxis.
3. State the prehospital emergency care for a patient suffering an anaphylactic

Instructor Preparation

Reading preparation for the lesson:

EMT Prehospital Care, Chapter 12, pages 546-552

Optional reading:

Schwartz GR (ed):Principles and Practices of Emergency Medicine. 2nd ed. Philadelphia, W.B. Saunders, 1986.

Suggested Learning Activities
Using a lecture format with the aid of slides, overhead transparencies or charts, provide a presentation on anaphylactic emergencies. **Provide case history examples of anaphylactic emergencies.**

Content

VII. Anaphylaxis overview **(Slide 12-47)**
- A. Allergic condition
- B. Antibody-antigen reaction
- C. Release of substances which can cause shock, bronchoconstriction and airway obstruction
- D. Can be extremely rapid and result in death within minutes

VIII. Pathophysiology **(Slide 12-48)**
- A. Antibody - antigen reactions **(Slide 12-49)**
  - 1. Antigen - substance which is recognized as foreign to the body
  - 2. Antibody - protein that combines with antigen to neutralize toxins or fight infection
  - 3. Helpful in fighting disease and toxic ingestions
  - 4. Take place all of the time
  - 5. Anaphylaxis - an antigen-antibody reaction gone "haywire"
- B. In anaphylaxis: **(Slide 12-50)**
  - 1. Reaction releases chemicals such as histamine
  - 2. Blood vessels dilate and capillaries leak
  - 3. Blood pressure falls, resulting in distributive shock
  - 4. Plasma leakage causes swelling of face, mouth, tongue and other airway structures
  - 5. Person must be previously exposed to antigen
  - 6. Antibodies are then formed
  - 7. Attach to specialized cells which release chemicals
  - 8. Reexposure activates anaphylactic response
  - 9. Common manifestations involve skin, respiratory, circulatory and gastrointestinal systems
- C. Common agents which cause anaphylaxis **(Slide 12-51)**
  - 1. Antibiotics and other drugs
    - a) Penicillin
    - b) Cephalosporins (Keflex, etc.)
    - c) Tetracycline, nitrofurantoin and local anesthetics, such as lidocaine and procaine
  - 2. Foods
    - a) Nuts, shellfish, eggs
    - b) Chocolate, cottonseed oil
    - c) Grains and beans
    - d) Food preservatives such as sulfites
  - 3. Insect stings
    - a) Yellow jackets, honey bees
    - b) Wasps and hornets
    - c) Fire ants
  - 4. Anaphylactoid ("anaphylactic like" reaction)
    - a) Dyes used in x-ray studies
    - b) Anti-inflammatory drugs such as aspirin, indomethacin (indocin) and aminopyrine.

Content

- D. The anaphylactic reaction **(Slide 12-52)**
  1. Antigens react with antibodies
  2. Specialized cells release histamine and other chemical substances
  3. Smooth muscle constriction
     a) Bronchial constriction, wheezing
     b) Abdominal cramps, vomiting and diarrhea
  4. Increased permeability
     a) Leakage of plasma and protein
     b) Edema and loss of blood volume
  5. Dilation of the arterial and venous vessels **(Slide 12-53)**
     a) Decreased peripheral resistance
     b) Fall in blood pressure
     c) Venous pooling of blood
     d) Decreased venous return
     e) Decreased cardiac output
     f) Hypotension
  6. Increased mucus secretions **(Slide 12-54)**
     a) Nasal congestion
     b) Sneezing
  7. Patients will die from airway obstruction and shock
  8. Reactions will vary from patient to patient

IX. Patient assessment

- A. History **(Slide 12-55)**
  1. May have history of previous reaction
  2. Patients may carry ID bands
  3. May carry medication to block the anaphylactic response (anaphylactic kit):
     a) Adrenaline
     b) Antihistamines
- B. Physical assessment **(Slide 12-56)**
  1. Skin and general signs
     a) Feeling of warmth
     b) Tingling of face, extremities and upper chest
     c) Itching and generalized flushing of skin
     d) Urticaria
     e) Hives and swelling of face and airway
     f) Nasal congestion, sneezing, itching around eyes
     g) Abdominal pain
     h) Sense of impending doom
  2. Respiratory signs **(Slide 12-57)**
     a) Dyspnea
     b) Throat tightness, hoarseness, stridor
     c) Cyanosis
     d) Accessory muscle use
     e) Suprasternal and intercostal retractions
     f) Wheezing and rhonchi
     g) Later stages
        (1) Breath sounds may be absent or diminished

Content

(2) Complete airway obstruction
(3) Respiratory failure
3. Cardiovascular signs **(Slide 12-58)**
a) Generalized "pink" appearance
b) Increase in pulse and respiratory rate
c) Skin may become pale and diaphoretic as the patient decompensates
d) Hypotensive
e) Altered mental state ranging from agitation to lethargy through coma

X. Treatment **(Slide 12-59)**
A. Administration of epinephrine
1. Block effects of reaction
2. Patient may carry kit to self administer
3. EMT may assist patient to administer epinephrine according to state and local protocols
4. Epinephrine subcutaneously
a) 0.3 mg. (0.3 ml.) of a 1:1000 solution
b) 1:1000 solution
c) Pediatric dose
.01 mg./Kg.
1:1000 solution
B. Subcutaneous injection (epinephrine) **(Slide 12-60)**
1. Assemble equipment **(Slide 12-61)**
2. Check medication **(Slide 12-62)**
3. Clear top of ampule of medication **(Slide 12-63)**
4. Break off top of ampule **(Slide 12-64)**
5. Withdraw solution **(Slide 12-65)**
6. Clear air bubbles from syringe **(Slide 12-66)**
7. Select site (mid deltoid) **(Slide 12-67)**
8. Prep site **(Slide 12-68)**
9. Inject at 45° angle with skin pinched **(Slide 12-69, 12-70)**
10. Check for blood **(Slide 12-71)**
11. Inject medication **(Slide 12-72)**
12. Remove needle **(Slide 12-73)**
13. Massage area
14. Properly dispose of needle and syringe
C. Use of Ana-Kit
1. Push plunger to clear air **(Slide 12-74)**
2. Turn plunger 1/4 turn clockwise **(Slide 12-75)**
3. Inject as above
D. EpiPen **(Slide 12-76)**
1. Given intramuscularly
2. Automatic mechanism when pressed against thigh
E. Airway, ventilation and oxygenation **(Slide 12-77)**
1. Complete airway obstruction
a) Abdominal, chest thrusts and finger sweeps are of no value
b) Rapid transport is the main priority

Content

c) Patients require cricothyroidotomy or tracheostomy
d) Ventilations during transport
(1) "Forced positive pressure"
(2) High concentration oxygen

2. Respiratory distress or failure **(Slide 12-78)**
a) High concentration oxygen
b) Patients who are hypoventilating should receive assisted ventilation

3. Cardiovascular support **(Slide 12-79)**
a) Hypovolemic or distributive shock
(1) Supine position with their legs elevated
(2) PASG according to local protocols
b) All procedures performed enroute to hospital
c) Avoid rough handling
d) Prevent loss of body heat
e) Vital signs every 5 minutes

4. Treatment of bites and stings **(Slide 12-80)**
a) Constricting band above injury
b) Tight enough to reduce venous return but not obstruct arterial flow
c) If present, carefully scrape stinger or venom sack away
d) Place an ice pack over bitten area

Chapter 12

Section 3

Poisons and Overdose

Objectives
(Slide 12-81)

At the conclusion of the chapter the students will be able to:

1. **Define poison.**
2 **List 4 ways for poison to enter body and give 2 examples of each.**
3. **State how to contact nearest poison control center.**
4. **List 3 circumstances when vomiting should not be induced in patients suffering from ingested poison.**
5. **State how to induce vomiting in adult and pediatric patient.**
6. **List the general steps of emergency care for victims of the following poison:**

Inhaled	**Injected**
Ingested	**Absorbed**

7. **Describe the physical characteristics of a pit viper and a coral snake.**
8. **List 4 signs or symptoms of a patient bitten by a pit viper.**
9. **List 4 signs or symptoms of a patient bitten by a coral snake.**
10. **List emergency care for snake bites.**
11. **List 3 examples of stinging marine animals.**
12. **Describe emergency care for marine animal stings.**
13. **List 6 signs/symptoms of a patient who has abused chemical substances.**
14. **List the general treatment procedures to be taken when caring for substance abuse patients.**

Instructor Preparation

Reading preparation for the lesson:

EMT Prehospital Care, Chapter 12, pages 552-578

Optional reading:

Goldfrank, L.R., Flomenbaum, M.E., Lewis, N.A., Weisman, R.S., Howland, M.A.: Goldfrank's Toxicologic Emergencies. 4th ed. New York, Appleton & Lange, 1990.

Suggested Learning Activities

Using a lecture format with the aid of slides, overhead transparencies or charts, provide a presentation on poisons and overdose.

Provide case history examples of poisoning emergencies.

Content

XI. Poisoning overview
- A. Definition **(Slide 12-82)**
  1. Poison - substance which through its chemical action usually kills, injures, or impairs an organism
  2. Toxicology - study of poisons
  3. Overdose - administration of drugs, taken in excess or in combination with other agents, to the point where poisoning occurs
  4. Types of poisoning **(Slide 12-83)**
     - a) Accidental
     - b) Intentional
     - c) Plants
     - d) Bites and stings
  5. Poison can enter the body through
     - a) GI tract (ingestion)
     - b) Airway (inhalation)
     - c) Skin (absorption)
     - d) Injection (including envenomation)
  6. Reasons to suspect a poisoning
     - a) Nausea and vomiting, abdominal pain, diarrhea
     - b) Dilation or constriction of the pupils
     - c) Excessive salivation or sweating
     - d) Abnormal respirations
     - e) Unconsciousness, and convulsions
     - f) Smells on breath
     - g) History from patient or bystanders
     - h) Physical evidence
  7. Cardinal rules **(Slide 12-84)**
     - a) Treat the patient, not the poison
     - b) Cardiorespiratory support
     - c) Rapid transport for cyanide or nitrites
     - d) Most cases require supportive care
     - e) Protect yourself and bystanders
     - f) Look for clues of trauma
     - g) Maintain a high index of suspicion
     - h) Look for patterns of multiple exposures
- B. Incidence **(Slide 12-85)**
  1. Over 5 million poisonings each year in the United States
  2. Over 10,000 deaths
  3. Most accidental poisonings occur in children under the age of 5
  4. In adolescent and older groups, suicide is often attempted by poisoning
  5. Recreational drug users and addicts may overdose by injecting drugs
  6. Industrial accidents
  7. Snakes, insects, arthropods, and sea creatures
  8. Over 250,000 potentially poisonous drugs and commercial products
- C. Poison control centers **(Slide 12-86)**
  1. Source of information on toxins, management, and antidotes

Content

2. Available by phone at all times to physicians, EMS personnel, and the public
3. Learn and remember the number
4. Poison centers can
    a) Provide access to experts
    b) Coordinate emergency response

D. Types of exposure **(Slide 12-87)**
    1. Ingestion (most common route), examples:
    a) Suicidal patient who takes pills
    b) Street alcoholic who drinks wood alcohol
    c) Toddler who drinks from open bottle of antifreeze
2. Injection
    a) Self administered (i.e., opioids)
    b) Insulin that a diabetic person inadvertently administers
    c) Bee stings and venomous snake bites
    d) Injected poisons have the fastest onset
3. Inhalations
    a) Carbon monoxide is the most common inhaled toxin
    b) Glue, freebasing cocaine, and smoking crack
    c) Cyanide, phosgene, and nitrous dioxides may be inhaled in industrial, or agricultural settings, or during fires
    d) Protective measures essential for EMT
4. Absorbed - cutaneous
    a) Insecticides such as organophosphates
    b) Corrosives such as acid or alkali
    c) Hydrofluoric acid can both chemically burn skin and be absorbed in circulation
    d) Cocaine, snorted through the nose, is absorbed by the membranes in the nasopharynx

E. General assessment and management **(Slide 12-88)**
1. Airway, ventilation and supplemental oxygen
    a) Smoke inhalation; oxygen is antidote
    b) Airway management for all unconscious patients
2. Decontaminate the victim
    a) Flush ocular and skin exposures
    b) Remove contaminated clothing
    c) Wear protective clothing
    d) When possible, decontaminate before transport
3. Gather history **(Slide 12-89)**
    a) What is the poison?
    b) How was it taken?
    c) Ingested, inhaled, absorbed or injected?
    d) When was it taken?
    e) How much was taken?
    f) What evidence supports the history?
    g) Multiple ingestions?
    h) History may be unreliable; ask family

Content

4. Perform a focused physical exam **(Slide 12-90)**
    a) Primary survey
    b) Vital signs
    c) Pupils
    d) Skin (for color, moisture, and temperature)
    e) Abdomen
    f) Mental status
    g) Gag reflex
        (1) Protect airway should vomiting occur
        (2) Vomiting is never induced without gag reflex
    h) Needle marks over the veins ("tracks")
    i) Signs of injury
5. Institute treatment **(Slide 12-91)**
    a) Prevent further absorption
        (1) Induce vomiting, except for
            (a) Caustics, hydrocarbons
            (b) Infants or patients with coma or no gag reflex
        (2) Activated charcoal
    b) Hasten elimination **(Slide 12-92)**
        (1) Cathartic
        (2) Hemodialysis or charcoal hemoperfusion
        (3) These techniques used after arrival at the hospital
    c) Treat signs and symptoms **(Slide 12-93)**
        (1) Antidote may be available; examples:
            (a) Oxygen - carbon monoxide poisoning
            (b) Naloxone - opiates
            (c) Snakebite - antivenom
        (2) Most given in hospital
6. Dealing with the poisoned patient **(Slide 12-94)**
    a) Suicidal patients
        (1) May be extremely depressed and despondent
        (2) Require active listening
        (3) May have left a note
        (4) May hide toxic products
    b) Parents
        (1) May feel guilt about leaving toxic substances around the home
        (2) Don't be judgmental
    c) EMT
        (1) Feelings of hopelessness
        (2) Sense of identity with similar age patient who has attempted suicide
        (3) Maintain a professional approach
        (4) Minimize potential for emotional responses interfering with care
        (5) Avoid antagonizing patient

Content

- (6) Be careful regarding how patients are labeled
- (7) Explain actions
- (8) Psychiatric consultation for intentional poisoning

d) Protective custody **(Slide 12-95)**
- (1) Patients refusing medical attention
- (2) Must not be abandoned
- (3) Encourage them to go to the hospital
- (4) Call police if necessary
- (5) Mental status and judgment may be impaired

XII. Ingested poisons

A. History **(Slide 12-96)**
1. What is the poison?
   a) Ask bystanders
   b) Ask patient
   c) Check physical evidence
2. How was it taken?
   a) All pills at once?
   b) Repeated intervals?
3. How much was taken?
   a) Dose
   b) Number of pills or volume of liquid
4. What evidence supports the history?
   a) Bring containers
   b) Bring substance
5. Has the patient vomited?
   a) Ipecac administered?
   b) Save sample of vomitus
6. Multiple ingestions?
7. History may be unreliable; ask family

B. Physical Exam **(Slide 12-97)**
1. Same as above
2. Primary survey
   a) Breath sounds
   b) Signs of compromise
3. Vital signs
4. Pupils
5. Skin (for color, moisture, and temperature)
6. Abdomen **(Slide 12-98)**
7. Mental status
8. Gag reflex
   a) Protect airway should vomiting occur
   b) Vomiting is never induced without gag reflex
9. Needle marks over the veins ("tracks")
10. Signs of injury

C. Prevention of absorption **(Slide 12-99)**
1. First assure ABCs

Content

2. Test for consciousness and gag reflex
3. Check for contraindications to vomiting
4. Induce vomiting - syrup of ipecac **(Slide 12-100)**
    a) Contains natural alkaloids
    b) Causes vomiting in 60% of patients, usually in 15 minutes, 90% within 30 minutes
    c) Dose for adults
        (1) 30 cc
        (2) Two tablespoons
    f) Dose for children over age 1
        (1) 15 cc
        (2) One tablespoon
    g) Infants aged 6-12 months should have vomiting induced in hospital
5. Give water or other liquid **(Slide 12-101)**
    a) After giving the ipecac, give water or other available liquid
        (1) Adults: two glasses (8-16 ounces)
        (2) Children: 4-8 ounces
    b) Serves to dilute the contents and provide a liquid which can be "vomited"
    c) Don't give excessive fluid, as it will tend to move the stomach contents into the intestine
6. Prepare to protect airway with suctioning **(Slide 12-102)**
7. Contraindications to inducing vomiting
    a) Unconscious or seizing patients
    b) Patients without a gag reflex
    c) Corrosive ingestions (give one or two glasses of water or milk)
    d) Certain hydrocarbons
        (1) Little chance for absorption
        (2) High risk of aspiration pneumonia
        (3) Consult poison control
    e) When ipecac may delay administration of antidote
8. Other methods of stomach emptying (usually in-hospital) **(Slide 12-103)**
    a) Gastric lavage
        (1) For unconscious patients or patients without a gag reflex
        (2) Airway protected by intubation
        (3) Insertion of a large oral gastric tube
        (4) Some systems use this instead of ipecac in field
        (5) Review local protocols
    b) Activated charcoal **(Slide 12-104)**
        (1) Adsorbent material that binds most toxins
        (2) Done after vomiting occurs
        (3) Keeps toxins within GI tract

(4) Dose - 1 gm per kilogram of body weight (minimum 50-100 gm for adults)
(5) Premixed liquid or powder mixed with water
(6) Sweeteners are added to make it palatable
(7) Almost never any harm

D. Enhance excretion - cathartic **(Slide 12-105)**
1. Sorbitol
2. Magnesium sulfate
3. Induce diarrhea, speed transit time through GI tract
4. Reduce chance for absorption
5. Given with or after charcoal
6. Do not administer to dehydrated or kidney failure patient

E. Types of ingestions **(Slide 12-106)**
1. Sedatives, hypnotics and anti-anxiety agents
a) Definitions
(1) Sedatives (allaying activity and excitement)
(2) Hypnotics (sleep inducing)
(3) Antianxiety (reduce anxiety)
b) Effects
(1) Respiratory depression
(2) Alteration of mental status from relaxation through stupor to coma
(3) Especially when used with alcohol
c) Management
(1) Assisting with ventilations
(2) Supplemental oxygen
(3) Protecting the airway
(4) Left lateral recumbent position
2. Opioids ("narcotics") **(Slide 12-107)**
a) Actions
(1) Special class of depressants
(2) Alter perception of pain
b) Signs and symptoms
(1) Depressed mental status and coma
(2) Respiratory depression
(3) Pinpoint pupils
(4) Track marks
c) Examples
(1) Morphine, heroin
(2) Demerol or meperidine
(3) Codeine
(4) Oxycodone (Percodan & Percocet)
d) Naloxone (Narcan) is antidote
(1) Rapidly reverses the respiratory depression and mental depression
(2) Paramedics commonly use in the field

Content

3. Psychiatric medications **(Slide 12-108)**
   a) Types
      (1) Phenothiazine tranquilizers
      (2) Tricyclic antidepressants
      (3) Monoamine oxidase inhibitors
      (4) Benzodiazepines (Valium, Lithium, others)
   b) Findings encountered
      (1) Muscle spasms
      (2) Dry skin
      (3) High and low body temperature
      (4) Hypotension and hypertension
      (5) Abnormal heart rhythms
      (6) Cardiac arrest
      (7) Fast and slow heart beats
      (8) Altered respirations - depressed
      (9) Altered mental status to coma
      (10) Seizures
      (11) Monoamine oxidase inhibitors
         (a) Hypertensive crisis when taken with foods high in tyramine (beer, wines, cheeses, broad beans)
4. Stimulants **(Slide 12-109)**
   a) Types
      (1) Amphetamines and methyphenidate (Ritalin)
      (2) Cocaine
         (a) Ingested to avoid arrest
         (b) Condoms burst in GI tract
      (3) Crack
      (4) Freebase
      (5) Phencyclidine (PCP or angel dust)
   b) Signs and symptoms
      (1) Excitability
      (2) Seizures
      (3) Tachycardia, hypertension
      (4) Chest pain can occur
      (5) Behavioral
         (a) Anxious, delirious, and paranoid. Psychotic and violent behavior
      (6) Sudden death from arrhythmias
      (7) Phencyclidine can cause coma
   c) Management
      (1) Cardiorespiratory support
      (2) Reassure the patient
      (3) Be non-threatening
      (4) Offer calm environment
      (5) Maintain verbal contact

Content

(6) Do not be judgmental
(7) Avoid restraints if possible

5. Alcohol **(Slide 12-110)**
   a) Effects
      (1) Most common drug abused in the United States
      (2) Mental status and respiratory depression when taken in high doses
      (3) Effect increases when taken with depressant drugs
      (4) Can be lethal by itself
   b) Signs and symptoms
      (1) Coma
      (2) Respiratory failure
      (3) Aspiration of vomitus
   c) Management
      (1) Airway management is essential
         (a) Position
         (b) Suction
      (2) Ventilation
      (3) Oxygenation
6. Drugs for heart and lungs **(Slide 12-111)**
   a) May be used for suicide attempt
   b) Wide range of findings
   c) Alterations in heart rate, rhythm and blood pressure
7. Analgesics **(Slide 12-112)**
   a) Salicylates (aspirin) and acetaminophen are commonly encountered
   b) Early after the overdose there may be few if any symptoms
   c) Aspirin
      (1) Increased respiration
      (2) Later coma can occur
      (3) May require hemodialysis
      (4) Fever
   d) Acetaminophen **(Slide 12-113)**
      (1) Causes no symptoms or mild GI discomfort in first 24 hours
         (a) Nausea and vomiting
         (b) Malaise
      (2) After 48 hours with severe doses
         (a) Liver damage can appear
         (b) Important that all patients receive evaluation by a physician
   e) Commercial and industrial products **(Slide 12-114)**
      (1) Caustics
         (a) Both acids and alkalis
         (b) Acid products
            i) Toilet bowel cleaners
            ii) Bleaches
            iii) Metal cleaners and battery acid

Content

(c) Alkalies
i) Drain cleaners (lye, Draino)
ii) Clinitest tabs (used by diabetics)
iii) Chemistry labs and industry
(d) Treatment
i) Diluted with one or two glasses of water or milk
ii) Do not neutralize
iii) Should not induce to avoid

8. Methanol and ethylene glycol **(Slide 12-115)**
a) Can initially present as mild inebriation
b) Untreated can lead to coma and death
c) Products
(1) Dry gas - methanol
(2) Windshield washing solution - methanol
(3) Fuel for warming food (Sterno) - methanol
(4) Antifreeze (ethylene glycol)
d) Effects **(Slide 12-116)**
(1) Binds with enzyme that breaks down ethanol
(2) Makes toxic byproducts
(3) Metabolic acidosis results
(4) Hyperventilation
e) Treatment **(Slide 12-117)**
(1) Give normal drinking alcohol, i.e., whiskey
(2) Binds to the same enzyme
(3) May be ordered prehospital in extreme cases
(4) Dialysis is needed in severe cases

9. Hydrocarbons **(Slide 12-118)**
a) Molecules made up predominantly of carbon and hydrogen
b) Materials containing hydrocarbons
(1) Gasoline, kerosene, cleaning fluids
(2) Spot removers
(3) Plastic cements
c) Types of ingestions
(1) Toddlers
(2) Suicide
(3) Gas siphoning
d) Effects, signs and symptoms
(1) CNS changes (euphoria, stupor, delirium, coma)
(2) Cardiac arrhythmias
(3) Severe pulmonary damage due to inflammatory reaction in lungs when aspirated
e) Management
(1) Larger size molecules
(a) Mineral oil
(b) Vomiting not induced
(c) Usually not absorbed to significant degree
(d) If aspirated can cause a severe pneumonia

Content

(2) Medium size molecules
(a) Kerosene, gasoline, or turpentine
(b) May benefit from vomiting when ingested in quantities greater than 1 ml/kg
(3) Smaller size molecules and special agents
(a) Benzene, toluene
(b) Halogen molecules (chloride, fluoride, etc.)
(c) Heavy metals
(d) Insecticides, and camphor
(e) Vomiting is indicated
(4) Poison center should be consulted

10. Insecticides - organophosphates **(Slide 12-119)**
a) Taken by toddlers and in suicide attempts
b) Effects
(1) Bronchoconstriction
(2) Muscle weakness
(3) Respiratory muscle paralysis
(4) Pulmonary secretions
c) Signs and symptoms
(1) Vomiting
(2) Salivation, sweating, lacrimation (tearing)
(3) Urination, diarrhea
(4) Pinpoint pupils
(5) Slow heart rate
(6) Garlicky odor may be noted
(7) Often masked by a hydrocarbon smell
d) Treatment
(1) Rapid access to antidotal therapy in severe cases
(2) Ventilatory support
(3) Supplemental oxygen
(4) Rapid transport
(5) Administration of atropine
(6) May be absorbed through the skin
(a) Should be flushed with water and washed with soap and water

11. Food poisoning **(Slide 12-120)**
a) Toxins produced by bacteria, and viruses
b) Causes
(1) Improperly cooked or canned foods
(2) Contamination of food with fecal bacteria by food - handlers
c) Suspected when two or more persons become ill after eating same foods
d) Symptoms - nausea, vomiting, and diarrhea (sometimes bloody)
e) Botulism
(1) The most severe type of food poisoning
(2) Begins with flu-like illness
(3) Severe weakness and paralysis

Content

(4) Ventilatory arrest
(5) Treatment requires respiratory support and ventilations
f) Poisonous mushrooms **(Slide 12-121)**
(1) GI disturbances, hallucinations, and delirium
(2) Amanita muscaria mushroom
(a) Excessive salivation, tearing
(b) Bradycardia
(c) May require drug treatment
(3) Occurs when persons looking for psychedelic effects or exotic edible mushrooms
(4) Care is supportive
(5) Important to bring samples, even fragments, to hospital for ID
12. Plants **(Slide 12-122)**
a) Common household and wild plants can cause adverse effects
b) Gastrointestinal
c) Circulatory
d) Neurological
e) Severe skin and mucous membrane irritation
f) Example: dieffenbachia
(1) Severe irritation and swelling in the mouth
(2) When chewed, crystals in leaf feel like ground glass
(3) Treatment in this case centers on airway management
XIII. Inhaled **(Slide 12-123)**
A. Rescue considerations and precautions
1. Safety of rescuers is first consideration
2. Rescuers should avoid inhalation of fumes
3. Self-contained breathing apparatus
4. Victims should be removed from environment first
B. Carbon monoxide **(Slide 124)**
1. Most common poisonous gas
2. Fires, charcoal burners, automobile exhaust fumes and inadequately ventilated stoves
a) Treatment
(1) 100% oxygen
(2) Hyperbaric treatment if available for extreme cases
C. Asphyxiants **(Slide 12-125)**
1. Include carbon dioxide, methane (cooking gas, gas oven deaths)
2. Displace oxygen, the victim becomes hypoxic
3. Carbon dioxide
a) Heavier than air
b) Collects in poorly ventilated areas (mine shafts, holds of ships)
4. Methane, ethane, and propane
a) Small hydrocarbon molecules
b) No color or odor to warn victim
c) Commercially odor is added
d) Explosion potential is high if a spark is generated

Content

5. Chemical asphyxiants **(Slide 12-126)**
    a) Carbon monoxide, cyanide and hydrogen sulfide
    b) Carbon monoxide exposure is significant at all fires
        (1) Cause of majority of fire deaths
        (2) Binds to hemoglobin
        (3) Impairs transport and delivery of oxygen
        (4) Gives little warning of its lethal effect
            (a) Victims might feel headaches and nausea
            (b) Judgment, coordination and motor ability are impaired
            (c) Victims may collapse during exertion
        (5) Fatal inhalations in less than a minute with high concentrations
        (6) Treatment is 100% oxygen
        (7) Extreme cases require treatment in hyperbaric chamber
    c) Cyanide **(Slide 12-127)**
        (1) Found in industry
            (a) Electroplating, photography, and metal cleaning
            (b) Fumigant on cargo ships
            (c) Fires with burning polyurethanes
        (2) Rapidly acting and affects ability of body to use oxygen
        (3) Clinical symptoms are nonspecific
            (a) Increased heart and breathing rate
            (b) Later, breathing and heart may slow
        (4) High concentration oxygen
        (5) Antidote
            (a) Ampule of amyl nitrite
            (b) Patient inhales fumes from ampule for 30 seconds every minute
            (c) New ampule every 3 minutes and rapid transport
    d) Hydrogen sulfide **(Slide 12-128)**
        (1) Smell of rotten eggs
        (2) Types of exposure
            (a) Petroleum and rubber processing industries
            (b) Sewers
            (c) Animal rendering plants and tanneries
            (d) Fertilizer plants and farming
        (3) Because of odor, victims usually flee from exposure
            (a) Over time, nose becomes insensitive
            (b) Workers are exposed to increasing levels
        (4) Treatment includes high concentration oxygen

D. Irritant gases **(Slide 12-129)**
    1. Cause inflammatory damage to airway and bronchoconstriction
    2. React with water in airway to cause toxic reactions to mucosa

Content

3. Ammonia, sulfur dioxide, and hydrogen chloride will react almost immediately
   a) Signs and symptoms
      (1) Tearing, coughing
      (2) Discomfort in the nose and throat
      (3) Victims are impelled to flee
   b) Damage is usually confined to the upper airway unless inhaled in closed space or by an unconscious victim
   c) Upper airway obstruction is of greatest immediate concern
4. Phosgene and nitrous dioxides **(Slide 12-130)**
   a) Less likely to react immediately in upper airway
   b) Warning irritation may not be present
   c) Victims will inhale for a longer period of time
   d) Enter lower airway where damage can occur over hours to days
   e) May have severe symptoms some time after removal from the smoke or gas exposure

E. Management of inhaled poisons **(Slide 12-131)**
1. Remove from source
2. Assess the need for basic life support
3. Assess the upper airway
   a) Look for hoarseness or stridor
   b) Rapid transport if signs of oral edema, since risk of airway closure
4. Give humidified oxygen

XIV. Absorbed poisons **(Slide 12-132)**
A. Skin is damaged by corrosive and caustic agents
B. Can cause severe chemical burns
C. Contaminated clothing is removed
D. Flushed with copious amounts of water
E. Eyes irrigated with water for at least 15-20 minutes
F. Dry powder (e.g., dry lime)
1. Brushed off the skin first
2. Flushed with water

G. Agents absorbed through the skin into the body
H. Insecticides are an example of absorbed toxin
I. Washed off the skin by flooding with water and soap and water
J. EMT must wear protective clothing to avoid splashing

XV. Injected poisons **(Slide 12-133)**
A. General principles
1. Cause most rapid onset of drug effect
2. Little can be done to eliminate
3. Often self-administered overdoses
4. Bites and stings

B. Commonly injected drugs **(Slide 12-134)**
1. Heroin
2. Amphetamine
3. Cocaine

C. Management same as ingested or inhaled, except no attempt to prevent absorption

Content

D. Insect bites and stings **(Slide 12-135)**
   1. Most severe reaction is anaphylaxis
   2. Other effects are usually local
   3. Remove constricting clothing and jewelry
   4. Brown recluse spider
      a) Found mostly in the South but can occur nationwide
      b) Local necrosis about the bite
      c) Has a dark color band on the dorsum shaped like a violin
      d) Venom causes **(Slide 12-136)**
         (1) Local pain
         (2) Spreads out from the bite site to surrounding skin
         (3) Painful red spot with a central blister
         (4) Darkened center, surrounding blanches and red outermost ring "patriotic bull's eye"
         (5) Few have fever, chills, weakness
         (6) Blood cells and clotting mechanisms disturbed
         (7) The treatment is hospital based
   5. Black widow spider **(Slide 12-137)**
      a) More common, found throughout the U.S.
      b) Characteristic black shiny body with a red hourglass shape on the abdomen
      c) Venom includes a neurotoxin
      d) In severe cases weakness and respiratory depression can occur
      e) Common signs and symptoms
         (1) Bite site: pain, swelling and mark
         (2) Abdominal pain, rigidity and tenderness
         (3) Lower extremity weakness
         (4) Fever and chills
         (5) Rigidity and spasm of large muscles
      f) Antivenom is available for severe cases
      g) Small children and debilitated adults are most susceptible to severe consequences
      h) Treat like snake bites
      i) Immobilize extremity
      j) Avoid unnecessary movement
   6. Fire ants **(Slide 12-138)**
      a) Southern parts of the United States
      b) Can cause multiple stings
      c) Sting can give rise to a raised papule
      d) Develops pus in 6-24 hours
      e) Care is supportive
   7. Scorpion and tarantula bites in the United States cause local pain but are usually not fatal

E. Snake Bites **(Slide 12-139)**
   1. Overview
      a) Venomous snakes in the United States
         (1) Pit vipers (rattlesnakes, water moccasins, copperheads)
         (2) Coral snakes

Content

- b) Pit vipers
  - (1) Cause local necrosis
  - (2) In severe cases, systemic effects occur and death may result
  - (3) Definitive care requires use of antivenom
- c) Coral snake
  - (1) No local necrosis
  - (2) Nervous system is affected when the poison is absorbed
  - (3) Onset of effects may be delayed up to 12 hours

2. Pit vipers **(Slide 12-140)**
   - a) How to recognize pit viper
     - (1) Elliptical pupils
     - (2) Pit (heat sensor) between the eyes and nostril
     - (3) Fangs
     - (4) Single row of subcaudal plates on the tail
     - (5) Bite has fang marks at site
     - (6) Swelling, pain, and redness at the site
   - b) Approaching the snake bite victim
     - (1) Move out of range, generally less than the length of the snake
     - (2) Larger snake, larger potential envenomation
     - (3) If possible, bring dead snake to the hospital
     - (4) Do not handle directly, dead head can cause reflex envenomation
   - c) Treatment
     - (1) Have the victim rest
     - (2) Immobilize the extremity with a splint
     - (3) If swelling is present, mark its edge to identify changes later
     - (4) Transport to the closest hospital able to care for snakebites
     - (5) If great distance to hospital or systemic effects are present
       - (a) Some authors recommend application of a venous tourniquet 4-6 inches above the site
       - (b) Know local protocols
     - (6) Do not use ice or cut the wound
     - (7) Do not attempt to suck out the venom
3. Coral snakes **(Slide 12-141)**
   - a) How to recognize coral snake
     - (1) Found in the southern United States
     - (2) Red, yellow and black bands
       - (a) "Red on yellow, kill a fellow"
       - (b) "Red on black, venom lack"
     - (3) Very small fangs
     - (4) Bite marks more noteworthy than fang marks
     - (5) Drop of blood expressed after envenomation
     - (6) Confirm fangs entered the skin
     - (7) Snake often holds on and "chews" for a few seconds
     - (8) Sensation as pulling off Velcro

Content

b) Signs and symptoms
(1) May be mild
(2) Minimal redness and swelling at bite site
(3) Contrast to pit viper
c) Approach to patient
(1) Same as pit viper, except
(2) Many advocate application of bandage to delay systemic adsorption
(3) Early antivenom administration
(4) Most recommend against the use of ice and cutting and sucking out venom
(5) Follow your local protocols

F. Marine animals **(Slide 12-142)**
1. Cause stings and punctures by spines
2. Stinging animals
a) Portuguese man-of-war
b) Anemones
c) Corals
3. Treatment
a) Flooding the affected area with sea water (never fresh water)
b) Washing with alcohol if available
c) Apply shaving cream, sand, or talcum powder to the area, then scrape it off
d) Avoid washing with fresh water
e) Punctures can occur from cone shells, urchins, stingrays and spiny fish
(1) Toxin introduced in the wound
(2) Inactivated with hot water (45 degrees C.)
(3) Soak 30 to 90 minutes or until pain relieved
(4) Immobilize affected area

XVI. Drugs of abuse **(Slide 12-143)**
A. One of the greatest problems in modern society
B. Repeated self-administration for sense of well-being or "high"
C. Ingestion, inhalation, or injection
D. Continued use develops tolerance to the drug effects
1. Greater doses are required to reach the same feeling of well being
2. May mix drugs to improve effect
E. Dependence **(Slide 12-144)**
1. Cannot sustain sense of well-being without drug
2. Psychological or physical
3. Symptoms occur if person stops using the drug
4. Addicted - compulsive behavior concentrated on obtaining the drug
F. Alcohol **(Slide 12-145)**
1. Most commonly abused drug in United States
2. Withdrawal can cause shakes, tremors and seizures
3. In severe cases, delirium tremors
a) Hyperactivity
b) Increased respiratory and pulse rates
c) Increased temperature, and hypertension
d) Hallucinations (insects crawling around)

e) Can cause death if untreated

Content

G. Other drugs of abuse include heroin, cocaine, LSD, PCP (angel dust), and many prescription drugs **(Slide 12-146)**

H. EMT's approach
1. Psychological care
2. Treat physical manifestation

Section 4

Communicable Diseases

Objectives
(Slide 12-147)

At the conclusion of the chapter the students will be able to:	
1.	**Define infectious or communicable disease.**
2.	**List 4 ways a communicable disease can be transmitted.**
3.	**Describe universal precautions.**
4.	**List steps EMTs must take in maintenance of equipment and vehicle post exposure to a communicable disease.**
5.	**List personal health measures an EMT can take to reduce personal risk.**

Instructor Preparation

Reading preparation for the lesson:

EMT Prehospital Care, Chapter 12, pages 578-595

Optional reading:

Schwartz GR (ed):Principles and Practices of Emergency Medicine. 2nd ed. Philadelphia, W.B. Saunders, 1986.

Centers for Disease Control: A curriculum guide for public safety and emergency response workers: Prevention of transmission of human immunodeficiency virus and hepatitis B virus. Atlanta, Centers for Disease Control, 1989.

Centers for Disease Control: Guidelines for prevention of transmission of human immunodeficiency virus and hepatitis B virus to health-care and public-safety workers: A response to P.L. 100-607 the health omnibus programs extension act of 1988. MMWR 38 (S-6):1-37, 1989.

Williams WW: CDC guidelines for infection control in hospital personnel. In Williams WW: Guidelines for prevention and control of nosocomial infections. Atlanta, Centers for Disease Control, Center for Infectious Diseases: Hospital Infections Program, reprinted February 1986.

Suggested Learning Activities

Using a lecture format with the aid of slides, overhead transparencies or charts, provide a presentation on emergencies involving communicable diseases.

Provide case history examples of emergencies involving communicable diseases.

Content

XVII. Overview **(Slide 12-148)**
- A. Communicable diseases are capable of being spread from one person to another
  - 1. Common cold
  - 2. Spread through sneezing and coughing
- B. Some are life threatening
- C. EMT must take precautions to prevent spread
- D. Diseases may be obvious or not be obvious
- E. EMTs need basic understanding
  - 1. How infections are spread
  - 2. Body's response to exposure
  - 3. Actions to take before, during and following care
- F. Infection control **(Slide 12-149)**
  - 1. Common sense actions to block spread of infections
  - 2. Part of everyday behavior, i.e., wearing a seat belt
- G. Routinely followed in hospitals
- H. Center for Disease Control (CDC) publishes guidelines

XVIII. What are infectious agents **(Slide 12-150)**
- A. Microorganisms (not visible to the naked eye) which are toxic to the body
- B. Include bacteria, viruses, fungi, and parasites
- C. Multiply and can cause direct and indirect damage
- D. Harmful microorganisms are said to be pathogenic
- E. Some are treated with medications which inhibit or kill microorganisms, examples **(Slide 12-151)**
  - 1. Antibiotics
    - a) Used to treat bacterial infections
    - b) Penicillin
    - c) Taken for pharyngitis (streptococcus bacteria)
  - 2. Antiviral drugs
    - a) Many viral infections have no "cure"
    - b) Most viruses are eliminated by immune system
  - 3. Antifungals for fungal infections, e.g., athlete's foot
  - 4. Antiparasitic drugs are effective for parasitic infections
- F. Many severe infections once established, have no or little effective treatment **(Slide 12-152)**
  - 1. Polio, rubella ("German measles")
  - 2. Measles, diphtheria, tetanus ("lockjaw")
  - 3. Pertussis ("whooping cough") and hepatitis B
  - 4. Vaccination or immunization is means to prevent infection
- G. If no immunization is available (e.g., AIDS)
  - 1. Prevention takes on the greatest of importance
  - 2. Infection control measures
- H. Not all microorganisms are harmful **(Slide 12-153)**
  - 1. Bacteria are normally found:
    - a) Intestine where they aid digestion
    - b) Upper respiratory tract
    - c) Skin surface

Content

2. Can be harmful if they enter part of body where they are not normally found
    - a) Intestine bacteria which spill into the peritoneal cavity
    - b) Bacteria in mouth, if aspirated into the lung, can cause pneumonia

XIX. How are communicable diseases spread? **(Slide 12-154)**

- A. Spread from a source to a host
- B. Source may be person, insect, object, or substance that carries or is contaminated by infectious agent
- C. Reservoir
    - 1. Source where agents live and multiply
    - 2. Cholera epidemic in 1850's was traced to polluted river Thames
    - 3. Bubonic plague was carried by rats and humans
    - 4. Typhoid fever was spread by "Typhoid Mary," a cook
- D. Incubation period
    - 1. Period between contact and occurrence of signs and symptoms
    - 2. During incubation period, host may or may not be infectious
- E. Communicable period
    - 1. Time during which a person can transmit infectious disease to others
    - 2. May be before, during or even after the symptoms
- F. Carrier
    - 1. Person who shows no signs of the disease yet harbors an infectious organism
    - 2. May be a source of infection to others (Typhoid Mary)
- G. Exposure **(Slide 12-155)**
    - 1. Coming in contact with an infectious agent with or without being infected
    - 2. Type of exposure necessary to transmit
    - 3. Measles
        - a) Highly contagious
        - b) Transmitted simply by being in same room with deseased person
    - 4. Hepatitis B or HIV, the AIDS virus
        - a) Not spread through "casual" contact
        - b) Requires body fluid to body fluid contact
    - 5. Not everyone who is exposed becomes sick
    - 6. Nosocomial infectious: diseases are spread
        - a) By health care workers
        - b) Within a health care setting
- H. Modes of transmission **(Slide 12-156)**
    - 1. Contact transmission
        - a) Most important and frequent cause of nosocomial infections
        - b) Divided into 3 subgroups
            - (1) Direct contact
                - (a) Direct transfer between host and an infected person
                - (b) Applying dressings or performing other patient care procedures
                - (c) Patient to patient
            - (2) Indirect contact
                - (a) Contact with a contaminated object
                - (b) Instruments, dressings or other material

Content

(c) Personnel can contaminate objects when assembling or handling equipment

(3) Droplet contact

(a) Coughing, sneezing, or talking by an infected person

(b) Droplets can enter eyes, nose, etc.

(c) Droplets usually travel no more than about 3 feet

(d) "Close contact" is used to mean within 3 feet

(e) Tuberculosis is spread this way

c) Can be several steps involved in contact transmission, for example:

(1) Patient with conjunctivitis will touch his hand to the infected eye

(2) Another person shakes another person's hand

(3) Person rubs his own eye

d) Hand washing is a very important infection control measure

2. Vehicle route **(Slide 12-157)**

a) Transmitted through contaminated items, i.e., blood

b) Contaminated blood can be the vehicle for the spread of hepatitis B

3. Airborne transmission

a) Dissemination of droplet nuclei (remain suspended in the air) or dust

b) Organisms are inhaled or deposited on the susceptible host

4. Vectorborne **(Slide 12-158)**

a) Transmitted by mosquito or other insect

b) Greater concern in developing countries

c) Examples

(1) Mosquito-transmitted malaria

(2) Lyme disease, spread by the deer tick

d) Control of disease is sometimes related to elimination of the vector

I. Factors influencing spread

1. Potency of agent **(Slide 12-159)**

a) Some organisms have greater infective potential than others, for example:

(1) Virus causing measles is very potent

(2) Hepatitis B virus more likely than HIV (AIDS virus) to cause infection of health workers

b) The greater the number of microorganisms transmitted to the host, the more significant the exposure

2. Mechanism of transmission

a) Route organism enters will affect potential for infection, for example:

b) Blood transfusion is a greater exposure than needle stick

Content

3. Type and duration of contact
   a) Wearing blood soaked clothing for an hour is more significant than a splash washed off soon after
   b) EMTs should record the type and duration of contact on incidence or occurrence reports
4. Resistance
   a) One's ability to fight off infection following exposure
   b) White blood cells can consume infectious agents and produce antibodies
   c) Antibodies block and bind invading organisms and the toxins they produce
   d) Lymph nodes filter out organisms brought through the lymphatic circulation
5. Immunity **(Slide 12-160)**
   a) Body is able to halt disease before the infecting agent can establish itself
   b) Beyond one's natural defense system, immunity can be achieved by several means
      (1) Congenital
         (a) Antibodies from the mother
         (b) Protection is temporary
      (2) Vaccination
         (a) Vaccines contain killed or weakened microorganisms
         (b) Stimulate the immune system
         (c) Not enough to cause disease
         (d) "Primes" the immune system so that the body can later respond to the infection
         (e) For example
            i) Smallpox has been eliminated from the planet
            ii) Polio, diphtheria
            iii) Tetanus, pertussis
            iv) Measles, mumps, rubella
            v) Haemophilus influenzae
      (3) Previous exposure
         (a) Acquire immunity from actually having that infection
         (b) One's immune status can be checked by measuring amount of antibody in blood
      (4) Passive immunity
         (a) Can be conveyed by injection of antibodies (immune globulin)
         (b) Injected antibodies fight the infection
6. High-risk individuals **(Slide 12-161)**
   a) Elderly
   b) Patients with respiratory and cardiac disease
   c) Diabetic patients
   d) Patients with immune system deficiencies such as Acquired Immune Deficiency Syndrome (AIDS)

Content

- e) Health care providers
  - (1) Due to frequent exposure
  - (2) Must take actions to reduce risk
  - (3) Should be vaccinated, i.e., against hepatitis B

7. Whether or not precautions were used **(Slide 12-162)**
   - a) Important for health professionals
   - b) EMTs can take several actions to prevent infecting patients
     - (1) Hand washing is a simple and most important step to prevent spread of disease
     - (2) Dressings applied to wounds should be sterile
     - (3) Equipment must be cleaned
     - (4) Bed linen should be replaced with every patient
     - (5) Maintaining one's personal health status
     - (6) Immunizations
     - (7) Wearing personal protective gear
     - (8) Practicing universal precautions
     - (9) Employing simple isolation procedures

XX. Specific Communicable Diseases **(Slide 12-163)**

- A. Many diseases are of concern to the EMT
- B. Diagnosing specific disease is beyond the bounds of prehospital care
- C. Certain conditions are important to understand to appreciate the range of possible diseases
- D. General signs and symptoms of infections **(Slide 12-164)**
  1. Fever and chills
  2. Absence of fever does not rule out infection
  3. Rashes
  4. Cough and sputum
  5. Flank pain typical of a kidney infection
  6. Severe headache or stiff neck with fever
  7. White blood cell count (in hospital)
- E. Blood-borne diseases **(Slide 12-165)**
  1. AIDS (Acquired Immune Deficiency Syndrome)
     - a) Described in 1982 as disease of unknown etiology
     - b) Results in a defect of cell mediated immunity
     - c) Important concepts
       - (1) Immunity to many bacterial infections is mediated through production of antibodies
       - (2) Immunity to fungi, parasites, and other unusual infections = cell mediated immunity
       - (3) AIDS affects cell mediated immunity; patients are prone to unusual infections
       - (4) Virus lives in blood, lymph tissue, and certain other body fluids
       - (5) Causes body to lose its natural defenses
       - (6) Open to attack from mild to life threatening illness
     - d) Related illness **(Slide 12-166)**
       - (1) Pneumonia in AIDS (due to Pneumocystic carini), is hardly ever seen in healthy individuals

(2) Karposi's sarcoma, a cancer, affects skin and the lining of blood vessels
(3) May spread throughout the body
(4) Virus found to infect the central nervous system, causing many neurological problems
(5) Healthy appearing individuals may be infected with the AIDS virus

e) Appropriate precautions must be used on all patients of all ages **(Slide 12-167)**

f) AIDS refers to individuals who have had a documented opportunistic infection

g) First stage of infection is generally asymptomatic and can continue for a decade

h) AIDS related complex, or ARC (second stage) **(Slide 12-168)**
(1) Weight loss
(2) Fatigue, lethargy
(3) Swollen lymph nodes, and chronic diarrhea

i) Patient can transmit HIV virus during all stages

j) Transmission via direct contact with body fluids **(Slide 12-169)**
(1) Sexual contact (anal, vaginal, oral)
(2) Needle sharing among IV drug abusers
(3) Transmission via transfusion of blood or blood products
(4) From mother to fetus
(5) Transfusion has now been virtually eliminated due to testing of blood
(6) Not transmitted by air or by casual contact
(7) Not transmitted by mosquitoes or other insects

k) Epidemiology **(Slide 12-170)**
(1) 176,047 reported cases of AIDS have been reported as of May 1991
(2) 111,815 patients have already died
(3) children under the age of 13 have been infected
(4) 1,161 children have died
(5) Suspect 1.2 million are infected
(6) Currently no cure or vaccine for the disease
(7) No known case of job-related transmission to prehospital providers

l) Recommendations **(Slide 12-171)**
(1) Practice safe sex
(a) Condoms during vaginal or oral sex
(b) Avoidance of anal sex
(c) Avoidance of sex with someone using IV drugs
(d) Avoidance of sharing intravenous drug needles
(2) Universal precautions for health workers
(a) Strict adherence to needle precautions
(b) Gloves, goggles, gowns and face masks
i) Routinely used where there is any potential for blood being splashed
ii) Change of clothing should always be available

Content

2. Hepatitis **(Slide 12-172)**
    a) Infection of the liver
    b) Caused by one of three different types of viruses
        (1) Hepatitis A spread by oral-fecal routes (infectious hepatitis)
        (2) Hepatitis B contacted in the same manner as AIDS and via saliva through a bite
        (3) Non-A, non-B type thought to be spread similar to hepatitis B
    c) Virus that causes hepatitis B is called HBV **(Slide 12-173)**
        (1) Is of concern to health workers
        (2) 25% of infected individuals develop acute hepatitis
        (3) 6-10% will become HBV carriers
        (4) Carriers are at risk of active liver disease and are infectious to others
        (5) About 300,000 new HBV infections in the U.S. each year
        (6) 12,000 are health care workers who contact the disease through their job
        (7) 200-300 health workers who contact hepatitis caused by HBV die each year
    d) Precautions **(Slide 12-174)**
        (1) Same personal practices as you would to avoid HIV
        (2) Follow-up for bites from an infected person
        (3) Vaccination against HBV is available (90% effective for 7 years)
        (4) Recommended for all EMTs
        (5) Passive and active immunity are available following possible exposure
        (6) Blood can be tested for antibodies against HBV.
    e) Risk after needlestick is much greater for HBV (6-30%) than for HIV (0.5%).

F. Respiratory secretions and airborne exposures
1. Meningitis **(Slide 12-175)**
    a) Infection of the meninges or covering of the central nervous system
    b) Caused by virus, bacteria, and other organisms
    c) Can present with or follow a respiratory infection
    d) Includes fever, headache, stiff neck, altered mental status
    e) Very close contact with respiratory secretions is of concern
    f) The antibiotic rifampin may be prescribed if the exposure to one type of meningitis is significant
2. Chickenpox **(Slide 12-176)**
    a) Very contagious and is spread by respiratory secretions and contact with the moist vesicles
    b) Same virus causes shingles
    c) If no prior exposure is known, EMT should take precautions to avoid close contact with patient

Content

3. Measles **(Slide 12-177)**
    a) Spread by respiratory droplets and contact with nasal secretions
    b) Highly contagious
    c) Vaccine is available
    d) EMTs should be immunized if they have no immunity
4. Rubella (German measles) **(Slide 12-178)**
    a) Respiratory droplets and contact with secretions
    b) Exposure should be avoided if possibly pregnant
    c) Health workers are urged to know their immunization status
5. Tuberculosis **(Slide 12-179)**
    a) Increasing in many parts of the country, in part because of AIDS
    b) Spread by droplets
    c) Patients with active tuberculosis can be given a mask to wear to block spread
    d) Checking for exposure is often part of a physical exam for health workers

G. Close Contact **(Slide 12-180)**
1. Herpes zoster (shingles)
    a) Localized infection along a dermatome
    b) Presenting first as pain, then as pustules
    c) Same virus that causes chickenpox
    d) If one has had chickenpox, then one is immune
2. Lice and scabies
    a) Can infect the head, body, or pubic area
    b) Close contact is required
    c) Usually first noted about the fingers
    d) Both cause itching and are cured by the same treatment

H. Fecal/Oral **(Slide 12-181)**
1. Diarrhea, if infectious, can be spread by the fecal/oral route
2. Hepatitis A can also be spread this way
3. Routine use of gloves to avoid direct contact with stool and handwashing are key to avoid exposure

XXI. Infection control **(Slide 12-182)**

A. Overview
1. Personnel health status through physical examination and review of immunization
2. Health status should be evaluated periodically
3. Health workers should not work if they have a contagious illness

B. Immunizations
1. Immunizations should be up to date
2. Records of immunizations and personnel health status should be available

C. Actions to block spread
1. Handwashing **(Slide 12-183)**
    a) Most important measure to block spread of infection
    b) Hands should be washed immediately:
        (1) If contaminated with blood, body fluids or potentially contaminated articles

Content

(2) After gloves are removed
(3) After patient contact and before caring for another patient

c) Use ordinary soaps
d) Do not wash hands in food preparation areas
e) Have waterless antiseptic hand cleanser available in ambulance

2. Aseptic technique **(Slide 12-184)**
a) When caring for open wounds
b) When using instruments that enter the skin or touch normally sterile parts of the body

3. Cleaning, disinfection, sterilization **(Slide 12-185)**
a) Ambulance and equipment are cleaned, disinfected or sterilized
b) Level is dictated by the intended use of the equipment
c) HIV is destroyed by many chemical disinfectants
(1) 70% alcohol, hydrogen peroxide
(2) Glutaraldehyde, quaternary ammonium chlorides
(3) Formalin, lysol, iodine
(4) Chlorhexidine gluconate/ethanol mix
(5) Household bleach (5.25% sodium hypochlorite) in dilutions between 1:100 and 1:10
(6) Capable of viral inactivation within one to ten minutes
(7) Soap and water will readily inactivate virus, as will exposure to drying

4. Universal precautions refer to approach to body substances and fluids that may carry the HIV or HBV virus **(Slide 12-186)**
a) EMT cannot always tell from outward appearance who is carrying infectious diseases
b) Must apply precautions to every (universal) situation
(1) Blood
(2) Semen
(3) Vaginal secretions
(4) Body fluids which surround
(a) Lungs, heart, brain
(b) Joints, abdominal organs
(c) Fetus
(5) Other fluids are not likely to contribute to blood borne infection
(a) Urine, feces, nasal secretions
(b) Sputum, sweat, tears and vomitus
(c) Other diseases may transmit through these routes

c) Personal protective gear **(Slide 12-187)**
(1) Consists of barriers to prevent direct contact with blood or other fluids
(2) Should be routinely available for EMTs
(3) Gloves **(Slide 12-188)**
(a) Heavy gloves (OSHA requirements) for handling sharp edges or broken glass
(b) Disposable, medical gloves for most situations
(c) Sterile, disposable gloves when delivering baby or caring for burn
(d) Utility gloves for cleaning

Content

(e) Don gloves when you anticipate the need for universal precautions
(f) CDC suggested procedures for use of gloves
i) Bleeding control
ii) Childbirth
iii) IV or blood drawing
iv) Suctioning
v) Intubation
(g) Change gloves between patients or whenever they are torn or soiled
(h) Avoid touching personal items such as combs when wearing gloves
(i) Reusable gloves which become contaminated
i) Wash with soap and water
ii) Wipe with disinfectant
iii) Hang in an inverted position to air dry
(4) Mask, goggles, gowns **(Slide 12-189)**
(a) When splash of blood is anticipated
i) Arterial bleeder
ii) Heavy bleeding or discharge of body fluids
(b) Use barriers to protect your eyes, mucous membranes and clothing
i) Mask (surgical mask)
ii) Goggles should be used with a faceshield
iii) Impervious gowns should be used to protect clothes
iv) Extra change of clothing should be available.
d) Needles and sharps **(Slide 12-190)**
(1) Needlesticks and other sharp objects represent highest risk of HIV or HBV
(2) Proper handling is of utmost importance
(3) Needles should never
(a) Be recapped, bent or broken by hand, removed from disposable syringes
(b) Otherwise manipulated
(c) Be allowed to touch any part of your body
(4) Place in a puncture resistant container for disposal at a later time
(5) Puncture resistant container should be as close to the site where a needle is used as possible
e) Isolation **(Slide 12-191)**
(1) With known or suspected contagious patient, prevent unnecessary exposure
(2) For example, with suspected measles patient
(a) Advise the triage nurse
(b) Bring the patient to the appropriate area
(c) Do not allow others to have unnecessary contact

Content

f) Decontamination and cleaning **(Slide 12-192)**
(1) Blood spills are cleaned as soon as possible
(2) Use gloves, boots over shoes, or face and eye protection as the situation dictates
(3) Place soiled towelling in a plastic bag to prevent contamination
(4) Clean surfaces with 1:100 solution of household bleach or other germicide
(5) Let the area dry
(6) Remove contaminated coverings and gloves last
(7) Place in the plastic bag
(8) Wash hands
g) Linen and clothing **(Slide 12-193)**
(1) Risk from contaminated linen and clothing negligible
(2) Place in a plastic or cloth bag for laundering
(3) Wash hands after handling
(4) Use gloves if it is heavily contaminated
(5) Can be washed with detergent and bleach in accordance with product recommendations
h) Disposal **(Slide 12-194)**
(1) Dispose of waste in accordance with local or state regulations
(2) Cleaning of vehicles
5. Post exposure follow-up **(Slide 12-195)**
a) If exposed, file a report with agency
b) Follow up with hospital to confirm the existence of an infectious condition
c) Hospital infection control programs track contacts of patients with certain infectious conditions
d) Diagnosis may be made after the EMT has left the patient
e) Hospitals will use prehospital record as one means to reach people

XXII. Summary **(Slide 12-196)**
A. Infection control practices are designed to block spread of infectious disease among patients, EMTs and the public at large
B. Must be practiced until it is a habit
C. Understanding of methods of disease transmission and diseases will help incorporate principles and techniques
D. Practice will lower risk to acceptable levels
E. EMT is a sophisticated partner in the care of patients who have infectious conditions
F. Continued updates in infection control are recommended

Chapter 12

MEDICAL EMERGENCIES

Examination

1. Insulin is produced in specialized cells in the:

   a. gall bladder
   b. liver
   c. pancreas
   d. appendix

2. Patients with an inadequate secretion of the hormone insulin have a disease called:

   a. hypo-insulin
   b. pancreatitis
   c. diabetes
   d. sclerosis of the liver

3. The larger molecule called _________ is composed of multiple molecules of glucose which are stored in the liver and the muscle:

   a. glycerine
   b. triglyceride
   c. hyperglucose
   d. glycogen

4. While most cells also use other sources of fuel, such as fats, the central nervous system depends almost exclusively on ______________.

   a. insulin
   b. glycogen
   c. glucose
   d. glucagon

5. The disease which occurs when there is a relatively prolonged insulin deficiency, which causes the blood glucose to rise and fatty acids to be produced in the blood is called:

   a. hypoglycemia
   b. diabetic ketoacidosis
   c. insulin dependency
   d. hyperacidity

6. The type of respirations that may be observed in a diabetic, characterized by deep and usually rapid respirations, are called:

   a. diabetic hyperventilation syndrome
   b. ketonic respirations
   c. Cheyne-Stokes breathing
   d. Kussmaul's respirations

7. Type I diabetics requires treatment with intramuscular:

   a. glucose
   b. glycogen
   c. orinase
   d. insulin

8. The most common and treatable diabetic problem encountered in prehospital care is:

   a. diabetic ketoacidosis
   b. Kussmaul's respirations
   c. hypoglycemia
   d. hyperglycemia

9. A patient with a known history of diabetes is found unconscious after jogging 2 miles. His wife states that he took his insulin this morning but has not eaten. He is probably suffering from:

   a. diabetic ketoacidosis
   b. Kussmaul's respirations
   c. hypoglycemia
   d. hyperglycemia

10. Which of the following is an appropriate treatments for unconscious patient with suspected hypoglycemia:

   a. administer oral glucose solutions and oxygen
   b. administer oxygen and dose of insulin
   c. administer oxygen and maintain the patients body temperature
   d. administer oral glucose solutions and transport rapidly

Match the type of diabetic emergency in column B with the signs and symptoms in column A (column B items can be used more than once).

Column A		Column B	
11.	increased thirst	a.	hypoglycemia
12	sweaty skin	b.	diabetic ketoacidosis
13.	pale skin		
14.	increased urination		
15.	abdominal pain (especially in children)		
16.	combative behavior		
17.	Kussmaul's respiration		
18.	fruity breath odor		
19.	rapid onset		

20. A drug that is given intramuscularly for hypoglycemia and may be carried at times by the patient is:

    a. glucose
    b. glucagon
    c. glycogen
    d. insulin

21. Which of the following drugs might a type II or noninsulin dependent diabetic take daily to stimulate the production of insulin:

    a. Orinase
    b. phenobarbital
    c. Dilantin
    d. glucagon

22. Shock secondary to anaphylaxis is:

    a. obstructive
    b. cardiogenic
    c. distributive
    d. neurogenic

Match the physiologic effect of anaphylaxis in column A to the signs and symptoms they cause in column B.

Column A		Column B	
23.	Constriction of bronchial smooth muscle	a.	hypotension due to decreased resistance
24.	Increased permeability of capillaries and fluid leakage	b.	swelling of the skin and stridor due to obstruction
25.	Dilation of the arteries	c.	sneezing and nasal congestion
26.	Increased mucus secretions in the respiratory tree	d.	wheezing breath sounds

27. An allergic reaction that results in vasodilation and capillary leakage and causes swelling of the face and airway are called:

    a. erythema
    b. purpura
    c. anaphylactis
    d. urticaria

28. The treatment for anaphylactic shock includes:

    a. administration of oxygen
    b. administration of epinephrine
    c. administration of IV fluids
    d. all of the above

29. The pediatric dose of epinephrine is usually administered subcutaneously at a dose of ______ mg/kg of body weight:

    a. 0.01
    b. 0.03
    c. 0.1
    d. 0.3

30. PASG may be useful in the treatment of shock secondary to anaphylaxis because the PASG:

    a. are the definitive treatment for anaphylaxis
    b. increase peripheral vascular resistance and improve the circulatory status of the patient
    c. decrease peripheral vascular resistance and allow the circulatory system to compensate appropriately
    d, negate the need for using epinephrine

31. When an anaphylactic reaction occurs secondary to a bite or sting in the arm you should place a constricting band:

    a. above the injury and tight enough to obstruct arterial flow
    b. above the injury and tight enough to obstruct venous return
    c. below the injury and tight enough to obstruct arterial flow
    d. below the injury and tight enough to obstruct venous return

32. If the stinger is still present at the site of the bite you should:

    a. leave the stinger alone
    b. stabilize the stinger in place with a 4 x 4
    c. scrape the stinger away
    d. place an ice pack over the stinger

33. A substance that through its chemical action usually kills, injures, or impairs an organism is defined by Webster's Dictionary as a(n):

    a. overdose
    b. toxic
    c. poison
    d. adverse reaction

34. A poison control center is:

    a. where all patients suffering from a poisoning must be taken
    b. a regional agency that studies the effects of poisoning on the body
    c. a regional agency available for phone consultation in the event of a poisoning
    d. a regional agency that decides what warning labels are required on products

Match the substance in column B with the type of poisoning in column A.

Column A	Column B
35. ingestion	a. carbon monoxide
36. inhalation	b. insecticide on skin
37. injection	c. methanol
38. absorption	d. scorpion sting

39. The first priority when dealing with a patient who has been poisoned by an intentional overdose of sleeping pills is to:

    a. treat the poison
    b. treat the patient
    c. respect the patient's desire to commit suicide and do nothing
    d. call the police, as a crime may have been committed

40. The first priority in the management of an unconscious suspected poison victim is to:

    a. induce vomiting
    b. provide cardiorespiratory support
    c. hasten elimination of the poison
    d. keep the patient awake

41. The most appropriate history that the EMT should take regarding a poisoning incident includes:

    a. what was taken, how much was taken, why was it taken
    b. what was taken, was it a suicide attempt, when was it taken
    c. was it a suicide attempt, what was taken, how much was taken
    d. when was it taken, what was taken, how much was taken

42. Inducing vomiting and giving activated charcoal are two methods of:

    a. hastening elimination
    b. neutralizing the poison
    c. preventing absorption
    d. providing an antidote

43. Regardless of the type of poison or the route of exposure, poison treatment centers around all of the following goals <u>except</u>:

    a. prevent further absorption
    b. treat signs and symptoms
    c. prevention of elimination
    d. hasten elimination

44. A medication given to induce diarrhea is called a(n):

    a. cathartic
    b. antidote
    c. oral suspension
    d. detoxinating agent

45. The correct dose of syrup of ipecac in an adult is:

a. 10 cc or two teaspoons
b. 15 cc or one tablespoon
c. 30 cc or two tablespoons
d. 60 cc or four tablespoons

46. The correct dose of syrup of ipecac for children over 1 year of age is:

a. 5 cc or one teaspoon
b. 15 cc or one tablespoon
c. 30 cc or two tablespoons
d. 60 cc or four tablespoons

47. Pinpoint pupils are the most common pupillary finding in:

a. cocaine overdoses
b. alcohol ingestion
c. narcotic overdoses
d. barbiturate overdoses

48. Respiratory arrest is a common complication of:

a. cocaine overdoses
b. alcohol ingestion
c. narcotic overdoses
d. PCP overdoses

49. The most common drug abused in the United States is:

a. crack cocaine
b. heroin
c. valium
d. alcohol

50. The acronym SLUD is used to remember sweating, lacrimation, urination, and diarrhea, which are all signs of a(n) __________ ingestion:

a. organophosphate
b. hydrocarbon
c. methanol glycol
d. ethylene glycol

51. The <u>first</u> and most important step in the management of an inhalation poisoning is:

a. removal from the toxic environment
b. administration of oxygen
c. positive pressure ventilation
d. cardiopulmonary resuscitation

52. All of the following are commonly injected drugs, <u>except</u>:

a. amphetamines
b. valium
c. cocaine
d. heroin

Match the type of snake in column B with the distinguishing features in column A.

Column A	Column B
53. round eyes	a. nonpoisonous
54. pit between eyes and nostrils	b. pit vipers
55. fangs	
56. elliptical eyes	

57. The treatment of coral snake bites includes:

a. suck out the venom and apply a constricting band
b. apply ice and administer oxygen as indicated
c. bring the dead snake to the hospital for positive identification and suck out the venom
d. bring the dead snake to the hospital for positive identification and splint the extremity

58. The treatment for punctures from cone shells or urchins includes:

a. immobilize the affected area and apply an ice pack
b. stimulate the affected area and immerse in cold water
c. immerse the affected area in hot water and immobilize the affected area
d. stimulate the affected area and immerse the affected area in hot water

59. A disease that is capable of being spread from one person to another is called a(n) __________ disease:

a. communicable
b. iatrogenic
c. parasitic
d. bacterial

Match the term in column B with the definition in column A.

Column A		Column B	
60.	coming in contact with but not necessarily being infected by a disease-causing agent	a.	carrier
		b.	nosocomial infections
61.	a source in which infectious agents can live and multiply	c.	communicable period
62.	time between contact with an infectious agent and the onset of signs and symptoms	d.	incubation period
		e.	reservoir
63.	a person who shows no signs of the disease yet harbors an infectious organism	f.	exposure
64.	infectious diseases that are spread by health care workers		
65.	time period during which a person can transmit an infectious disease to others		

66. Droplet contact, such as that spread by tuberculosis, usually involves an area no more than _____ feet from the infected person?

a. 2
b. 3
c. 4
d. 5

67. A vector borne transmission is spread by:

a. droplets
b. airborne contamination
c. insects
d. contaminated drinking water

68. HIV infection is transmitted through:

a. airborne routes
b. direct contact with infected carrier
c. urine and fecal exposure
d. body fluid to body fluid

69. The use of gloves and personal protection devices by every EMT when there is a possibility of contact with a patient's bodily fluid is referred to as:

a. general precautions
b. personal protective precautions (PPP)
c. barrier precautions
d. universal precautions

70. All of the following diseases are preventable with vaccines, except:

a. hepatitis B
b. measles
c. rubella
d. AIDS

71. Surface areas of transport vehicles that have come in contact with the patient's blood should be cleaned and decontaminated by using:

a. hypochlorite solution
b. air drying method
c. water
d. none of the above

72. The primary national agency that publishes guidelines which help standardize infection control practices across the country is the:

a. DOH
b. DOT
c. CDC
d. EPA

73. Penicillin is an example of a(n):

a. antihistamine
b. antibiotic
c. analgesic
d. anticonvulsant

74. Natural antibodies are carried by infants which provide protection against many common diseases this is called congenital:

a. resistance
b. barriers
c. immunity
d. protections

75. AIDS stands for:

a. allergic infectious disease syndrome
b. active infectious disease syndrome
c. acquired immune deficiency syndrome
d. active infectious disease syndrome

76. AIDS is transferable via:

a. food
b. body fluid to body fluid contact
c. skin to skin contact
d. skin to saliva contact

77. AIDS is a disease that compromises the ___________ system.

a. circulatory
b. endocrine
c. immune
d. central nervous

78. Common high risk modes of transmission for AIDS include all of the following, <u>except:</u>

a. sexual contact
b. needle sharing
c. food sharing
d. blood transfusion

79. The type of hepatitis that is spread by oral and fecal routes is called ______________ or infectious hepatitis.

a. hepatitis A
b. bacterial hepatitis
c. hepatitis B
d. HBV

80. An infection of the covering of the central nervous system that can be caused by virus, bacteria, and other organisms is called:

a. encephalitis
b. perineuritis
c. pleuritis
d. meningitis

Chapter 12

Skill Performance Sheet

Inducing Vomiting with Syrup of Ipecac

Student's Name______________________________ Date__________

Performance Standard	Performed	Failed
Check that the patient is responsive		
Check for a gag reflex		
Administer ipecac: (Adult - 30 cc, Child over 1 - 15 cc)		
Administer 1-2 glasses of water		
Place patient in sitting position		
Have suction at the ready		
Transport and observe		

Comments____

____

____

____

Instructor ___________________ Circle One: Pass Fail

Chapter 13

OBSTETRICAL EMERGENCIES

Materials and Equipment for Lesson

1. Anatomy slides, overhead transparencies, drawings or flipcharts
2. Handouts
   - Anatomy and physiology
   - Labor and delivery
   - Complications of labor and delivery
   - Trauma in pregnancy
3. Slide projector, overhead projector, flipchart and/or blackboard

Section 1

Anatomy and Physiology

Objectives
(Slide 13-1)

At the conclusion of the chapter the students will be able to:

1. List the location and function of the following anatomical structures:

Uterus	**Umbilical Cord**
Cervix	**Amniotic Sac**
Vagina	**Perineum**
Fetus	**Ovaries**
Placenta	**Fallopian Tubes**

2. Define the following terms:

Miscarriage/Abortion	**Presenting part**
Bloody show	**Position**
Crowning	

3. Define the three stages of labor.

4. List four physiologic changes that occur during pregnancy.

5. Describe the pathophysiology, signs and symptoms and prehospital treatment of the following conditions:
   - **Ecclampsia/Preeclampsia**
   - **Ruptured Ovarian Cyst**
   - **Ectopic pregnancy**
   - **Pelvic Inflammatory Disease**

5. List three indications of imminent delivery

6. List steps involved in predelivery preparation of the mother.

7. List the steps of care in a normal delivery.

8. Describe the postpartum care of the baby.

10. Describe how/when to cut the cord.

12. Describe the postpartum care of the mother.

13. List special considerations for multiple births.

14. Define a premature baby and list the special considerations for care.

15. Describe the procedures for:

Breech extraction	**Excessive bleeding in the mother**
Prolapsed cord	**Care of the pregnant trauma victim**
Arm/leg presentation	**Care of the rape victim**

Instructor Preparation

Reading preparation for the lesson:

EMT Prehospital Care, Chapter 13, pages 596-641

Suggested Learning Activities

Using a lecture format with the aid of slides, overhead transparencies or charts, provide a presentation on obstetrical emergencies.

Provide case history examples of obstetrical emergencies.

Content

I. Anatomy and Physiology of the Female Reproductive System
   A. Location, structure and function of organs **(Slide 13-2)**
      1. Uterus **(Slide 13-3)**
         a) Cervix
         b) Fundus
         c) Internal and external os
         d) Endometrium, myometrium, perimetrium
         e) Implantation
         f) Mucous plug
      2. Ovaries **(Slide 13-4)**
         a) Ovulation
         b) Menstruation
      3. Fallopian tubes **(Slide 13-5)**
         a) Fertilization occurs in the tubes
II. Blood Supply to the Uterus **(Slide 13-6)**
   A. Ovarian and uterine arteries
      1. Arteries arise directly from the aorta
   B. Venous drainage to the vena cava
III. Pregnancy
   A. 40 weeks of pregnancy **(Slide 13-7)**
      1. Three trimesters
            (1) Most birth defects occur in the 1st trimester, except for cocaine related growth defects
            (2) During the third trimester fetus acquires body fat and the liver and lungs mature
      2. Gestation and gestational age
   B. Placenta **(Slide 13-8)**
      1. Place where nutrients are exchanged
      2. Placental barrier
   C. Amnion **(Slide 13-9)**
      1. Amniotic fluid
         a) Functions as a cushion and to maintain temperature
         b) Meconium fluid
            (1) Danger of aspiration
            (2) 20% of babies with meconium fluid will have respiratory distress
   D. Umbilical cord **(Slide 13-10)**
      1. Umbilical vein carries oxygenated blood and nutrients to the baby
      2. Two umbilical arteries carry waste products away from baby
IV. Physiologic Changes of Pregnancy **(Slide 13-11)**
   A. Hematologic and Cardiovascular changes **(Slide 13-12)**
      1. Plasma volume increases almost 50%
      2. RBC volume increases only 32%
      3. Physiologic "anemia of pregnancy"
      4. Heart rate increases 15-20% **(Slide 13-13)**
      5. Blood pressure decreases in 2nd and third trimesters

Content

6. Classic signs of shock
7. Maternal shock carries an 80% chance of fetal mortality **(Slide 13-14)**
    a) Increased blood volume but decreased redistribution capability with blood loss
    b) First redistribution is constriction of the uterine artery
8. Supine hypotensive syndrome **(Slide 13-15)**
    a) Elevating the legs will not help
    b) Left lateral recumbent position is best **(Slide 13-16)**
    c) Use of a wedge or manual displacement of the uterus when cervical/spinal immobilization is needed **(Slide 13-17)**

B. Pulmonary changes
1. Tidal volume increases 50%
2. Respiratory rate does not change
3. Increased oxygen consumption
4. Elevation and stretching of the diaphragm
    a) Causes a decreased residual capacity
    b) More prone to hypoxia
    c) Dyspnea, shortness of breath more common

C. Gastrointestinal changes **(Slide 13-18)**
1. Progesterone slows the GI tract and relaxes the cardiac sphincter
    a) Assume the stomach is full
        (1) Prone to aspiration
2. Appendix moves to RUQ
3. Stretching and crowding of abdominal contents masks pain and makes diagnosis difficult
4. Uterus forms protective barricade, so traumatic injury less common

D. Genitourinary changes **(Slide 13-19)**
1. Bladder becomes an abdominal organ by the 12th week of pregnancy
    a) No longer protected by the bony pelvis
    b) Urine becomes trapped, bladder remains full
        (1) More prone to "burst balloon" rupture
        (2) Bladder, kidney infections more common
            (a) Fever, low back and flank pain common symptoms with infection
            (b) Infection may mimic or cause premature labor

V. Labor and Delivery

A. Three Stages of Labor **(Slide 13-20)**
1. First Stage of Labor -- Begins with first contraction and ends when cervix is fully dilated
    a) Three phases of the First Stage **(Slide 13-21)**
        (1) Early labor (0 to 3 or 4 cm)
            (a) Mild, irregular contractions
            (b) Effacement occurs **(Slide 13-22)**
        (2) Active labor (4-7 cm)
            (a) Contractions become painful, may last a minute, and become more regular, about 5 minutes apart
            (b) May begin to have bloody show

Content

(3) Transition (8-10 cm)
(a) Contractions closer, last up to 90 seconds, occur every 2 to 3 minutes and become very painful
(b) Nausea, vomiting and diaphoresis common
b) First stage in a primigravida may last 14 hours or more
(1) Not all labors will follow textbook rules
(2) Multigravidas may dilate rapidly because the cervix and muscles of the perineum have already been stretched
(3) False labor may be as painful as real labor
2. Second Stage of Labor -- Begins with full dilatation of the cervix and ends when the cervix is fully dilated
a) Pelvic cavity **(Slide 13-23)**
(1) Contains four joints, most nearly immovable
(a) 2 sacroiliac joints
(b) The symphysis pubis
i) Loosens slightly during pregnancy
(c) The sacrococcygeal (hinge) joint
(2) Bones welded together and capable of very little expansion
(3) The pelvic inlet **(Slide 13-24)**
(a) Heart-shaped entrance to the pelvis
(b) Limited by sacral promontory
(c) Transverse diameter is the longest diameter of the inlet
i) The baby will usually enter the pelvis facing the mother's left or right side
(4) The pelvic outlet **(Slide 13-25)**
(a) Diamond-shaped outlet through which the baby must emerge
(b) Limited by the ischial tuberosities
(c) Anteroposterior diameter is the longest diameter of the outlet
i) The baby's head must turn in order to negotiate the pelvic outlet. Most babies are born facing the mother's head or back
(5) Moulding of the baby's head may occur in order for the baby to fit through the pelvis **(Slide 13-26)**
(6) Abnormally shaped pelvis or large baby may delay birth or make vaginal delivery impossible
b) Presentation **(Slide 13-27)**
(1) Vertex
(2) Frank breech
(3) Footling breech
(a) Cervix may not be fully dilated when foot emerges
(4) Shoulder presentation
(5) Chin presentation
(6) Brow presentation

Content

(7) Malpresentation
(a) Prolapsed cord more prevalent
(b) Breech more dangerous in premature births because the head is proportionately much larger than the body
(8) As presenting part descends, mother will have an urge to push
(a) Patient should be examined during a contraction, since the presenting part may recede between contractions until crowning occurs **(Slide 13-28)**
c) Mechanics of Childbirth **(Slide 13-29)**
(1) Descent and Flexion -- The baby enters the pelvis facing the mother's right or left side. As the baby descends, it meets resistance, so the chin becomes sharply flexed upon the baby's chest
(2) Internal Rotation -- The baby turns to enter the pelvic outlet, so that it is now facing the mother's front or back.
(3) Extension -- The baby has to follow a longer path in the back of the pelvis than in the front because the pelvis is on a bent plane, leaving the vagina curved upwards. The head must extend to travel through the lower pelvis.
(4) External Rotation (Restitution) -- After the head is born, it must turn towards the mother's left or right side to realign with the shoulders.
(5) Expulsion -- Delivery of the shoulders and body.
3. The Third Stage of Labor -- Begins with delivery of the baby and ends when the placenta is expelled
a) Decrease in size of the uterus causes the inelastic placenta to separate from the wall of the uterus
b) Signs of placental separation:
(1) Uterus assumes a constant round shape instead of flattening between contractions
(2) Lengthening of the umbilical cord
(3) Gush of blood
c) Expect 50-200 cc blood loss
B. Assessment of the Labor Patient
1. History (Questions to ask)
a) Is this your first pregnancy?
b) What time did you start having regular contractions and how far apart are your contractions now?
c) Has your water broken? If so, what color is the fluid?
d) Do you have an urge to move your bowels?
e) Have you had any vaginal bleeding or bloody show?
f) When is your expected date of confinement? (sometimes referred to as EDC, due date, date of delivery)
g) Have you had any problems with this pregnancy, such as placenta previa?
h) Do you have any medical problems, such as diabetes, heart disease?

Content

(1) Babies born to diabetic mothers may be too large to deliver and become hypoglycemic shortly after birth **(Slide 13-30)**
(2) Mother with heart disease may not be allowed to push or may require antibiotics during delivery (mitral valve prolapse)

C. The Premature Infant **(Slide 13-31)**
1. Defined as 38 weeks or less
2. Less subcutaneous fat, less cartilage in the ears, no whorls on the soles of the feet
3. Greater amount of vernix
4. Lack pulmonary surfactant, so prone to respiratory distress
a) Nasal flaring
b) Sternal or intercostal retractions
c) Tachypnea
d) Nasal flaring
e) Cyanosis of mucous membranes
5. Poor temperature regulating ability; prone to acidosis after glucose reserves used up in attempt to maintain temperature
a) Heat on in ambulance
b) Dry thoroughly and wrap in clean, dry blanket, covering head
c) 100% oxygen and PPV if needed
d) Do not allow babies 34 weeks or less to nurse; lack ability to coordinate sucking and swallowing and may aspirate
e) More prone to intracranial hemorrhage and other injuries; handle very gently
f) Immature immune system; avoid exposing to infection
g) Radio ahead to hospital

D. The Postmature Infant **(Slide 13-32)**
1. Like the premature, has very little subcutaneous fat
2. No vernix
3. Wrinkled, waterlogged, peeling skin
4. Treat like premature

E. Physical Exam
1. Check patient during contraction, since presenting part may recede between contractions
2. Place on stretcher for delivery
3. Load stretcher onto ambulance in reverse position

VI. Management of Normal Labor and Delivery
A. Prep perineum if there is time
B. Prepare Obstetric Kit using sterile technique **(Slide 13-33)**
C. Prevent explosive delivery with gentle pressure on baby's head; have mother pant-blow to refrain from pushing **(Slide 13-34)**
D. When head is out, check for cord around neck
1. If loose, gently slip off **(Slide 13-35)**
2. If tight, clamp and cut carefully between clamps (1-34)
E. Gentle traction upward and then downward if necessary to deliver anterior and posterior shoulders

Content

F. Suction baby's mouth; if meconium fluid, suction after head is born (before body is delivered) **(Slide 13-36)**
G. Clamp and cut cord **(Slide 13-37)**
H. Check severed cord site for bleeding **(Slide 13-38)**
I. Dry baby and place on clean towel; have partner take over care of baby
J. After placenta delivers, remove dirty linen, place peri-pad on mother and cover her with blanket
K. Fundal massage if needed to control bleeding

VII. Resuscitation of the Newborn
- A. Evaluate respirations, heart rate and color, in that order **(Slide 13-39)**
- B. Try stimulating twice
- C. PPV with 100% oxygen if resuscitation required: **(Slide 13-40 to 13-43)**
  - 1. Not breathing or heart rateless than 100
    - a) First breath must be greater pressure than normal to simulate first breath of life (force fluid out of alveoli)
  - 2. Heart rate less than 60 or 60-80 but not increasing
  - 3. Cyanosis of mucous membranes (lips, gums, tongue)
- D. Chest compressions if heart rate less than 60 or 60-80 but not increasing **(Slide 13-44)**
- E. If breathing and heart rate over 100: **(Slide 13-45)**
  - 1. Slowly withdraw oxygen if color good
  - 2. Continue 100% oxygen if cyanotic or pale
  - 3. Continue to stimulate occasionally

VIII. Apgar Score **(Slide 13-46)**

IX. Newborn Survey
- A. Explain normal phenomena and check for birth injuries before giving baby to mother
  - 1. Milia **(Slide 13-47)**
  - 2. Moulding **(Slide 13-48)**
  - 3. Cephalhematoma **(Slide 13-49)**
  - 4. Cleft lip **(Slide 13-50)**
  - 5. Check for hidden cleft palate **(Slide 13-51)**
    - a) Do not allow baby with cleft palate or lip to nurse
  - 6. Brachial plexus damage **(Slide 13-52)**
  - 7. Fractured clavicle
  - 8. Spinal cord defect **(Slide 13-53)**

X. Maintaining a Warm Environment **(Slide 13-54)**
- A. When newborn becomes chilled, he uses large amount of oxygen and glucose reserves
  - 1. Anaerobic metabolism
  - 2. Lactic acid production = acidosis
  - 3. Hypoglycemia

XI. Third Stage Care of the Mother
- A. Transport immediately if baby is requiring resuscitation or if mother is bleeding heavily **(Slide 13-55)**
- B. Allow placenta to deliver by its own weight

Content

C. Do not pull on cord:
1. Cord may tear
2. Extra lobe of placenta **(Slide 13-56)**
3. Improper implantation of cord **(Slide 13-57)**
4. Placenta accreta (placenta grows into myometrium)

D. Check fundus for good contraction; should be at or below the umbilicus and bleeding should not be much heavier than menstrual bleeding **(Slide 13-58)**
1. Fundal massage to control bleeding
2. Nursing baby will release oxytocin which contracts uterus; may help to control bleeding
3. If a long distance to hospital, check fundus and bleeding at least every half hour

XII. Complications of Labor and Delivery

A. Prolapsed Cord **(Slide 13-59)**
1. Cord becomes compressed between the presenting part and the vagina or pelvis
2. Occurs more commonly with malpresentation (breech, shoulder) or when membranes rupture before the head has descended into the pelvis
3. Elevate <u>the presenting part</u>, not the cord
4. Elevate the mother's hips and displace uterus to the left
5. High concentration oxygen
6. Rapid transport; notify hospital

B. Breech Delivery **(Slide 13-60)**
1. Transport unless buttocks are emerging
2. Breech births usually longer and more dangerous than vertex
    a) Complications include prolapsed cord, premature separation of placenta, meconium aspiration, fractured clavicle, damage to brachial plexus, and head and neck injuries (fractured skull, intracranial hemorrhage, etc.)
    b) Breech does not make a good dilating wedge
    c) Buttocks smaller diameter than head; may emerge before cervix is fully dilated
    d) More dangerous in premature; head of premature is proportionately much larger than buttocks
    e) Meconium usually present from pressure on abdomen
    f) Prolapse of umbilical cord more common
    g) If body is delivered and head remains entrapped, uterus contracts and placenta may separate
3. Aim for slow, controlled delivery **(Slide 13-61)**
    a) Delivery may be easier if mother is moved to edge of stretcher with knees sharply bent
    b) Allow breech to deliver up to scapula by its own weight
    c) Gently pull loop of cord after umbilicus is born, to prevent tearing of cord
    d) May need to assist in external rotation of shoulders **(Slide 13-62)**
        (1) External rotation must occur to deliver shoulders

Content

(2) Downward traction to deliver anterior shoulder; upward traction for posterior
(3) Reach in a finger to hook out each arm if they do not deliver spontaneously
(a) Too much traction when arms are extended over head may damage brachial plexus
e) After shoulders are delivered, back will again be facing up **(Slide 13-63)**
f) Head must be flexed (chin on chest) to deliver **(Slide 13-64)**
(1) If head does not deliver spontaneously, place two fingers in mouth and pull chin onto chest
(2) Suprapubic pressure may be needed
(3) If head does not deliver in three minutes, provide an airway by making a "V" with your fingers and pressing the vaginal wall away from the baby's nose
(a) There will be pressure on the umbilical cord, and the placenta will start to separate at this time
i) Elevate hips
ii) High concentration oxygen
iii) Rapid transport

C. Shoulder Dystocia **(Slide 13-65)**
1. Head delivers but shoulders become wedged in pelvis
2. Suprapubic pressure
3. McRobert's maneuver
a) Flex mother's knees sharply against either side of her chest to straighten spine and enlarge pelvis
4. If still unable to deliver, suction baby's mouth and transport rapidly, giving oxygen to mother

D. Abruptio Placenta **(Slide 13-66)**
1. Premature separation of the placenta
a) 25% recurrence rate
b) Cocaine use, history of hypertension or other vascular disease increases risk
c) Separation may be partial, with little effect on baby, or complete, causing fetal death
d) May be concealed or may present with dark vaginal bleeding
(1) Uterus is painfully hypertonic, with no relaxation between contraction
(2) If concealed, uterus may enlarge; mark fundus with felt tip pen
e) Give oxygen and transport on left side

E. Placenta Previa **(Slide 13-67)**
1. Placenta grows over the cervical os
2. Painless third trimester bleeding (bright red blood)
3. Rapid transport on left side, oxygen, PASG with legs inflated if large blood loss

F. Ruptured Uterus **(Slide 13-68)**
1. Causes 5% of maternal deaths

Content

2. Greatest risk: overdistended uterus (multiple gestation, hydramnios), aging uterus with history of several previous births, previous cesarian section or other uterine surgery
3. Presents with acute abdominal pain, tearing sensation, vaginal bleeding; contractions have stopped and uterus may be palpated beside the fetus. Often confused with abruptio placenta
4. May be complicated by ammonitic fluid embolism
    a) Dyspnea, chest pain, cyanosis, shock
    b) Interferes with clotting mechanism; often leads to DIC **(Slide 13-69)**
5. Rapid transport on left side with oxygen and PASG (leg compartments) if signs of shock

G. Premature Rupture of Membranes
1. Early rupture of the membranes before head is engaged may cause prolapsed cord
2. Rupture of membranes more than 24 hours before delivery can lead to infection

3. Pathway for bacteria is open; may cause amnionitis

H. Postpartum Hemorrhage **(Slide 13-70)**
1. Blood loss greater than 500 cc following delivery
2. Early Postpartum Hemorrhage
    a) Occurs in the first 24 hours (most common in first hour after delivery)
    <u>b) Most common cause is uterine atony</u>, often brought on by retained placental tissue. May also be caused by: **(Slide 13-71)**
        (1) Uterine rupture
        (2) Placenta accreta
        (3) Coagulation defects
        (4) Genital lacerations
        (5) Inverted uterus
        (6) Prolapsed uterus
        (7) Displacement of the uterus by a full bladder, preventing contraction of the uterus
3. Late postpartum hemorrhage **(Slide 13-72)**
    a) Occurs 6-10 days postpartum
    <u>b) Most common cause is retained placental tissue</u>. May also be caused by:
        (1) Infection
        (2) Opening of episiotomy or cesarian scar
4. Symptoms of postpartum hemorrhage: **(Slide 13-73)**
    a) Massive vaginal bleeding
    b) Soft, boggy uterus above the level of the umbilicus
5. Treatment of postpartum hemorrhage: **(Slide 13-74)**
    a) Massage uterus until it becomes a firm, hard ball at or below the level of the umbilicus

Content

b) If the uterus is inverted, place a gloved fist into the inverted fundus and attempt to reinsert the uterus through the cervical ring. Apply counterpressure to the fundus with your other hand by pushing on the abdomen. Elevate hips and transport rapidly

c) PASG if in shock

d) Lactated Ringer's/large gauge (16 or 18) IV

e) Breast-feeding by the mother will release oxytocin, causing the uterus to contract. May help to control bleeding, but mother may be weak from blood loss and strain of delivery, so she should not be left unattended

I. Preeclampsia and Eclampsia **Slide 13-75)**

1. Toxemia of pregnancy with elevated blood pressure (>140 diastolic or >90 systolic), proteinuria and edema, all occurring after the 20th week of pregnancy
2. Occurrence of a seizure constitutes eclampsia
3. Occurrence:
    - a) 1 out of 10 pregnancies affected by preeclampsia
    - b) Second leading cause of maternal death in the United States
    - c) Primigravidas
4. Risk factors: **(Slide 13-76)**
    - a) Primigravida
    - b) Obesity/malnutrition
    - c) Pre-existing vascular disease (diabetes, heart disease, hypertension, kidney disease)
    - d) Multiple gestation (twins)
    - e) Genetic history
5. Vasospasm of preeclampsia affects all major organs, may cause widespread damage and symptoms: **(Slide 13-77)**
    - a) Visual disturbances and photophobia (retinal edema)
    - b) Epigastric pain (stretching and bleeding beneath liver capsule)
    - c) Oliguria (kidney damage)
    - d) Headache, hyperreflexia, stroke (cerebral edema)
    - e) Blood clots, bleeding
        - (1) DIC, low platelets
        - (2) Patient is actually hypovolemic; fluid has shifted to third space
        - (3) Hemoconcentration leads to hypercoagulation
    - f) Placental abruption (vasospasm causes poor placental circulation, infarcts and abruption)
    - g) Pulmonary edema
    - h) Heart failure
6. Treatment for preeclampsia/eclampsia **(Slide 13-78)**
    - a) Delivery of baby is only "cure"
    - b) Magnesium Sulfate (MGSO4)
        - (1) Central nervous system depressant
        - (2) Inhibits parathyroid hormone, causes hypocalcemia

Content

(3) Magnesium toxicity causes hyporeflexia, depressed level of consciousness, difficulty swallowing, respiratory depression or arrest, cardiac asystole

(4) First sign of toxicity is loss of deep tendon reflexes

(a) When transporting patients on MGSO4, check reflexes, blood pressure, respiratory rate at least every 15 minutes

c) Baby born to mother on Magnesium Sulfate may also show signs of magnesium toxicity (respiratory depression, poor muscle tone). Be prepared to resuscitate.

J. Disseminated Intravascular Coagulopathy **(Slide 13-79)**

1. Occurs when there is widespread destruction of tissue (preeclampsia, abruption, missed abortion, preeclampsia, amniotic fluid embolism). Clotting factors are released into the bloodstream; may present with massive emboli or uncontrollable hemorrhage

2. Treatment is rapid transport with oxygen while attempting to control hemorrhage. Minimize injection sites if IV line is started.

K. Vaginal bleeding **(Slide 13-80)**

1. Assessing vaginal bleeding

a) Amount

(1) Pad count may not give true picture; amount of blood absorbed by different types of pads differs by as much as 200 cc

(2) Bleeding is often noted in toilet bowl, where amount seems much greater than it is

b) Color

(1) Dark bleeding vs bright bleeding may distinguish between placenta previa and abruption

(2) Record color exactly, i.e., pink stain, brown spotting

c) Clots

(1) Note the presence or absence of clots or placental tissue

L. Abortions **(Slide 13-81)**

1. Definitions:

a) Induced abortion - voluntary termination of pregnancy

b) Spontaneous abortion - miscarriage before the 20th week of gestation

c) Stillbirth - loss of fetus after 20th week gestation

d) Complete abortion - passing all the products of conception

e) Incomplete abortion - passing some, but not all of the products of conception (often means the fetus has been passed but the placenta retained)

f) Missed abortion - retention of fetus in utero 4 or more weeks after fetal death has occurred

g) Septic abortion - abortion with pelvic or peritoneal infection

h) Threatened abortion - vaginal bleeding and mild contractions in a pregnant patient with no dilatation of the cervix

i) Inevitable abortion - profuse vaginal bleeding with dilatation of the cervix and rupture of the membranes

Content

2. Management of threatened abortion or stillbirth **(Slide 13-82)**
    a) Elevate hips to relieve pressure on cervix
    b) Treat for shock if necessary
    c) Resuscitate premature infant if not macerated

M. Ectopic pregnancy **(Slide 13-83)**
1. Pregnancy occurring outside of uterine cavity; 90% are tubal but may occur elsewhere
2. Leading cause of 1st trimester deaths in non-white women; causes more than 11% of all maternal deaths in United States
3. Major cause of infertility (inability to conceive)
4. Predisposing factors: **(Slide 13-84)**
    a) History of pelvic inflammatory disease (30%)
    b) Endometriosis
    c) Genetic defect causing narrowing of fallopian tubes
    d) Adhesions; previous pelvic surgery
    e) Failed tubal ligation
    f) Failed use of IUD
    g) Previous ectopic pregnancy
5. Symptoms: **(Slide 13-85)**
    a) Amenorrhea
    b) May have positive pregnancy test, abdominal swelling and knowledge of pregnancy
    c) Sudden onset of poorly localized lower abdominal pain that may radiate to or be felt only in shoulder area (shoulder pain caused by irritation of diaphragm)
    d) May have vaginal or rectal pain
    e) Nausea and vomiting may be present
    f) Often mistaken for appendicitis
6. Ruptured ovarian cyst may mimic ectopic pregnancy **(Slide 13-86)**
7. Treatment for ectopic pregnancy or ruptured ovarian cyst is rapid transport with treatment for shock if symptoms occur
8. Major cause of infertility and ectopic pregnancy

N. Pelvic inflammatory disease **(Slide 13-87)**
1. Sexually acquired infection of uterus, fallopian tubes, adjacent structures
2. Causative organisms:
    a) Most common are gonorrhea or chlamydia
    b) Staphylococcus
    c) Streptococcus
3. Incidence: **(Slide 13-88)**
    a) May follow procedures that dilate cervix (i.e. D and C), suction abortion, insertion of an IUD (women with IUD more susceptible)
    b) Most common in sexually active women ages 15-24
    c) Virtually nonexistent in pregnant women
4. Symptoms: **(Slide 13-89)**
    a) First symptom usually painful intercourse
    b) Dull, aching, bilateral and continuous abdominal pain
    c) Foul smelling vaginal discharge
    d) Vaginal bleeding and fever (more than 50% of cases)
    e) Nausea and vomiting if bowels are involved

Content

f) Toxic shock may evolve **(Slide 13-90)**
(1) Caused by Staphylococcus, an organism often found on the skin which releases toxins when it enters the bloodstream
(2) May be introduced via a tampon, surgical packing, infected mosquito bite or untreated boil
(3) Symptoms are flu-like, with fever, joint pain, watery diarrhea and typical sunburn-like rash on face

XIII. Trauma in Pregnancy **(Slide 13-91)**
A. Motor vehicle accidents most common cause
1. Injury less severe if wearing restraint, especially shoulder/lap combination
B. Physiologic changes of pregnancy make treatment of pregnant trauma victim unique with special considerations (see section on physiologic changes of pregnancy) and injuries not often seen in the non-pregnant victim: **(Slide 13-92)**
1. Abruption (usually occurs within 24 hours of injury)
2. Ruptured uterus
3. Burst balloon bladder rupture (from urine trapped in bladder which is now partially an abdominal organ)
4. Premature labor
C. Treatment priorities: **(Slide 13-93)**
1. Assume the stomach is full
a) Airway and suction nearby
b) Aggressive airway management
2. Prevent shock: Maternal shock = 80% chance of fetal mortality
3. PASG without abdominal compartment inflated
4. Left lateral recumbent position
a) If spinal immobilization is in effect, apply wedge under right flank or manually displace uterus to the left side to prevent vena caval compression

XIV. Asthma in pregnancy **(Slide 13-94)**
A. Treat with humidified oxygen via face mask at 5 L/min
B. If patient becomes cyanotic, use non-rebreather with reservoir
C. Transport in position of comfort, usually upright

XV. Rape **(Slide 13-95)**
A. Gentle, compassionate manner is essential
B. Attempt to preserve evidence:
1. Have patient avoid shower, douche, brushing teeth, urinating, defecating or changing clothes
C. Assess for other injuries and treat accordingly

XVI. Perineal injuries **(Slide 13-96)**
A. Occurrence:
1. Rape
2. Gymnastics, ice skating, skiing, bicycle injuries
3. Vulvar lacerations, hematomas
4. Periurethral tears
B. Treatment **(Slide 13-97)**
1. Control bleeding with direct pressure
2. Do not pack vagina
3. Ice pack to site may reduce pain and help to control bleeding

OBSTETRICAL AND GYNECOLOGIC EMERGENCIES

Examination

Match the answer in column A with the best symptoms or definition from column B.

Column A		Column B	
1.	missed abortion	a.	missed period and sudden onset of abdominal pain referred to shoulder with vaginal bleeding and signs of shock
2.	pelvic inflammatory disease (PID)	b.	marked by sharp, tearing pain and an abrupt cessation of labor pains
3.	abruptio placentae	c.	painless, bright red vaginal bleeding
4.	placenta previa	d.	dead fetus retained in uterus
5.	disseminated intravascular coagulation (DIC)	e.	rigid uterus, bleeding may be dark, no break between contractions
6.	ruptured uterus	f.	fever, abdominal pain and vaginal discharge
7.	ruptured ectopic pregnancy	g.	disruption of the normal clotting mechanism with uncontrollable hemorrhage as a result

8. What is the largest diameter of the pelvic outlet?

   a. transverse
   b. anteroposterior
   c. oblique
   d. lateral

9. The release of a mature egg from the female ovary is called:

   a. menstruation
   b. conception
   c. fertilization
   d. ovulation

10. A major function of the fallopian tubes is the:

    a. carrying of eggs from ovary to the uterus
    b. site of implantation of a normal pregnancy
    c. connecting point between the cervix and the vagina
    d. site of egg production

11. The part of the body where eggs are stored and become mature and where female hormones are produced is the:

    a. fallopian tube
    b. uterus
    c. ovary
    d. cervix

12. The section of the uterus that must be effaced and dilated during labor is the:

    a. body
    b. cervix
    c. fundus
    d. myometrium

13. The lining of the uterus into which the embryo implants and that is shed during menstruation is the:

    a. myometrium
    b. endometrium
    c. perimetrium
    d. cervometrium

14. The uppermost part of the uterus is the:

    a. cervix
    b. fundus
    c. endometrium
    d. crown

15. The organ through which nutrients and waste products are exchanged between the baby and the mother is the:

    a. uterus
    b. placenta
    c. liver
    d. cervix

16. The umbilical cord contains:

    a. one vein and one artery
    b. one vein and two arteries
    c. two veins and one artery
    d. two veins and two arteries

17. The first stage of labor:

    a. begins with full dilation of the cervix and ends when the baby is born
    b. lasts from the onset of contractions until the cervix is completely dilated
    c. ends at the onset of transition
    d. should never last more than 1 hour

18. In the transition period of labor, you can expect:

    a. contractions 2-3 minutes apart lasting 60-90 seconds
    b. sweating and nausea
    c. delivery of the placenta
    d. a and b only
    e. all of the above

19. True labor is differentiated from false labor by:

    a. intensity of contractions
    b. regularity of contractions
    c. dilation of the cervix
    d. amount of bloody show

20. All of the following are parts of the mechanism of childbirth <u>except</u>:

    a. flexion
    b. composition
    c. internal rotation
    d. expulsion

21. During the second stage of labor:

    a. the mother often has an urge to move her bowels
    b. postpartum hemorrhage may occur
    c. you can expect to deliver the placenta
    d. labor contractions stop

22. During a normal vertex delivery, as soon as the baby's head is born, you should:

    a. immediately tell the mother to push before the cervix closes
    b. ask the mother to pant while you check to see if there is a cord wrapped around the baby's neck
    c. examine the baby's mouth to see if he or she has a cleft lip
    d. dry the baby's head

23. Your <u>first</u> action after the baby is out is to:

    a. clamp the cord
    b. suction the baby's mouth and nose with a bulb syringe
    c. dry the baby thoroughly
    d. deliver the placenta

24. If a baby's head is born and you find that the umbilical cord is wrapped tightly around the baby's neck, you should:

    a. give the mother oxygen and transport rapidly
    b. stretch the cord over the baby's head to unwind it
    c. clamp the cord close together in two places and cut between the clamps
    d. try to push the head back inside a little bit to ease tension around the baby's neck

25. McRobert's maneuver, sharply flexing the mother's knees back toward either side of her abdomen, straightens the spine and may be useful:

    a. when the placenta will not deliver
    b. in the pregnant trauma victim
    c. when the head is born but the shoulders seem to be stuck
    d. in a postpartum hemorrhage

26. In a vertex delivery with meconium-stained fluid, the mouth should be suctioned:

    a. only after the nose is suctioned
    b. as soon as the head is born, before delivering the rest of the baby
    c. only after you check the heart rate
    d. the mouth should not be suctioned because you will contaminate the mouth with bacteria

27. When you find that the baby's leg is projecting out of the vagina in a laboring patient, you should:

    a. grasp the leg firmly and pull until you can reach the other leg
    b. transport rapidly while giving oxygen to the mother
    c. try to push the leg back inside the vagina
    d. press on the mother's fundus and ask her to push

28. After a baby is born and the cord is cut, you notice lengthening of the umbilical cord and contractions of the uterus. This would indicate:

    a. laceration of the vagina
    b. the onset of a postpartum hemorrhage
    c. the placenta is about to be delivered
    d. uterine rupture

29. Allowing the mother to nurse a healthy, full-term newborn after birth:

    a. should never be done in the ambulance
    b. can help to contract the uterus
    c. can relieve cyanosis in a newborn
    d. supplies the baby with the calories it needs

30. If the placenta does not spontaneously deliver within 15-20 minutes after the baby is born, you should:

    a. ask the mother to push while you pull on the cord
    b. proceed to the hospital
    c. ask the mother to stand; gravity may deliver the placenta
    d. perform McRobert's maneuver

31. All of the following are normal in the newborn <u>except</u>:

    a. a heart rate of 156
    b. a white, creamy film on the baby's skin
    c. tiny white spots covering the nose and chin
    d. limpness or apparent weakness in one or both arms

32. When resuscitating a newborn, the heart rate is counted for:

    a. a full minute
    b. 6 seconds
    c. only after the Apgar score is done
    d. 30 seconds

33. All of the following are symptoms of respiratory distress in the newborn <u>except</u>:

    a. grunting
    b. nasal flaring
    c. cyanosis of the hands and feet
    d. sternal retractions

34. All of the following are <u>improper</u> actions when resuscitating a newborn <u>except</u>:

    a. hyperextending the neck before ventilating
    b. quickly drying the baby immediately after birth
    c. giving chest compressions with the heel of one hand
    d. ventilating the baby at a rate of 80 breaths/min

35. Positive pressure ventilation for a newborn should be done at a rate of:

    a. 20-30 breaths/min
    b. 40-60 breaths/min
    c. 80-100 breaths/min
    d. 120-140 breaths/min

36. The concentration of oxygen for positive pressure ventilation of a newborn should be:

    a. 90-100%
    b. 40-50%
    c. never give oxygen to a newborn

37. Chest compressions in the newborn should be:

    a. 1/2-3/4 inch at 100 beats/min
    b. 1/2-3/4 inch at 120 beats/min
    c. 1-2 inch at 150 beats/min
    d. 1-2 inch at 120 beats/min

38. A newborn is breathing at birth, so you check the heart rate. It is 85. Your next action would be to:

    a. evaluate the baby's color
    b. begin positive pressure ventilation with 100% oxygen
    c. begin cardiac compressions
    d. give 100% free-flow oxygen

39. When resuscitating a newborn, cardiac compressions should be discontinued once the baby's heart rate has reached:

    a. 50 beats/min
    b. 80 beats/min
    c. 90-100 beats/min
    d. compressions should not be performed at all if the baby has a heart rate

40. An infant born with a cleft palate:

a. will probably also be brain damaged
b. should not be allowed to nurse
c. should not be shown to the mother
d. all of the above

41. Allowing the newborn to become chilled can:

a. help to establish respirations if the baby does not cry
b. cause hypoglycemia and acidosis
c. stimulate a more rapid heart rate as the baby tries to stay warm
d. help to keep the baby awake so that it can nurse

42. A common complication of abdominal trauma in the pregnant patient is:

a. placenta previa
b. ruptured bowel
c. abruptio placentae
d. all of the above

43. In general, the position for transport of a pregnant patient in her third trimester is:

a. supine
b. prone
c. on her left side
d. on her right side

44. The reason for transporting a pregnant woman on her left side is:

a. you always want to have the mother facing you in the ambulance
b. most babies are facing the mother's right side late in pregnancy, and pressure on the back of the baby's head can dangerously lower the heart rate
c. to prevent damage to the liver
d. the vena cava is right of the midline and you do not want to compress it between the spinal column and the weight of the baby

45. During normal pregnancy, the blood pressure:

a. should not change
b. becomes slightly higher than it was before pregnancy
c. becomes much higher than it was before pregnancy
d. becomes lower than it was before pregnancy

46. A baby born to a diabetic mother:

    a. is prone to hypoglycemia after delivery
    b. is prone to hyperglycemia after delivery
    c. is not usually affected by the mother's disease
    d. will probably be born with diabetes

47. A baby born to a diabetic mother is likely to be:

    a. larger than normal
    b. smaller than normal
    c. average size

48. Maternal hypertension is defined as:

    a. systolic greater than 180 or diastolic greater than 100
    b. systolic greater than 160 or diastolic greater than 100
    c. systolic greater than 150 or diastolic greater than 90
    d. systolic greater than 140 or diastolic greater than 90

49. Preeclampsia becomes eclampsia when:

    a. hypertension and edema are both present
    b. the blood pressure exceeds 180/100
    c. a seizure occurs
    d. all of the above

50. All of the following are predisposing factors to ectopic pregnancy <u>except</u>:

    a. history of PID
    b. previous ectopic pregnancy
    c. adhesions from previous surgery
    d. high blood pressure

51. If you examine a laboring patient and find the umbilical cord bulging out of the vagina, you should:

    a. clamp and cut the cord so that the baby can be delivered
    b. try to elevate the presenting part with a gloved hand so it does not compress the cord
    c. gently place the cord back inside the vagina
    d. place a moist pressure dressing over the vagina

52. Prolapsed cord is often associated with:

    a. placenta previa
    b. abruptio plancentae
    c. abnormal presentation, such as breech or shoulder
    d. preeclampsia

Chapter 13

Skill Performance Sheet

Normal Childbirth

Student's Name______________________________ Date__________

Performance Standard	**Performed**	**Failed**
EMT #1 washes hands, if possible		
Apply gloves using sterile technique and prepare sterile field		
Apply gentle pressure on baby's head with flat hand		
Once head is delivered, check for cord around baby's neck		
If cord cannot be slipped over the head, clamp and cut cord if around neck		
Suction mouth if there is meconium-stained fluid		
Ask mother to push and gently deliver shoulders with downward traction for upper shoulder and upward traction for lower shoulder		
Suction baby with bulb syringe		
Place baby on dry towels		
Deliver placenta		
Massage uterus as necessary		
Place placenta in bag		
Deliver mother and baby to hospital while keeping warm		

Comments____

____

Instructor ___________________ Circle One: Pass Fail

Skill Performance Sheet

Resuscitation of the Newborn

Student's Name____________________________ Date_________

Performance Standard	Performed	Failed
Dry infant and place on clean towel in a warm place		
Place head in "sniffing position"		
Suction mouth and nose with bulb syringe		
Evaluate breathing		
If infant not breathing, stimulate by rubbing back and slapping feet		
If not breathing, provide positive pressure ventilation (40/min)		
Evaluate heart rate after 30 seconds of ventilation		
If heart rate is less than 80, begin chest compressions at a rate of 120 compressions per minute		
If heart rate is between 80 and 100, continue positive pressure ventilation, but do not perform compressions		
After 30 seconds of chest compression, check heart rate		
If heart rate below 80, continue CPR		

Comments____

____

____

____

Instructor __________________ Circle One: Pass Fail

Chapter 14

PEDIATRIC EMERGENCIES

Materials and Equipment for Lesson

1. Anatomy slides, overhead transparencies, drawings or flipcharts
2. Handouts
   - Pediatric emergencies
   - Local laws pertaining to reportable incidents
3. Slide projector, overhead projector, flipchart and/or blackboard

Objectives
(Slide 14-1)

At the conclusion of the chapter the student will be able to:

1. List two developmental differences for the following ages of children and two factors on how this alters your approach to the patient.
- **Infant**
- **Toddler 15 months - 3 years**
- **Small child 4 -8 years**
- **Preadolescent 9-12**
- **Adolescent**

2. List one of the differences in anatomy and physiology of infants and children with respect to each the following:
- **Respiratory function**
- **Respiratory rate**
- **Pulse rate**
- **Blood pressure**
- **Metabolic considerations**
- **Neurological differences**
- **Response to hypovolemia and shock**

3. List the steps of the primary and secondary survey for a pediatric patient.

4. List three signs and symptoms and the prehospital treatment for each of the following conditions:
- **Croup**
- **Epiglottitis**
- **Foreign body obstruction**
- **Bronchiolitis**
- **Asthma**
- **Pneumonia**
- **Foreign bodies in lower airway**
- **Near drowning**
- **SIDS**
- **Febrile child**
- **Seizures**

5. List five findings associated with child abuse.

6. List the steps of the approach to the pediatric trauma patient.

Chapter 14

Instructor Preparation

Reading preparation for the lesson:

EMT Prehospital Care, Chapter 14, pages 643-677

Suggested Learning Activities
Using a lecture format with the aid of slides, overhead transparencies or charts, provide a presentation on pediatric emergencies.
Provide case history examples of pediatric emergencies.

Content

I. Overview **(Slide 14-2)**
- A. Child patients present several challenges
  - 1. Emotional aspects of EMTs, family, bystanders and child
  - 2. Unwilling and uncooperative patient
  - 3. Communication problems
  - 4. Key differences between adults and children
- B. Children are not small adults, differences: **(Slide 14-3)**
  - 1. Developmental
  - 2. Anatomical
  - 3. Physiologic
  - 4. Types of emergencies
  - 5. Response to accidents and illness

II. Epidemiology -- common causes of death **(Slide 14-4)**
- A. Accidents and respiratory conditions after first year
  - 1. Accidental death 23,000
    - a) Motor vehicles (50%)
    - b) Falls (25-30%)
    - c) Drowning (10%)
    - d) Poisoning and assaults (15%).
  - 2. Causes of respiratory arrests in children **(Slide 14-5)**
    - a) Asthma
    - b) Trauma
    - c) Drug ingestion
    - d) Drowning
    - e) Smoke inhalation
    - f) Sudden infant death syndrome [SIDS]
    - g) Infection
- B. Cardiac arrest is rarely due to heart disease **(Slide 14-6)**
  - 1. Congenital heart disease or cardiomyopathy is exception
  - 2. Usually follow a respiratory insult
  - 3. After prolonged hypoxia
  - 4. Bradyarrhythmias into asystole
  - 5. Ventricular fibrillation rare
  - 6. Better chance of brain recovery after hypoxia than do adults

III. Differences Between Children and Adults
- A. Overview **(Slide 14-7)**
  - 1. Unable to understand the nature of their problem or rationale of treatment
  - 2. Pain and fear may make them uncooperative
  - 3. Two patients; child and the parent
    - a) Primary attention to child
    - b) Parents may be anxious, fearful and impatient
    - c) Gain cooperation and mobilize energy of parents
  - 4. Control your reactions
    - a) Panic may suggest a more serious problem
    - b) Calm, objective and understanding approach is essential

Content

B. Developmental differences **(Slide 14-8)**
   1. Infant -- birth to 1 year
      a) Minimal language capability
      b) Responds to facial expressions and tone of voice
      c) Interact with parents before child
      d) Infants often demonstrate anxiety with strangers
      e) Collect history from the parents
      f) Examine in sight of parents or in their arms
      g) Minimal touching to reduce anxiety
      h) Provide warm emotional and physical environment
      i) Toe to head approach
   2. Toddlers -- 15 Months to 3 years **(Slide 14-9)**
      a) So called "terrible twos" -- may refuse to cooperate
      b) Easily distracted during assessment
      c) Are individual and assertive
      d) Fear pain and separation from parents
      e) Difficult to explain
         (1) Soothing tone of voice
         (2) Examine on the mother's lap
         (3) Approach them at eye level
         (4) Distract with colorful toy or puppet
         (5) Examine toe to head
         (6) If possible, don't undress
         (7) Let them play with stethoscope and BP cuffs
   3. Small Child -- 4 to 7 Years Old **(Slide 14-10)**
      a) Curious and communicative
      b) World of intense play fantasy "magical thinking"
      c) Strong fear of pain and separation
      d) Take a few moments to play with the child
      e) Talk to the parents first
      f) Be honest during treatments
      g) Don't overexplain
   4. Preadolescent -- 9 to 12 year old **(Slide 14-11)**
      a) Struggle between adulthood and childhood
      b) Many personal fears and fear of disfigurement
      c) Demonstrate that you consider their opinion important
      d) Explain procedures and treatment
   5. Adolescent **(Slide 14-12)**
      a) Same as above
      b) See themselves as adults
      c) Under the stress may feel helpless and childlike
      d) Respect space, answer questions, respect shyness
      e) Allow them to retain as much control as possible
      f) Don't be confrontational
      g) Keep the child and parent together
      h) Be calm at all times

C. Anatomy and physiology differences **(Slide 14-13)**
   1. Better ability to compensate in the early phases
   2. Less reserve
   3. Airway

Content

a) Small caliber airways at all levels
b) Tongue is large relative to the airway
c) Greater potential for obstruction
d) Glottis anterior and superior
e) Large, u-shaped epiglottis
f) Cricoid ring is the narrowest part of upper airway
g) Membranous tube rather than firm cartilage
h) Clinical application **(Slide 14-14)**
(1) Place head in sniffing or neutral position to open airway
(2) Lifting the tongue away from the airway -- especially important
(3) Small obstructions can result in blockage
(4) Obligate nose breathers (infants)
(5) Suctioning can improve status
(6) Humidification of oxygen can also help

4. Respiratory Function **(Slide 14-15)**
a) Respiratory rate faster
(1) Gradually decreases with age
(2) Infants - 30 breaths/min avg
(3) 5 year olds - 25 breaths /minute avg
(4) 10 year olds - 20 breaths /minute avg
(5) Be generally familiar with the range
b) Respiratory volumes vary with age
(1) Do not overventilate
(2) Observe chest rise
(3) More prone to gastric distention
c) Very compliant chest walls, when stressed:
(1) Use accessory muscles
(2) Supraclavicular, substernal, and intercostal retractions
(3) Nasal flaring
d) Respiratory effort and fatigue
(1) Experience respiratory fatigue more rapidly than adults
(2) Experience a sudden deterioration
(3) Beware when the patient lies down
(4) Positive pressure may be needed
(5) Anxiety/anxious behavior-sign of hypoxia
e) Clinical application
(1) Humidified oxygen and warmth will extend compensatory period
(2) No contraindication to high concentration oxygen outside newborn period

5. Pulse Rate and Blood Pressure **(Slide 14-16)**
a) Average pulse decreases with age **(Slide 14-17)**
(1) Newborn to 3 months: average 140
(2) 3 months to 2 year: average 130
(3) Be generally familiar with range and variance
b) Blood pressure increases with age **(Slide 14-18)**
(1) Use appropriate cuff size
(a) Width of the cuff should cover approximately two thirds of the length of the upper arm

(b) Bladder should cover approximately 75% of the arm's circumference
(c) Small cuff= falsely high
(d) Large= falsely low
(2) ACS definition of shock for children
(a) Systolic BP of less than 70 mm Hg
(b) Tachycardia
(c) Cool skin

6. Metabolic Considerations **(Slide 14-19)**
a) Keeping child warm is a simple and valuable measure
b) Children have a higher baseline metabolic rate
c) Larger heads and skin surface area relative to adults
d) Increased heat and moisture loss
e) Increased heat loss through respirations
f) Can exhaust the glycogen supply during illness
g) Lower energy reserves
h) Infants less than 6 months of age cannot shiver
i) Keeping the child warm and well oxygenated extends the grace period

7. Neurological Differences **(Slide 14-20)**
a) Pediatric patients are more likely to suffer head injury
b) Infant can become hypovolemic with head injury
c) More prone to apneic episodes with head trauma
d) Have greater chance of recovery from brain hypoxia or head trauma

8. Response to Hypovolemia and Shock States **(Slide 14-21)**
a) Hypovolemic shock is the most common type of shock in childhood
(1) Acute dehydration
(a) Possible in any sick child
(b) Due to increased metabolic needs and poor intake
(c) Vomiting and diarrhea will hasten dehydration
(d) The smaller the child, the more vulnerable
(e) Signs of dehydration **(Slide 14-22)**
i) Early signs
a) Decreased urine output
b) Dry mucosa
ii) Late signs
a) Sunken fontanelles
b) Skin tenting
c) Delayed capillary refill
d) Hyperventilation
e) Altered mental status
f) Thready pulse
g) Hypotension (very late)
(2) Hemorrhage **(Slide 14-23)**
(a) Average blood volume is 80cc/kg
i) 10 kg-1 year old infant= 800cc of total blood volume
ii) 200cc blood loss= 25% of blood volume

Content

(b) Healthier compensatory mechanisms
i) Can maintain BP until nearly 40% of blood volume is lost
ii) Hypotension a later finding than in adults
iii) Hypotension = severe shock
iv) Also susceptible to other less common causes of shock
a) Distributive shock with sepsis
b) Anaphylaxis
c) Spinal cord shock
d) Obstructive shock from tension pneumothorax and cardiac tamponade
e) Rarely suffer cardiogenic shock

IV. Assessment of The Pediatric Patient
A. General components (same as adult) **(Slide 14-24)**
1. Dispatch review
2. Scene survey
3. Primary survey
4. Secondary survey [vital signs, history and physical exam]
B. Variations in approach **(Slide 14-25)**
1. Toe to head survey in infants and small children
2. Airway maneuvers
3. Evaluating and interpreting vital signs
C. Primary survey **(Slide 14-26)**
1. "From the doorway" observations
a) "Is this child significantly ill?"
b) "Am I dealing with a respiratory problem?"
c) Activity and playfulness
d) Color
e) Respiratory effort
f) Temperature
g) Example:
(1) Screaming 3 year old child
(2) Running about and is combative and uncooperative
(3) Parents are hysterical and upset
(4) You assess the following
(a) Airway is patent and functional--pink and screaming
(b) Circulatory function is adequate--upright and moving about
(c) No severe infectious process--active and crying
2. Physical Signs **(Slide 14-27)**
a) Related to the age and development
b) General Signs **(Slide 14-28)**
(1) General level of activity -- is the child:
(a) Limp? Anxious/agitated?
(b) Drowsy? Normal?

Content

(2) For infants **(Slide 14-29)**
- (a) Does baby make eye contact with mother?
- (b) Will eyes follow a toy?
- (c) Aware of and interacting with environment
- (d) Should be appropriately upset
- (e) Be wary of a child who is "too good" or quiet during exam

(3) Weight and nutritional status **(Slide 14-30)**
- (a) Does the child appear too thin or wasted?
- (b) Evidence of adequate nutritional and fluid intake?
- (c) Does the child feel warm or is there a history of fever?
- (d) Signs of dehydration present?
  - i) Poor skin turgor
  - ii) Sunken eyes
  - iii) Dry mucous membranes
  - iv) Sunken fontanelle in the infant

(4) Skin color **(Slide 14-31)**
- (a) Pallor
- (b) Jaundice
- (c) Flushing
- (d) Cyanosis
- (e) Lift shirt
  - i) Mottling of the trunk--inadequate perfusion
  - ii) Cold environment may normally cause mottling

(5) Respiratory Signs **(Slide 14-32)**
- (a) Respiratory rate (in relation to age)
- (b) Signs of increased work to breathe
  - i) Accessory muscles
  - ii) Supraclavicular, intercostal or substernal retractions
  - iii) Position of child (tripod position?)
  - iv) Nasal flaring (seen predominantly in infancy)
- (c) Nasal congestion
- (d) Breath sounds
  - i) Wheezing or cough
  - ii) Stridor
  - iii) Grunting
- (e) Key Respiratory Findings To Note In Children **(Slide 14-33)**
  - i) Retractions
    - a) Visible because of the compliance or flexibility of the chest wall
    - b) Inward depression of muscular areas
  - ii) Stridor
    - a) High pitched noise usually heard at inspiration
    - b) Caused by obstruction to airflow in the upper airway

Content

c) Severe airway obstruction may result in stridor at inspiration and expiration
d) Audible without a stethoscope

iii) Wheezing
a) High pitched "musical" sound
b) Narrowing of the lower airways
c) Caused by edema or bronchiole constriction

iv) Cough
a) Productive vs. nonproductive
b) Determined by presence of mucus or phlegm

v) Cyanosis
a) Low oxygen saturation of hemoglobin
b) Late signs of hypoxia
c) AMS may appear before cyanosis
d) May be absent with anemic children

D. Secondary survey
1. Taking a history **(Slide 14-34)**
a) Follows the same format as in the adult
(1) Chief complaint
(2) History of present illness
(3) Past medical history
(4) Medications and allergies
b) For the infant **(Slide 14-35)**
(1) Any problems during pregnancy or birth
(2) Was the baby premature
(3) The younger the child, the more reliance on the parent's history
c) Use terms appropriate for the age and vocabulary of the child
d) Consider factors related to development
2. Physical Examination **(Slide 14-36)**
a) Listen to lungs early
(1) Warm stethoscope
(2) Quality of air movement
(3) Abnormal breath sounds
(4) Remembering the faster normal respiratory and heart rates
b) Tricks to help assess child's respiratory status **(Slide 14-37)**
(1) Ask him to blow at a pen as if it were a birthday candle
(2) Place your stethoscope near the nose to appreciate air movement
(3) Rhonchi may be transmitted via upper airway
c) Other Considerations **(Slide 14-38)**
(1) Fontanelles
(a) Normal infant (sitting up), level with skull or only slightly depressed
(b) Dehydrated = depressed even when the baby is lying down

Content

(c) Increased intracranial pressure = bulging fontanelle
i) Most common concern is meningitis
ii) Subdural hematomas are possible
iii) Strain of crying can cause the fontanelle to bulge
(2) Stiff neck
(a) Key indicator of meningitis
(b) May be difficult to assess
i) Get the child to follow a toy or your keys
ii) May not be present in small children
(3) Rashes
(a) Common in children
(b) Allergic reactions and viral illness
i) Measles
ii) Rubella [German Measles]
iii) Varicella (chickenpox)
iv) Nonspecific viral illness
(c) Also seen with bacterial illness (meningococcemia)
(d) Specific diagnosis is often difficult

V. Respiratory disorders **(Slide 14-39)**
A. Most common cause of death in children
B. Airway, ventilation and oxygenation are the most important part of pediatric resuscitation
C. Children normally have strong hearts
D. Control or treat the respiratory system and the heart will follow
E. Important to differentiate types of airway obstruction **(Slide 14-40)**
1. Upper airway
a) Foreign body
b) Croup
c) Epiglottitis
2. Lower airway
a) Diseases affecting middle and lower bronchioles and alveoli
b) Asthma, bronchiolitis and foreign body obstruction
c) May progress to respiratory failure and arrest
d) Usually do so over a longer period of time

VI. Upper airway disease **(Slide 14-41)**
A. Overview
1. Major diseases -- croup, epiglottitis and foreign body
2. All run the risk of complete obstruction
3. Distinction must be made between infectious causes and foreign body since the management varies
4. Obstructed airway maneuvers are of no value for croup and epiglottitis. Moreover, stimulation of pharynx and epiglottis must be avoided since it can cause closing of the airway
B. Croup **(Slide 14-42)**
1. Accounts for majority of stridor in childhood
2. Croup is very common, and epiglottitis is uncommon
3. Viral infection affecting the larynx, trachea, and bronchi
4. Airway narrowing, especially at the level of the cricoid ring

Content

5. Classic presentation **(Slide 14-43)**
    a) Upper respiratory infection or cold
    b) Child may be hoarse
    c) Cough that sounds like a barking seal
    d) Low grade fever
    e) Varying degrees of inspiratory stridor
    f) Worse at night or upon awakening
    g) Most common from ages 6 months to six years
    h) Majority less than three years old
6. Management **(Slide 14-44)**
    a) Humidified oxygen
    b) May appear to be cured by humidification or by cool night air
    c) Many cases are asymptomatic by the time they reach the hospital
    d) Severe cases can result in complete airway obstruction

C. Epiglottitis **(Slide 14-45)**
1. Infectious swelling of the epiglottis
2. Caused by a bacterial infection
3. Rapid onset of approximately 10-12 hours
4. Usually affects children aged 2-6
5. Can occur in older children and adults
6. Signs and symptoms **(Slide 14-46)**
    a) High fever
    b) Sore throat and dysphagia (difficulty in swallowing)
    c) Inspiratory stridor
    d) Tripod position **(Slide 14-47)**
        (1) Sitting upright
        (2) Leaning forward
        (3) Weight distributed on hands
        (4) Mouth open, tongue protruding
        (5) Chin thrust forward
    e) Restlessness
    f) Drooling
    g) Flushed face
    h) Signs of dehydration
7. Management **(Slide 14-48)**
    a) Potentially life threatening emergency
    b) Stimulation of pharynx may cause reflex spasm of epiglottitis resulting in airway obstruction
    c) Gentle, calm handling, staying away from the child's airway
    d) Let child stay in mother's arms even during transport
    e) Humidified 0_2 but if child is alert and resists
        (1) Do not force mask in place
        (2) Mother may try to hold the mask near child's airway
    f) With cyanosis, lethargy, inadequate ventilation
        (1) Attempt positive pressure ventilation
        (2) Bag-valve-mask ventilation can be effective in most patients

Content

VII. Foreign Body Airway Obstruction
- A. Overview **(Slide 14-49)**
  - 1. Patient will usually be a previously healthy child with a history of choking
  - 2. Infant is someone less than 1 year of age
  - 3. Child is someone between 1 and 8 years old
  - 4. Age parameters are a guide
    - a) Small 13 month old may be treated as an infant
    - b) Large 11 month old may be treated as a child
- B. Main considerations **(Slide 14-50)**
  - 1. Is the obstruction partial or complete?
  - 2. Is immediate intervention needed or can the patient clear obstruction with coughing?
  - 3. Is the obstruction caused by an infectious process or a foreign body?
- C. Patient assessment (general) **(Slide 14-51)**
  - 1. Primary survey and history
  - 2. Level of consciousness
  - 3. Air exchange
    - a) Ability to speak or cry
    - b) Ability to ventilate
  - 4. Infectious cause **(Slide 14-52)**
    - a) Recent upper respiratory infections
    - b) Fever and barking cough
    - c) History of choking after eating or playing with small objects
  - 5. Do not manipulate or attempt to examine the airway (epiglottis)
  - 6. Alert child **(Slide 14-53)**
    - a) Can speak and cough
    - b) Stridor and a rapid respiratory rate
    - c) Keep the child and parents calm
      - (1) Allow child to remain in parent's arms
      - (2) Position of comfort
    - d) Humidified oxygen
      - (1) Without agitating the child
      - (2) Face mask, nasal cannula, or holding mask near nose and mouth
    - e) Transport quickly
    - f) Management regardless of croup, epiglottitis or foreign body
  - 7. Complete obstruction or partial obstruction with poor air exchange
    - a) Partial with poor air exchange **(Slide 14-54)**
      - (1) Decreasing mental status
      - (2) Severe retractions without air movement
      - (3) Cyanosis
      - (4) Rapid respiratory rate and pulse
      - (5) If you suspect an infectious cause
        - (a) Positive pressure ventilation
        - (b) Rapid transport
      - (6) If you suspect foreign body, proceed with protocol for complete obstruction

Content

- b) Complete **(Slide 14-55)**
  - (1) Child cannot speak or cry
  - (2) Inability to ventilate unconscious child

D. Management

1. Complete foreign body obstruction (Conscious Infant)
   - a) Support on your arm and thigh **(Slide 14-56)**
   - b) Face down with the head toward your palm and slightly dependent
   - c) Four back blows should be administered between the scapula **(Slide 14-57)**
   - d) Each blow given with intent of removing the object
   - e) Turn the infant supine **(Slide 14-58)**
   - f) Administer four chest thrusts, 1 finger breadth below nipple line **(Slide 14-59)**
   - g) Continue until the obstruction is removed or the infant becomes unconscious
2. Infant who becomes unconscious with complete obstruction **(Slide 14-60)**
   - a) Perform a tongue-jaw lift **(Slide 14-61)**
   - b) Visualize the airway **(Slide 14-62)**
   - c) Perform a finger sweep, only if you can see the foreign body
   - d) Attempt to ventilate
   - e) If you cannot ventilate, repeat **(Slide 14-63)**
     - (1) Back blows
     - (2) Chest thrusts
     - (3) Finger sweep [when visualized]
     - (4) Ventilations
     - (5) Repeat until you can ventilate or during transport to the hospital
3. Infant found unconscious with complete airway obstruction **(Slide 14-64)**
   - a) Inability to ventilate
   - b) Reopen airway and attempt a second ventilation
   - c) Still unable to ventilate
   - d) Administer four back blows
   - e) Four chest thrusts
   - f) Finger sweep
   - g) Rapid transport if unable to clear
4. If the airway is cleared **(Slide 14-65)**
   - a) Check the pulse and respirations
   - b) If pulse present with no respirations, provide positive pressure ventilation
   - c) If no pulse perform CPR
5. Child obstructed airway
   - a) Conscious patient **(Slide 14-66)**
     - (1) Assess by asking, "Are you choking?"
     - (2) Administer Heimlich maneuver just above the umbilicus and well below xiphoid process **(Slide 14-67)**
     - (3) Thrusts are directed inward and upward

Content

(4) Each thrust is given with the intent of dislodging the obstruction
(5) Thrusts are continued until obstruction is removed or patient becomes unconscious
b) Conscious patient who becomes unconscious **(Slide 14-68)**
(1) Perform finger sweep while maintaining tongue jaw lift (if obstruction visualized) **(Slide 14-69)**
(2) Attempt to ventilate using head tilt-chin lift maneuver
(3) Administer 6 to 10 abdominal thrusts with heel of hand
(4) Finger sweep **(Slide 14-70)**
(5) Attempt to ventilate **(Slide 14-71)**
(6) If ventilations are effective, assess pulse and breathing and administer CPR if needed
c) Unconscious airway obstruction
(1) Recognized by inability to ventilate the unconscious patient
(2) Reopen airway and attempt to ventilate
(3) If unable to ventilate, proceed with 6 to 10 abdominal thrusts, finger sweep and ventilation sequence

VIII. Other upper respiratory problems **(Slide 14-72)**
A. Upper respiratory infections
B. Most are the common "cold"
C. Sore throats with inflammation of the pharynx and tonsils
D. Secretions in nasal passage can narrow the infant's and child's airway
E. Upper respiratory problem may precede croup and epiglottitis or severe tonsillitis
F. Call for help should cause search for complicating factors
1. Dehydration
2. Exhaustion
3. Severe complications

IX. Lower airway disease
A. Bronchiolitis **(Slide 14-73)**
1. Viral illness affecting infants
2. Usually 2 to 6 months of age but up to 2 years
3. Causes edema and mucus production in lower and smaller airways
4. Follows an upper respiratory infection
5. Often occurs in the winter
6. Results in impeded air flow
7. Wheezing, rhonchi and rales can be heard
B. Asthma **(Slide 14-74)**
1. Overview
a) Common, recurrent condition, which affects children and adults
b) Causes bronchospasm with mucus and edema
c) Narrowing and obstruction of the lower airways
d) Increased resistance to airflow, primarily during expiration
e) Wheezing, usually bilaterally
f) Expiration is prolonged
2. Triggering mechanisms **(Slide 14-75)**
a) Infections of the respiratory tract
b) Allergies

Content

c) Withdrawal of some medications (such as stopping steroids)
3. Home treatments
a) Nebulizers with mist of bronchodilator drugs
b) Alupent, epinephrine and bronchosol
c) Theophylline and steroids
4. Severe asthma **(Slide 14-76)**
a) Patients can die from asthma
(1) Obstruction is so complete that no effective air exchange takes place
(2) When they become exhausted
b) May be no wheezing whatsoever
c) Patient may be unable to speak
d) Increased resistance may be encountered during positive pressure ventilations
5. Treatment **(Slide 14-77)**
a) For conscious alert child
(1) Provide oxygen by mask or nasal cannula
(2) Allow mother to hold child
b) Child who becomes lethargic and wants to lie down
(1) Provide positive pressure ventilation
(2) High resistance to flow should be anticipated
(3) Maintain an effective seal
(4) Rapid transport may be lifesaving

C. Pneumonia **(Slide 14-78)**
1. Will often follow simple upper respiratory infection
2. May be viral or bacterial
3. Complaint or history of fever and cough
4. Dehydration may be present
5. Abdominal pain, due to irritation of the diaphragm
6. Rales may present a day or more after fever and cough
7. With or without wheezing
8. Pleuritic pain may be noted
9. Treat with humidified oxygen and ventilatory support as needed

D. Foreign bodies in the lower airway **(Slide 14-79)**
1. Peanuts, food, plastic, metal and teeth can be inhaled and lodge in the lower airways
2. Most likely on right side due to straight mainstem bronchus
3. Cough, initially nagging and unproductive
4. Wheezing may be heard on one side
5. If undiagnosed for long period **(Slide 14-80)**
a) Fever and mucus production
b) Productive cough
6. Cannot be removed by the complete airway obstruction technique
7. Bronchoscopy (visualization with an instrument) or surgical intervention is needed
8. Treatment in the field is directed at respiratory support

X. Respiratory failure and arrest **(Slide 14-81)**
A. Airway
1. Head tilt-chin lift
a) Preferred method for opening airway

Content

b) Infants
(1) Do not hyperextend
(2) Neutral or slightly extended ("sniffing") position
c) Children
(1) Slight extension may be useful
(2) Avoid kinking airway
2. Jaw thrust without head tilt **(Slide 14-82)**
a) Thumbs on cheek bone
b) Fingers at angle of the jaw
c) Lift jaw without tilting neck
B. Breathing **(Slide 14-83)**
1. If need for positive pressure is established, provide two initial breaths
2. Same as adult with the following modifications
a) Rate
(1) Infant, one breath every three seconds
(2) Child, one breath every four seconds
b) Use volumes in proportion to the size of the patient
3. Technique **(Slide 14-84)**
a) Breaths should be gentle
b) Given smoothly over a 1 to 1.5 second period to avoid gastric distension
c) Bag-Valve-Mask can be used
(1) Airway resistance may cause air leakage at pop-off valve
(2) Disarm with tape to assure adequate ventilation
(3) Mask and oropharyngeal airway should be selected according to the size of the patient
d) With rescue breathing, cover the infant's nose and mouth
e) Suction as needed
f) If chest does not rise, adjust the airway position and try again
g) If still unsuccessful, follow airway obstruction procedures
4. When to ventilate **(Slide 14-85)**
a) Alteration of consciousness
b) Cyanosis or mottling
c) Very fast or slow respiratory rates relative to age
d) Labored breathing
e) Retractions
f) The child who does not resist positive pressure will most likely need it
g) When in doubt, ventilate
5. Children that are responsive in respiratory distress should receive humidified high flow O_2
XI. Near drowning **(Slide 14-86)**
A. Epidemiology
1. Over 5,000 children die each year of drowning
2. Most vulnerable population age is 18 months to three years
3. In addition to falling into swimming pools
a) Bathtubs, laundry pails
b) Wells and rain barrels

Content

4. Adolescents are also a high risk group due to
    a) Decreased supervision
    b) Increased risk taking behavior
    c) Co-existing alcohol and drug use

B. Pathophysiology **(Slide 14-87)**
1. Children fare much better than adults, especially in a cold water immersion
2. Numerous children have survived prolonged ice water immersion
3. Pathophysiology of drowning
    a) Same as for adults
    b) Infants and children have an exaggerated diving reflex
    c) Shunts blood to the body core and slows down metabolism
4. Drowning patients should be given the benefit of the doubt and transported while providing CPR
5. If shallow water, consider the possibility of cervical spine injury **(Slide 14-88)**
    a) Maintain in-line immobilization of the spine
    b) Spine board can be used during the removal
    c) When conditions permit, rescue breathing should be started in the water
    d) High concentration oxygen can be added
    e) Maintain the body temperature

XII. Sudden Infant Death Syndrome (SIDS)

A. Epidemiology **(Slide 14-89)**
1. Leading cause of death from one month to one year
2. Each year about 8,000 infants die from SIDS in the United States
3. Incidence is 2 per 1,000 live births
4. Vast majority of children die while asleep and are found dead by their parents **(Slide 14-90)**
5. Large majority of calls occur in the early morning
6. Many children are in perfect health or have minor respiratory infection
7. Not associated with newborn period
8. Majority of cases occur before six months
9. Peak at 10 to 14 weeks of life
10. Higher incidence in late fall and winter

B. Significant risk factors include: **(Slide 14-91)**
1. Low socio-economic group
2. Adolescent mother
3. Crowded living conditions
4. Drug use during pregnancy
5. Black mother (three fold increase in risk)
6. Native American (five fold increase in risk)
7. Risk factors associated with the birth **(Slide 14-92)**
    a) Prematurity, especially if baby was on a respirator
    b) Multiple birth grouping (twins, triplets, etc.)
    c) If sibling of SIDS victim, risk increases 5 to 10 times
    d) Near SIDS event, defined as an unexplained apneic event

Content

C. Suspected causes **(Slide 14-93)**
   1. Immaturity of the neurologic system
   2. Poor control of the respiratory system
   3. Airway compromise resulting in prolonged apnea

D. EMT at the scene **(Slide 14-94)**
   1. Scene will be emotionally charged
   2. Two circumstances you may encounter
      a) Infant found in respiratory and cardiac arrest after a length of time
      b) Parents observed a period of apnea which was transient and baby appeared fine
   3. Infant is not breathing and/or pulseless
      a) Perform CPR
      b) Transport
   4. Infant is breathing **(Slide 14-95)**
      a) Observe signs of thwarted sleep apnea
      b) Is or was the child cyanotic?
      c) Was there evidence of shallow respirations?
      d) Was there evidence of respiratory or cardiac arrest?
      e) Continued need for CPR?
      f) Monitor the infant enroute
      g) Administer humidified O_2
      h) Keep infant warm
   5. Additional observations **(Slide 14-96)**
      a) Infant responsive or dazed?
      b) Breathing labored or irregular?
      c) Color pale, blue, flushed, or mottled?
      d) Infant limp, hypertonic [muscle spasm] or
      e) Exhibiting jerking movements?
      f) Blood or vomitus on the bedsheet?
   6. Decision making **(Slide 14-97)**
      a) Unless clear signs of death [rigor mortis] initiate resuscitation and transport
      b) Avoid delay at the scene
      c) Twin sibling should be brought to hospital
   7. Psychological aspects **(Slide 14-98)**
      a) Parents feel better knowing everything possible, was done
      b) Parents may experience denial, grief and guilt
      c) Confusion with abuse
         (1) Victims may have mottling in dependent areas
         (2) May be confused as bruises associated with child abuse
         (3) Never be judgmental
         (4) If you suspect abuse, report it to physician at the emergency department
         (5) Do not question the parents in a suspicious manner
         (6) Professional and tactful behavior is very important in helping parents cope with loss

Content

XIII. Febrile child
- A. Overview **(Slide 14-99)**
    1. Fever is common in children
    2. Minor illness with fever is most common presenting complaint
    3. Common misconceptions
        - a) Fever itself is dangerous
        - b) The higher the fever the more the risk of causing a seizure
    4. About 5% of children will experience a febrile seizure
    5. High fevers can be associated with a simple viral illness or serious infection
    6. Febrile child should be transported to the emergency department
- B. Treatment **(Slide 14-100)**
    1. Common practice to cool down a febrile child
    2. Usually not necessary and may be dangerous
    3. EMTs should not dispense or suggest medication
    4. Aspirin is discouraged with fever because of Reye's syndrome
        - a) Poorly understood syndrome
        - b) Involves liver and brain
        - c) Marked by coma and profound hypoglycemia
        - d) Follows one week after chickenpox or influenza
        - e) Linked to aspirin use in children
    5. Cooling, if done **(Slide 14-101)**
        - a) Tepid water soaks
        - b) Towels or sheets can cool quickly
        - c) Given risk of hypothermia, you should weigh carefully the use of this option

XIV. Seizures **(Slide 14-102)**
- A. Common and controllable medical emergency of childhood
- B. May frighten parents and results in emotional response
- C. Usually not life threatening unless it occurs while swimming, climbing, etc.
- D. As long as the airway is maintained, child can tolerate grand mal seizure in excess of 20 minutes
- E. Review of the common definitions **(Slide 14-103)**:
    1. Seizure: isolated event from an abnormal electrical discharge of cells in the brain
    2. Epilepsy: tendency to have recurrent seizures
    3. Convulsions: seizure with a change in muscle/motor activity
    4. Generalized convulsions: involving entire body associated with loss of consciousness (LOC)
    5. Focal Seizure: involving one area of body not necessarily associated with an altered mental state
    6. Petite Mal: extremely brief periods of LOC without loss of muscle tone which is more common in children
- F. Febrile seizure **(Slide 14-104)**
    1. Most common with pediatric patients
    2. Often seizure is first sign of an illness

Content

3. Brief, less than 5 minutes, associated with fever and tonic/clonic generalized convulsion
4. Most likely to be in the postictal phase
5. Considered complex if **(Slide 14-105)**
    a) Greater than 15 minutes in duration
    b) If there is focality
    c) Multiple episodes within 24 hours
    d) Status epilepticus (5% of seizures in children)
6. Transport every child with a seizure as there may be a serious underlying cause
7. Ten percent of children with meningitis present with seizures
8. Meningeal signs, such as a stiff neck, may not be present in small children

G. Causes of seizures in children **(Slide 14-106)**
1. Infections: encephalitis, meningitis, roseola, shigella
2. Metabolic: hypoglycemia, hypoxia, fever, hyponatremic, hypocalcemia
3. Toxic: lead, aminophylline, lidocaine, cocaine, nicotine, phenothiazine
4. Drug withdrawal, especially from prescribed anticonvulsants
5. Structural: trauma, bleed, mass lesion, brain scar
6. Vascular anomalies and tumors (cause 47% in adults and 3% in children)
7. Infections, toxins and metabolic cases (are more common in children than in adults)

H. Complications of seizures **(Slide 14-107)**
1. Respiratory
    a) Decreased respiratory drive
    b) Airway obstruction by the tongue
    c) Risk of aspiration
    d) Ineffective respiratory muscles during seizure
2. Metabolic
    a) Rise of body temperature from persistent muscular activity
    b) Depletion of glycogen stores and blood glucose
3. Central nervous system, damage from
    a) Prolonged electrical activity of the brain
    b) Respiratory and metabolic complications

I. Management **(Slide 14-108)**
1. Protect the patient from self-injury
2. Maintain the airway, if necessary, with the jaw thrust maneuver
3. Supplement oxygen
    a) Mask over the mouth and nose of the breathing patient
    b) Bag valve mask when necessary
4. Do not force any objects into the mouth
5. If febrile, you may want to attempt cooling using tepid water
6. History **(Slide 14-109)**
    a) Ascertain history of previous seizures
    b) Other medical problems
    c) Medications

d) Witnesses noticed the onset of the seizure
(1) Focal
(2) Toxic ingestion
(3) Duration of seizure and time of onset
7. Physical examination **(Slide 14-110)**
a) ABC's
b) Tongue biting
c) Type of seizure
d) Level of consciousness
e) Evidence of trauma, abuse or dehydration

XV. Trauma **(Slide 14-111)**
A. Number one killer of children one to fourteen years old
B. Number two killer of infants
C. Many more suffer debilitating injuries
D. A significant number of accidents are preventable
E. Prevention **(Slide 14-112)**
1. Car seats, seat belts
2. Bicycle helmets
3. Educating the public
4. Window guards
5. Water safety
6. Smoke detectors, fire prevention **(Slide 14-113)**
7. Supervision of children
8. Child-proof caps on medication
9. Adjusting household water heaters (not greater than 130 degrees)
10. EMTs should play an active role in community health education and prevention
F. Mechanisms of pediatric injury **(Slide 14-114)**
1. Less protected than adults
2. Bones are more resilient
3. Forces are more easily transmitted to internal organs
4. Skeleton clues to internal damage may be less obvious
5. Vital organs are within a small space **(Slide 14-115)**
6. Transmitted force can affect many organs
7. Increases the chances of multisystem injury
8. Child responds with initial compensatory mechanisms which can mask signs of blood loss
9. Serial examinations are necessary
G. Motor vehicle accidents **(Slide 14-116)**
1. Youngest individual in car is most vulnerable
2. If unrestrained or held in parent's arms, literally becomes a missile
3. Commonly victims of pedestrian accidents
a) More likely to experience injury to the vital organs from bumper
b) Most of these accidents occur in urban areas
c) Males, 4 to 12 years of age, represent the largest group of pedestrian victims
H. Bicycle injuries **(Slide 14-117)**
1. Often reckless on bicycles
2. Underestimate chance of injuries

Content

3. Rarely wear helmets
4. Struck by motorists
5. Common injuries
   a) Abrasions, fractures and head injury
   b) Of abdomen from the bicycle handle

I. Head trauma **(Slide 14-118)**
1. Leading cause of death in children
2. With early attention, greater number of children can be saved than of adults
3. Hypoxia and hypotension must be prevented and treated
4. Evidence of internal bleeding dictates rapid hospital intervention
5. Glasgow Coma Score is modified for age
6. Pupil and motor findings are elicited rapidly and repeatedly

J. Neck injuries **(Slide 14-119)**
1. Predominant in relatively large heads with small necks and weak cervical musculature
2. Best immobilization is combined use of high-cut rigid cervical collar and back board
3. Infants and small children are apt to suffer from high cervical spine injuries which can result in respiratory arrest

K. Head and multisystem trauma **(Slide 14-120)**
1. Children with head trauma also have a high rate of other organ or multisystem trauma. Accordingly, all children found with a head injury following a motor vehicle accident or fall should be evaluated and treated as victims of multisystem trauma. The presence of head injury may make it difficult to assess other organs, so a high degree of suspicion is necessary.

L. Chest trauma **(Slide 14-121)**
1. Chest wall allows transmission of energy to intrathoracic structures
2. Cardiac or pulmonary contusion without obvious external evidence
3. Transsection of the aorta is rare
4. Low pulmonary reserve volume will make other conditions worse
5. Tension pneumothorax will shift markedly within mediastinum **(Slide 14-122)**
6. Compression of the vessels, poor venous return to the heart, and obstructive shock
7. Rupture of the diaphragm
   a) Occurs in children from severe motor vehicle accidents and falls
   b) High abdominal pressure bursts the diaphragm
8. Rupture in the trachea, bronchus, or esophagus can result in respiratory compromise
9. Gastric distension
10. Respiratory compromise from pulmonary contusions

M. Abdominal trauma **(Slide 14-123)**
1. Thin abdominal walls
2. Little protection, organs subject to hemorrhage
3. Distension may be noted with severe hemorrhage
4. Child can suddenly deteriorate after a period of compensation
5. Should be transported as soon as possible
6. Monitoring of vital signs and treatment of shock enroute

Content

N. Musculoskeletal trauma **(Slide 14-124)**
1. Pliable bones break in different places
2. Basic approach to injuries is the same as for an adult
3. Traction may injure the pediatric growth plate
4. Traction is sometimes not used for femur fractures in children (check local protocols)
5. Child can bleed severely from a pelvic or femur fracture
6. If hypotension develops use the PASG

XVI. Child abuse **(Slide 14-125)**
A. Child abuse is a major problem
B. Only SIDS and accidents are responsible for more pediatric deaths
C. More than 100,000 children a year suffer permanent disability
D. Majority of children are under three years of age
E. Children are often subjected to recurrent beatings
F. Physical Abuse **(Slide 14-126)**
1. Accounting for 80% of reported cases of child abuse
2. Soft tissue, skeleton, CNS, viscera, teeth, sensory organs, poisoning
3. Four B's of active physical abuse
a) Battered
b) Bruised
c) Broken
d) Burned
4. Soft tissue injury **(Slide 14-127)**
a) Non-accidental bruises
b) Contusions on all parts of the head and neck area, trunk including the flanks, buttocks, and extremities can be found
c) Children normally bruise over bony prominences or on one surface in a fall
d) Bruising over head and truck but not extremities is suspicious
e) Marks left by belts, bite marks, electric cord
f) Multiple bruises in various states of healing
5. Burns **(Slide 14-128)**
a) Unusual patterns of burns should also trigger suspicion of abuse
b) Burns with sharp demarcations are rarely seen in accidents
c) Note burns that have shape or pattern
d) Any burn or injury to genitalia should be noted
6. Head **(Slide 14-129)**
a) Injury to the CNS carries a grave prognosis
b) 15% of reported cases of child abuse
c) Number one cause of mortality and permanent morbidity
d) Infants suffer significant subdural hematoma from being shaken
e) Presentation **(Slide 14-130)**
(1) Vomiting, agitation, seizures and coma
(2) Initially have nonspecific findings like poor feeding
(3) Chronic CNS injury associated with other systemic evidence of child abuse
(4) Any fracture in an infant is suspicious
(5) Multiple fractures, especially in various states of healing

G. Sexual abuse **(Slide 14-131)**
1. Harder to diagnose and harder to accept

Content

2. Abuser usually being someone known and close to the child
3. Crosses all socioeconomic lines
4. Physical findings are often scant
    a) External genital trauma
    b) Difficulty walking
    c) Sexually transmitted diseases
5. Children will be reluctant to admit because of
    a) Fear, guilt
    b) Unwillingness to break up family
6. Take seriously a child's statement that someone is bothering him or her
7. Children cannot usually make up details about sexual advances

H. Child neglect **(Slide 14-132)**
1. Subtle forms of abuse
2. Deprived of
    a) Adequate food, clothing, shelter
    b) Education
    c) Medical care, dental care
    d) Emotional nurturing
    e) Appropriate supervision
    f) These are children at risk for various self-inflicted injuries such as the unsupervised small child who accidentally sets his apartment on fire when playing with matches. These children are as at high a risk of growing up with severe emotional and developmental problems as is a child of physical abuse.

XVII. Obtaining the history **(Slide 14-133)**

A. Careful observation without accusation or confrontation

B. Possible abuse
1. Parents' story not consistent with injury, i.e.
    a) Nine month old with an obvious extremity deformity. Parents claim he fell off the couch.
2. History changes depending on who obtains the history.
3. Witnesses give contradictory histories.
4. Parent is reluctant to give history.
5. Delay in obtaining medical attention
    a) Timing of injury not consistent with finding, i.e. claim of recent injury with bruises of various stages of healing. **(Slide 14-134)**
6. Parent's response not appropriate to severity of injury
7. Child exhibiting inappropriate agitation with you or the family
8. Obvious alcohol or drug abuse by parents is evident
9. Pay attention to the environment, the sanitary state of home
10. Evidence of a struggle

C. Obtain if possible **(Slide 14-135)**
1. Time of the incident, witnesses
2. History of recent illness
3. Condition of child's clothing

D. Behavior **(Slide 14-136)**
1. May be overly friendly or withdrawn

Content

2. May be inappropriate in responses
3. Be concerned about the child who is too good
4. Be aware of your own emotional response
    a) Do not ask questions in an accusatory tone
    b) Try not to be judgmental

E. Reporting laws **(Slide 14-137)**
1. Vary from state to state
2. You may not be legally mandated to report
3. You are morally and professionally responsible to set things in motion
4. Laws are written so that the reporter is protected from litigation for reporting suspected abuse
5. Mandated reporters
    a) Physicians and nurses
    b) Would be held legally responsible for failure to report

Chapter 14

PEDIATRIC EMERGENCIES

Examination

1. Cardiopulmonary arrest in children is rarely due to _______________:

    a. motor vehicle accidents
    b. drug ingestion
    c. heart disease
    d. SIDS

2. The most common cause of death in children outside of the newborn period is:

    a. SIDS
    b. trauma
    c. congenital heart disease
    d. cancer

Match the developmental stage of the child in column B with the age group in column A.

Column A		Column B	
3.	infant	a.	imaginative thinking
4.	toddler (15 months to 1 year)	b.	want to see themselves as adults
5.	young child (4 to 7 years old)	c.	minimal language capability but responds to facial expressions
6.	preadolescent (9 to 12 years old)	d.	child is easily distracted, they see themselves as individuals, yet they fear pain and separation from their parents
7.	adolescent	e.	has many personal fears and a strong fear of disfigurement

8. Cardiac arrest in children usually follows a respiratory event and the body reacts in the following order:

   a. hypoxia, decreased ventilation, cardiac collapse, low blood oxygen
   b. hypoxia, acidosis, cardiac collapse, decreased ventilation
   c. hypoxia, decreased ventilation, low blood oxygen, cardiac collapse
   d. hypoxia, low blood oxygen, cardiac collapse, decreased ventilation

9. The secondary survey portion of your physical assessment for a sick infant should be done:

   a. in a head-to-toe fashion after listening to lung sounds
   b. in a head-to-toe fashion before listening to lung sounds
   c. in a toe-to-head fashion after listening to lung sounds
   d. in a toe-to-head fashion before listening to lung sounds

10. The narrowest part of the upper airway in infants is the:

    a. epiglottis
    b. trachea
    c. thyroid cartilage
    d. cricoid cartilage

11. Kinking and obstruction of the infant's airway may result from:

    a. hypoextending the neck
    b. hyperextending the neck
    c. laying the infant on his back
    d. ventilating too forcefully

12. The age group which breathes predominantly through the nose is the:

    a. infant
    b. toddler
    c. young child
    d. adolescent

13. Newborns have an average respirator rate of approximately _____ breaths per minute:

    a. 16
    b. 20
    c. 30
    d. 40

14. During ventilation you must be careful to closely observe __________ to determine the effectiveness of ventilation.

    a. pupil response
    b. skin color
    c. capillary refill
    d. chest rise

15. High concentration oxygen therapy for children in respiratory distress, in any age group:

    a. is contraindicated
    b. may cause blindness
    c. is very appropriate if needed
    d. is never needed

16. The American College of Surgeons considers a systolic blood pressure of less than __ mm Hg with tachycardia and cool skin an indicator of shock in children.

    a. 50
    b. 70
    c. 80
    d. 90

17. Early signs of dehydration in children include:

    a. tachycardia, hypotension, decreased urination
    b. decreased urination, tachycardia, skin tenting
    c. dry mucosal membranes, thready pulse, hypotension
    d. tachycardia, less urine output, dry mucosal membranes

18. A very late sign of dehydration in children is:

    a. sunken fontanelles
    b. hypotension
    c. sunken eyes
    d. lack of tears

Match the description of respirations in column B with the respiratory finding of the child in Column A.

Column A		Column B	
19.	retractions	a.	crowing, high pitched sound made on inspiration suggestive of an upper airway obstruction
20.	stridor	b.	protective reflex mechanism used to remove foreign material from the airway
21.	wheezing	c.	inward depression of muscular areas and their attached ribs
22.	cough	d.	high pitched musical sound caused by narrowing of the lower airways
23.	cyanosis	e.	sign of low oxygen saturation of the hemoglobin in the blood

24. The physical finding of a stiff neck in a child, termed nuchal rigidity, is a key indicator of:

   a. spinal trauma
   b. foreign body lodged in the trachea
   c. febrile seizures
   d. meningitis

25. A viral infection affecting the larynx, trachea, and bronchi that can cause airway narrowing, especially at the level of the cricoid ring, is called:

   a. bronchiolitis
   b. pharyngitis
   c. croup
   d. epiglottitis

26. Which of the following are signs of croup:

   a. a hoarse voice, drooling, a high fever
   b. drooling, a barking cough, sudden onset
   c. wheezing, drooling, a hoarse voice
   d. a low grade fever, a hoarse voice, barking cough

27. Epiglottitis is most common from ages _______ to _______.

    a. six months to two years
    b. six months to four years
    c. one year to three years
    d. two to six years

28. Epiglottitis is an acute bacterial infection of the epiglottis that has a rapid onset of approximately __ to __ hours.

    a. 1 to 2
    b. 2 to 4
    c. 10 - 12
    d. 24 - 72

29. Which of the following is not a common sign of acute epiglottitis:

    a. high fever, drooling, sore throat
    b. sore throat, drooling, dysphagia
    c. difficulty in swallowing, drooling, stridor
    d. barking cough, low fever, thirsty

30. The child with _________ will frequently be sitting upright and leaning forward resting the chin on the arms in the so-called "tripod position."

    a. croup
    b. epiglottitis
    c. wheezes
    d. airway obstruction

31. When faced with a child who has a <u>complete airway obstruction</u> from acute epiglottitis or croup, you should:

    a. administer back blows, attempt ventilations, rapid transport
    b. attempt ventilations, administer chest thrusts, keep the child warm
    c. attempt ventilations, initiate rapid transport, keep the child warm
    d. administer back blows, administer chest thrusts, perform a blind finger sweep

32. The correct order of treatment for an unconscious infant with a complete airway obstruction, after you have attempted ventilations and repositioned the head is:

    a. 4 chest thrusts, 4 back blows, blind finger sweep
    b. 4 back blows, 4 chest thrusts, blind finger sweep
    c. 4 back blows, 4 chest thrusts, look in the mouth and perform a finger sweep if you see an obstruction
    d. 4 chest thrusts, 4 back blows, look in the mouth and perform a finger sweep if you see an obstruction

33. A child with a foreign body airway obstruction is coughing forcefully. Your initial management for this child is:

    a. a deep finger sweep to the upper airway
    b. back blows and chest thrusts
    c. transport only
    d. positive pressure ventilation

34. Which of the following signs are associated with a partial airway obstruction with poor air exchange:

    a. a weak ineffective cough, stridor, cyanosis
    b. stridor, a strong cough, severe retractions
    c. cyanosis, severe retractions, a strong cough
    d. child is talking, a strong cough, cyanosis

35. The correct position for a chest thrust, while treating an infant with a complete foreign body airway obstruction is:

    a. 1 finger breadth above the xiphoid
    b. 1 finger breadth below nipple line
    c. nipple line
    d. the upper half of the breast bone

36. When a conscious child with a complete airway obstruction becomes unconscious you should <u>first</u>:

    a. attempt to ventilate and observe for chest excursion
    b. perform a jaw lift, examine the airway and perform a finger sweep, if you visualize a foreign body
    c. administer 4 back blows and 4 chest thrusts
    d. check for a brachial pulse to establish the need for cardiac compressions

37. The viral illness affecting infants that causes edema and mucus produuction in the lower and smaller airways is:

    a. asthma
    b. bronchiolitis
    c. epiglottitis
    d. pneumonia

38. The common and recurrent condition that causes bronchospasm with mucus and edema production is:

    a. asthma
    b. bronchiolitis
    c. epiglottitis
    d. pneumonia

39. The condition which often follows a simple upper respiratory infection that is usually accompanied by a complaint of fever, cough and sometimes pleuritic chest pain is:

    a. asthma
    b. bronchiolitis
    c. epiglottitis
    d. pneumonia

40. Any child in severe respiratory distress who becomes sleepy and lies down should receive:

    a. positive pressure ventilation
    b. humidified oxygen administration
    c. nebulized oxygen
    d. oxygen via nasal catheter

41. The proper rate of ventilations for an infant in respiratory arrest is 1 breath every:

    a. 2 seconds
    b. 3 seconds
    c. 4 seconds
    d. 5 seconds

42. The proper rate of ventilations for any child over 8 years of age in respiratory arrest is 1 breath every:

    a. 2 seconds
    b. 3 seconds
    c. 4 seconds
    d. 5 seconds

43. The procedure of applying gentle pressure on the cricoid cartilage to help prevent gastric distention is referred to as:

    a. a cricothyroidotomy
    b. Sellick maneuver
    c. Sylvester method
    d. Adam's maneuver

44. Anatomically, foreign bodies that enter the lower airway are more likely to enter the _______ mainstem bronchus.

    a. right
    b. left

45. When caring for a young drowning victim found in shallow water, you should automatically treat the child as if he had:

    a. kidney damage
    b. a cervical spine injury
    c. diabetes
    d. a bacterial infection

46. SIDS is the leading cause of death in which age group?

    a. newborn to 1 month
    b. 1 month to 1 year
    c. 1 year to 4 years
    d. 4 years to 8 years

47. Which of the following are considered risk factors of SIDS:

    a. low socioeconomic group, postmature baby, adolescent mother
    b. adolescent mother, drug use during pregnancy, low socioeconomic group
    c. drug use during pregnancy, mother over 30 years of age, low socioeconomic group
    d. postmature baby, drug use during pregnancy, adolescent mother

48. A common cause of seizures in small children is:

    a. overdose
    b. fever
    c. aspiration
    d. vomiting

49. The most common internal organ injured in children is the:

    a. heart
    b. lungs
    c. spleen
    d. liver

50. While examining injuries sustained to a 9 moth old you find yellow/brown and red/blue bruises. The mother and father have different explanations of how the injury occurred. You should suspect:

    a. hemophilia causing internal bleeding
    b. this is a normal situation as all children get bruises
    c. the child was inquisitive and fell
    d. child abuse

Chapter 14

Skill Performance Sheet

Child Mouth to Mouth Breathing

Student's Name________________________________ Date__________

Performance Standard	**Performed**	**Failed**
Open airway with appropriate maneuver (head tilt-chin lift or jaw thrust)		
Assess breathing (look, listen and feel)		
Seal mouth around the patient's mouth and pinch nose		
Give two smooth breaths while observing chest rise (1-1.5 seconds per breath)		
Take mouth away between breaths		
Check carotid pulse (pulse is present)		
Give one breath every 4 seconds		

Comments____

____

____

____

Instructor ____________________ Circle One: Pass Fail

Skill Performance Sheet

Infant Mouth to Mouth and Nose Breathing

Student's Name____________________________ Date_________

Performance Standard	Performed	Failed
Open airway with appropriate maneuver (head tilt-chin lift or jaw thrust)		
Assess breathing (look, listen and feel)		
Seal mouth around the patient's mouth and nose		
Give two smooth breaths while observing chest rise (1-1.5 seconds per breath)		
Take mouth away between breaths		
Check brachial pulse (pulse is present)		
Give one breath every 3 seconds (in adult)		

Comments____

____

____

____

Instructor __________________ Circle One: Pass Fail

Chapter 14

Skill Performance Sheet

Child One Rescuer CPR

Student's Name__________________________ Date_________

Performance Standard	**Performed**	**Failed**
Open airway with appropriate maneuver (head tilt-chin lift or jaw thrust)		
Assess breathing (look, listen and feel)		
Seal mouth around the patient's mouth and pinch nose		
Give two smooth breaths while observing chest rise (1-1.5 seconds per breath)		
Take mouth away between breaths		
Check carotid pulse (pulse is present)		
If no pulse, locate correct hand position		
Maintain vertical position and provide 5 compressions (80-100/minute) while continuing to maintain head tilt		
Provide two ventilations		
After 10 cycles of 5:1, give two ventilations and check for pulse		
If no pulse continue 5:1 cycle		

Comments____

____

____

Instructor ________________ Circle One: Pass Fail

Pediatric Emergencies

Skill Performance Sheet

Infant One Rescuer CPR

Student's Name____________________________ Date_________

Performance Standard	Performed	Failed
Open airway with appropriate maneuver (head tilt-chin lift or jaw thrust)		
Assess breathing (look, listen and feel)		
Seal mouth around the patient's mouth and nose		
Give two smooth breaths while observing chest rise (1-1.5 seconds per breath)		
Take mouth away between breaths		
Check brachial pulse (pulse present)		
Locate correct finger position (1 finger below nipple line)		
Maintain head tilt		
Provide compressions at a rate of 100 per minute (1/2 to 1 inch)		
Perform 10 cycles at 5:1 ratio		
Check pulse		
If no pulse continue CPR		

Comments____

____

____

Instructor _________________ Circle One: Pass Fail

Chapter 14

Skill Performance Sheet

Child Conscious Complete Airway Obstruction

Student's Name______________________________ Date__________

Performance Standard	**Performed**	**Failed**
Confirm obstruction by asking "Are you choking?"		
Apply manual abdominal thrusts		
Repeat thrusts until effective or until the patient becomes unconscious		

Comments____

____

____

____

Instructor ___________________ Circle One: Pass Fail

Skill Performance Sheet

Child Complete Airway Obstruction Conscious Patient That Becomes Unconscious

Student's Name__________________________ Date_________

Performance Standard	**Performed**	**Failed**
Perform finger sweep (only if object is visible)		
Open airway and attempt to ventilate		
Apply 6 to 10 abdominal thrusts		
Perform finger sweep (only if object is visible)		
Attempt to ventilate		
Repeat sequence of thrusts, finger sweeps and ventilation until effective		

Comments____

____

____

____

Instructor ________________ Circle One: Pass Fail

Chapter 14

Skill Performance Sheet

Child Unconscious Complete Airway Obstruction

Student's Name____________________________ Date_________

Performance Standard	Performed	Failed
Check for unresponsiveness		
Position the patient supine		
Open airway		
Attempt to ventilate (obstructed)		
Open airway and reattempt ventilation (obstructed)		
Perform 6 to 10 abdominal thrusts		
Perform finger sweep (only if object is visible)		
Attempt to ventilate		
Repeat sequence of thrusts, sweeps and ventilation until effective		

Comments____

____

____

____

Instructor __________________ Circle One: Pass Fail

Skill Performance Sheet

Infant Conscious Complete Airway Obstruction

Student's Name______________________________ Date__________

Performance Standard	**Performed**	**Failed**
Confirm obstruction by observing infant (consider infectious cause of obstruction)		
Perform 4 back blows		
Perform 4 chest thrusts (same position as chest compression but at slower rate)		
Repeat sequence of back blows and thrusts until effective or until the infant becomes unconscious		

Comments____

____

____

____

Instructor __________________ Circle One: Pass Fail

Chapter 14

Skill Performance Sheet

Infant Conscious Complete Airway Obstruction That Becomes Unconscious

Student's Name______________________________ Date__________

Performance Standard	**Performed**	**Failed**
View airway and perform finger sweep (only if object is visible)		
Open airway and attempt to ventilate (obstructed)		
Perform 4 back blows		
Perform 4 chest thrusts		
View airway and perform finger sweep (only if object is visible)		
Open airway and attempt to ventilate		
Repeat sequence of back blows, thrusts and ventilation until effective		

Comments____

____

____

____

Instructor ___________________ Circle One: Pass Fail

Skill Performance Sheet

Infant Unconscious Complete Airway Obstruction

Student's Name______________________________ Date__________

Performance Standard	**Performed**	**Failed**
Check for unresponsiveness		
Position the patient supine		
Open airway		
Attempt to ventilate (obstructed)		
Open airway and reattempt ventilation (obstructed)		
Perform 4 back blows		
Perform 4 chest thrusts		
View airway and perform finger sweep (only if object is visible)		
Open airway and attempt to ventilate		
Repeat sequence of back blows, thrusts and ventilation until effective		

Comments____

____

____

____

Instructor ____________________ Circle One: Pass Fail

Chapter 15

PSYCHOLOGICAL ASPECTS OF EMERGENCY CARE

Materials and Equipment for Lesson

1. Slides or overhead transparencies
2. Handouts
   - Psychiatric emergencies
   - DNR policies
   - Restraint procedures
5. Slide projector, overhead projector and/or blackboard

Psychological Aspects of Emergency Care

Objectives
(Slide 15-1)

At the conclusion of the chapter the student will be able to:	
1.	List six factors in effective communication with patients.
2.	List three special considerations in dealing with each of the following patients: Elderly patients / Blind patients Sick or injured child / Confused patients Deaf patients / Mentally retarded patients
3.	Provide three examples of situational reactions.
4.	List six symptoms of depression.
5.	List seven risk factors of suicide.
6	Describe the basic management of the suicidal patient.
7.	List five symptoms of the potentially violent patient.
8.	List six general guidelines in the evaluation and treatment of behavioral disorders.
9.	List the steps of management with the potentially violent patient.
10.	Describe four typical negative responses to death that may be exhibited by the EMT.
11.	List seven symptoms of job-related stress.

Chapter 15

Instructor Preparation

Reading preparation for the lesson:

EMT Prehospital Care, Chapter 15, pages 679-687
Local DNR protocols

Suggested Learning Activities
Using a lecture format with the aid of slides, overhead transparencies or charts, provide an overview of psychiatric emergencies.
Demonstrate the basic technique for restraining a patient.
Discuss emotions experienced by the EMT, patient and family at emergency or death.

Content

I. Overview **(Slide 15-2)**

A. Emergency Medical Services System Act of 1973 included behavioral emergencies among the seven disease categories

B. Recognized as a seriousness problem faced in prehospital emergency care

C. Remains an area of medicine which is highly subjective

D. Careful judgment and experience is valuable

E. Danger of bias toward or negative reactions to victims of psychatric problems

F. Field experience is vital for the EMT to be truly effective

G. Types of emergencies (type vs. cause) **(Slide 15-3)**

1. Type of behavior (rage, anxiety, suicide)
2. Cause (psychosis, hypoglycemia, head trauma)
3. Do not always occur in isolation
4. May be an emotional component superimposed on an acute organic illness

II. Scope of the problem **(Slide 15-4)**

A. Medical care often focuses efforts toward diseases which are understandable, measurable, and treatable

1. Emphasis is placed on heart attacks and pneumonia
2. Majority of their training focuses on medical and traumatic conditions
3. Dangerous message
    a) Heart attacks are "real" problems
    b) Behavioral problems are not as important
4. Behavioral emergencies require professionalism and compassion

B. Statistics **(Slide 15-5)**

1. Depression present in at least 5% of the population in the US
2. 10% to 20% of adults experiencing at least one episode of clinical depression at some time in their life
3. 60% of patients have underlying emotional disturbances which cause or contribute to the depression
4. About 25,000 people kill themselves each year
5. Depression is the most common mental disorder in elderly patients **(Slide 15-6)**
6. Rate of suicide in men over 65 at least three times that of the general population
7. More than 10,000 persons over 60 kill themselves each year
8. Young person attempts suicide every 90 seconds in the US
    a) Successful every 90 minutes
    b) From 1950 to 1980, the suicide rate in the adolescent age group tripled
9. Overall, suicide is the 10th leading cause of death in the US
10. Many victims sought medical attention prior to suicide
11. Suicide and depression are readily treatable

C. Pitfalls **(Slide 15-7)**

1. Health care professionals
    a) More interest with a pain from an organ
    b) Less interested in pain from life

Content

c) Tend to discount symptoms in patients who
   a) Are difficult
   b) Demanding, angry, hysterical
   c) Intoxicated or "crazy"
   d) Ordinary human reaction which leads to dangerous medical judgment
2. Many physical diseases present with behavioral manifestations
3. Many behavioral problems present with physical complaints
4. Health care personnel should recognize and treat, and not to judge
5. EMT and patient encounter often occurs in an atmosphere which is highly charged

III. Principles of communication **(Slide 15-8)**
   A. Focus attention on patient
   B. Introduce yourself
   C. Be truthful
   D. Use terms the patient can understand
   E. Maintain a nonthreatening, calm posture
   F. Speak slowly and clearly
   G. Explain what you are doing to the patient **(Slide 15-9)**
   H. Address the patient with proper respect
   I. Allow the patient ample time for response to questions
   J. Help to assure that the patient is comfortable
   K. Be aware that the patient may hide symptoms from you
   L. Maintain a professional and calm demeanor at all times
   M. Anticipate problems with communication
   N. Always assume that the patient understands what you say

IV. Special problems in communication
   A. Elderly patients **(Slide 15-10)**
      1. Treat with special respect
      2. Move patient with extra care
      3. Be sensitive to the spouse's concerns
   B. The sick or injured child
      1. Allow the parent to accompany the child
      2. Bring objects which help child feel more secure
      3. Interact with both the parent and child
      4. Be honest with the child
   C. Deaf patients
      1. Look directly at patient's face and speak in normal, slow voice
      2. Use short, written questions, if necessary
      3. Be patient
      4. Explain what you are doing to the patient
   D. Blind patients
      1. Maintain physical contact
      2. Describe in detail what you are doing
      3. If patient has a Seeing Eye dog, bring dog with the patient, or arrange for care of the dog

Content

- E. Patient who speaks another language **(Slide 15-11)**
  1. Use a translator if patient does not speak English
  2. Be patient
- F. Confused patients
  1. Use simple terms
  2. Give simple explanations
  3. Reinforce orientation and simple explanations
  4. Allow patient ample time to respond
  5. Assume that the patient can understand what you say
- G. Mentally retarded patients
  1. Give simple explanations and reinforcement
  2. Determine capability of patient to understand
  3. Distinguish mental from physical disability
  4. Assume that the patient can understand what you say

V. Types of behavioral disorders

- A. Situational reactions **(Slide 15-12)**
  1. Emotional responses
     - a) Sudden illness
     - b) Death in the family
     - c) Other difficult personal experience
  2. Anxiety
     - a) Increased nervousness, tension
     - b) Pacing, hand wringing and trembling
     - c) Expression of fear
  3. Paranoia
     - a) Patient feels threatened by his environment
     - b) Care should be taken due to suspicious nature of patient
  4. Hysteria
     - a) Crying or screaming
     - b) Refuses to communicate
     - c) Beating fists repeatedly against a wall
     - d) Throwing himself or herself to the ground
  5. Denial
     - a) May manifest denial
     - b) Helpful in dealing with severe stress
  6. Withdrawal
     - a) Patient may not communicate
     - b) Avoids answering questions
- B. Personality disorders **(Slide 15-13)**
  1. Profile
     - a) Character traits that interfere with success in work or relationships
     - b) Characteristically very manipulative
     - c) Shift the responsibility and blame onto others
     - d) Will not acknowledge problem
     - e) Tends to be self-centered and selfish
     - f) Patient will demand time and attention, oblivious to more seriously injured patients

Content

2. Approach to patient **(Slide 15-14)**
    a) Do not become angered
    b) Ignoring or belittling will only anger patient
    c) Be positive with the patient
    d) Establish limits in a positive and professional manner

C. Depression and suicide **(Slide 15-15)**
1. Symptoms of depression
    a) Loss of sleep, appetite, sex drive
    b) Loss of pleasure in satisfying activities
    c) Feelings of sadness, guilt, hopelessness
    d) Physical symptoms
2. Risk factors for suicide **(Slide 15-16)**
    a) Single
    b) Socially isolated
    c) Unemployed
    d) Prior psychiatric history
    e) Recent loss of loved one **(Slide 15-17)**
    f) Alcoholism or drug abuse
    g) Male
    h) Impulsive behavior
    i) Chronic or terminal illness
    j) Loss of job or status
3. Management of the suicidal patient **(Slide 15-18)**
    a) Bring patient to the hospital
    b) Protect the patient from doing further harm
    c) Remove harmful objects from vicinity of patient
    d) Keep constant watch on patient
    e) Bring pills, bottles, or other material which may assist in managing the patient
    f) Assess the patient for potential violence

D. Psychosis **(Slide 15-19)**
1. Description
    a) Implies disordered thought
    b) Distorted perceptions of reality
    c) Hallucinations and inappropriate responses to environment
2. Recognition **(Slide 15-20)**
    a) Oriented to time and place
    b) May hear voices which command the patient to perform certain acts
    c) Bizarre thoughts
    d) Has difficulty in communicating
    e) Speaks incoherently or rambles
    f) History will have to be obtained from bystanders, friends, or family members

E. Organic brain syndromes **(Slide 15-21)**
1. Presentation
    a) Disordered thought
    b) Disoriented to place and time
    c) Confusion, difficulty with attention

Content

d) Varying levels of alertness
e) Patient might be incontinent
f) Auditory hallucinations
g) Visual, tactile, or olfactory hallucinations

2. Causes **(Slide 15-22)**
   a) Tumor, trauma, infection
   b) Degeneration (such as senile dementia)
   c) Low blood sugar, shock, or drug intoxication
   d) Distinction between psychosis and organic brain syndrome is quite difficult
   e) Safer to assume organic cause until proven otherwise

F. Violent behavior **(Slide 15-23)**

1. Overview
   a) May overlap with any of the behaviors noted above
   b) Patient endangers himself or herself or others
   c) Caused by a variety of organic and functional problems
   d) Patient loses control and strikes out at his or her environment
   e) Can often be averted by dealing with the source of feelings
2. Recognition of potentially violent patient **(Slide 15-24)**
   a) Angry voice
   b) Pressured speech
   c) Pacing
   d) Expressions of violence
   e) Psychiatric patients
   f) Drug intoxication
   g) Situational frustration
   h) Metabolic causes, i.e., hypoglycemia
   i) Look for evidence of cause
3. Evaluation and treatment of behavioral disorders **(Slide 15-25)**
   a) Assess orientation of the patient
   b) Medical priorities first
   c) Be the patient's advocate
   d) Treat the patient with respect
   e) Take the patient's complaints seriously **(Slide 15-26)**
   f) Remain cool, calm, and professional
   g) In confused patients, keep explanations simple
   h) Get the patient to the hospital
   i) Gather as much information at the scene as possible
4. Management of violent patient **(Slide 15-27)**
   a) Protect yourself
   b) Detect potential for violence before it occurs
   c) Keep cool and calm
   d) Understand the patient's source of frustration
   e) Have one person be in charge
   f) Watch the patient at all times
   g) Provide medical care, such as is possible
   h) If necessary, assist police in subduing patient

Content

VI. Stress and Crisis Events
- A. Death **(Slide 15-28)**
  - 1. EMT should be prepared for a variety of emotional responses
    - a) Denial to guilt
    - b) Grief, anger, hysteria
    - c) Withdrawal, or physical reactions
  - 2. Treatment of the patient is of first priority **(Slide 15-29)**
    - a) Be honest and keep the family informed
    - b) Answer questions honestly as possible
    - c) Emotional responses (crying) should be encouraged
    - d) Adhere to family's wishes to be alone or see the body
    - e) Mutilated parts should be covered
    - f) Encourage the family to seek follow-up
    - g) EMT should be supportive
  - 3. Decision to resuscitate **(Slide 15-30)**
    - a) Family may call ambulance long after patient died
    - b) CPR should be initiated, unless
      - a) Signs of rigor mortis
      - b) Dependent lividity
- B. Terminal illness
  - 1. Emotional aspects **(Slide 15-31)**
    - a) EMT must be aware of inner feelings of helplessness
    - b) EMT may distance himself from the patient
    - c) Patients are sometimes treated as an object
    - d) EMT must allow for the patient to express his or her feelings **(Slide 15-32)**
      - a) Denial
      - b) Anger
      - c) Depression
      - d) Peace or relief
      - e) Acceptance
    - e) Calm, supportive role and sensitive management go a long way
    - f) Family
      - a) May have had time to adapt
      - b) Emotions tend to be less charged
      - c) Full range of emotions may manifest
  - 2. Communication **(Slide 15-33)**
    - a) Patient may indicate that he or she is dying
    - b) EMT should not deny the patient his or her expressions
    - c) Acknowledgment of such expressions appropriate
    - d) Patient will need warmth and communication
    - e) Honest and direct approach is important
    - f) Compassion and kind word and acknowledgment
  - 3. Management **(Slide 15-34)**
    - a) Primarily directed toward comfort
    - b) Assess patient's and family's awareness is regarding the patient's illness
    - c) Family may know that the patient has terminal lung cancer
    - d) The patient may not know **(Slide 15-35)**
    - e) EMT should not inform the patient of the diagnosis

Content

f) The family should be allowed to be with the patient
g) If the patient or the family refuses treatment
   a) Contact medical control for guidance
   b) May be appropriate to withhold treatment
   c) Local guidelines vary
h) EMT should record the patient's final words

C. Victims of crime **(Slide 15-36)**
1. Rape, assault, attempted murder
2. Provoke a number of reactions in the EMT
3. Great sympathy to disgust and anger
4. Calm, supportive, nonjudgmental approach
5. Cooperating with law enforcement should not interfere with care
6. Varied patient responses **(Slide 15-37)**
   a) Violence, disbelief, hysteria
   b) Extreme agitation in response to the event
   c) Quiet and withdrawn
   d) Severely depressed
   e) Profound sense of guilt
7. Medical care deserves priority **(Slide 15-38)**
8. Allow the patient to ventilate feelings
9. Do not ask patient to reveal details not related to treatment
10. In cooperation with law enforcement personnel
   a) Try not to move or touch things in environment except as necessary to evaluate and treat
   b) EMT should note whether clothes are torn prior to removing or cutting off

D. EMTs response to death **(Slide 15-39)**
1. Can be quite difficult for health care provider's field
   a) Represents ultimate failure in patient care
   b) Be aware of responses to unsuccessful resuscitation
   c) Resolve and maturity are needed to cope

E. Stress **(Slide 15-40)**
1. EMT must have outlet for dealing with feelings
   a) Sharing with colleagues, close friend or spouse
   b) Professional counselling
   c) Should not deal with feelings in front of patients and families
   d) Many situations are overwhelming **(Slide 15-41)**
      a) Death of a child
      b) Patient of similar background, age, or profession
      c) Disasters
      d) Chaos
      e) Sights of mutilation
      f) Feelings of being overwhelmed leave their mark on our emotions
      g) Debriefing
         (a) Where feelings can be discussed with peers and counsler
         (b) Hopefully, some feelings can be resolved

Content

2. Key symptoms of stress **(Slide 15-42)**
    a) Nightmares
    b) Inability to control one's temper
    c) Feelings of extreme sadness
    d) Symptoms of depression
    e) Feelings of guilt or denial
    f) Becoming accusatory **(Slide 15-43)**
    g) Wishing to leave a scene quickly
    h) Avoid dealing with family stress
    i) Feelings of not being appreciated
    j) Feelings of apathy toward work
    k) Unable to accept criticism
    l) Alcohol and drugs as an outlet
3. Response **(Slide 15-44)**
    a) Recognize and admit reactions and feelings
    b) Discussion with a coworker, the medical director, or a counselor

Chapter 15

PSYCHOLOGICAL ASPECTS OF EMERGENCY CARE

Examination

1. Depression is said to be present in at least _____ of the population:

   a. 5%
   b. 10%
   c. 20%
   d. 25%

Indicate which of the following methods of communication are effective vs. non-effective.

Column A		Column B	
2.	focus your attention at the family of the patient	a.	effective
3.	deal with the family, not the patient	b.	non-effective
4.	speak clearly		
5.	never explain treatments, it will frighten the patient		
6.	never use the patient's name, rather refer to them as sir or Ma'am		

7. Which of the following age groups of persons are more likely to commit suicide:

   a. small children
   b. persons in their 20's
   c. middle aged persons
   d. elderly persons

8. When caring for a sick or injured *child* who is afraid to go in the ambulance, your best approach would be to:

   a. encourage the child to bring along a favorite toy, doll or blanket, have the parents accompany the child, assure the child that no one will him at the hospital
   b. assure the child that no one will hurt him at the hospital, talk only to the parents, have the parents accompany the child
   c. talk only to the parents, let the patents then deal with the child, encourage the child to bring along a favorite toy, doll or blanket
   d. have the parents drive separately, assure the child that no one will hurt him at the hospital, encourage the child to bring along a favorite toy, doll or blanket

9. When caring for a deaf patient, you should always remember to:

    a. speak loudly
    b. look directly at the patient when you speak
    c. obtain the history from a family member
    d. never allow a deaf patient to refuse medical aid

10. It is preferable that patients who speak another language or who speak minimal English should be interviewed:

    a. at the hospital
    b. by the EMT using hand gestures as appropriate
    c. through a translator
    d. by using a bilingual EMS dictionary

11. While comforting for all patients, it is imperative to maintain physical contact with the __________ patient:

    a. deaf
    b. elderly
    c. blind
    d. non-English-speaking

12. A patient who witnessed a friend killed in an automobile accident is sitting on the sidewalk, refusing to talk or interact with the EMT. This is an example of:

    a. paranoia
    b. denial
    c. withdrawal
    d. anxiety

13. Your patient feels threatened by the environment and may believe that someone "is out to get them". This is an example of:

    a. paranoia
    b. denial
    c. withdrawal
    d. anxiety

14. Increased nervousness, tension, pacing, hand-wringing and trembling best describe the behaviors associated with:

    a. paranoia
    b. denial
    c. withdrawal
    d. anxiety

15. A patient is agitated, upset, crying uncontrollably and punching the wall. This is an example of:

    a. paranoia
    b. denial
    c. withdrawal
    d. hysteria

16. Character traits that interfere with a person's ability to function successfully in work or personal relationships are referred to as:

    a. personality disorders
    b. insanity
    c. psychotic episodes
    d. depression

17. A patient complains of sleep loss and feels that life is hopeless. This patient may be suffering from:

    a. denial
    b. anxiety
    c. insanity
    d. depression

18. Statistics indicate that patients with the following qualities are more likely to successfully commit suicide:

    a. married, female, alcoholic, unemployed
    b. married, male, alcoholic, unemployed
    c. single, female, alcoholic, unemployed
    d. single, male, alcoholic, unemployed

19. A patient who has been suffering from depression and is now very content and even happy:

    a. is not at risk to commit suicide
    b. is exhibiting traits of someone who may be about to commit suicide
    c. is considered to be cured
    d. will not commit suicide until signs of depression reappear

20. You are treating a 75 year old patient named Mrs. Janet Jones. The patient is very fearful. Which of the following is the best way of speaking with this patient?

    a. Hello Dear, how are you?
    b. Hello Ma'am, how are you?
    c. Hello Mrs. Jones, how are you?
    d. Hello Mom, how are you?

21. Response such as: guilt, grief, anger, hysteria, denial, withdrawal, or physical reactions are common reactions to:

    a. phobias
    b. pain
    c. organic illness
    d. death

22. Which of the following is <u>not</u> a likely cause of violent behavior:

    a. hypoglycemia
    b. hysteria
    c. organic brain syndrome
    d. Valium overdose

23. The first priority when faced with an emotionally disturbed patient is to:

    a. transport the patient to a psychiatric hospital
    b. consider possible medical causes
    c. give sedation and restrain the patient
    d. get permission from the police to restrain the patient

24. The EMTs first priority with a potentially dangerous patient is:

    a. self protection
    b. the patient's protection
    c. the legal implications
    d. restraining him or her

25. A good strategy when encountering a child who is refusing oxygen is to:

    a. have the parent hold the child down and administer oxygen via face mask
    b. offer a choice such as a simple face mask or nasal cannula
    c. tell the child it is a toy that he/she can wear to the hospital
    d. do not transport the patient as "quality care" has not been rendered

Chapter 16

LIFTS AND MOVING PATIENTS

Materials and Equipment for Lesson

1. Slides or overhead transparencies
2. Handouts
   - Lifting and moving patient
   - Body mechanics
   - Skills sheets for lifting
3. Slide projector, overhead projector and/or blackboard
4. COT stretcher, blankets and sheets
5. Spine boards, straps and cervical collars
6. Stair chair, scoop stretcher and stokes basket

Lifting and Moving Patients

Objectives
(Slide 16-1)

At the conclusion of the chapter the students will be able to:

1. **Describe effective body mechanics during lifting.**
2. **List the steps of performance for the following emergency evacuation techniques:**
   - **Clothes drag**
   - **Blanket drag**
   - **Assisting an ambulatory patient**
   - **Firefighter drag**
   - **Firefighter carry**
   - **Extremity carry**
3. **Describe the common uses and basic transfer procedures for each of the following devices:**
   - **Wheeled Cot Stretcher**
   - **Portable Stretcher**
   - **Scoop Stretcher**
   - **Spine Boards**
   - **Stair Chair**
   - **Long Spine Board**
   - **Kendrick Extrication Device**
   - **Short Spine Board**
   - **Stokes Basket**
4. **List the steps of performance for the following techniques:**
   - **Log Roll**
   - **Rapid Extrication Procedure**
   - **Standing takedown**
5. **Describe the ideal transport approach for the following patients:**
   - **Dyspnea or Chest Pain**
   - **Unconscious Medical Patient**
   - **Abdominal Pain**
   - **Automobile accident victims**
   - **Injured pedestrians**
   - **Head Injury**
   - **Pregnant Patients**

Chapter 16

Instructor Preparation

Reading preparation for the lesson:

EMT Prehospital Care, Chapter 16, pages 688-714
Skill sheets for lifting and moving

Suggested Learning Activities

Using a lecture format with the aid of slides, overhead transparencies or charts, provide an overview of lifting and moving patients.

Demonstrate the basic techniques for lifting and moving patients.

Discuss examples of different situations and have students suggest transport method.

Content

I. Overview **(Slide 16-2)**
- A. Each situation requires unique strategy for lifting and moving
- B. Factors affecting choice
    - 1. Available manpower
    - 2. Terrain
    - 3. Hazards
    - 4. Condition of the patient
- C. General principles **(Slide 16-3)**
    - 1. Trauma patient should be immobilized with a short spine before moving, exceptions:
        - a) Danger to patient or others
        - b) Patient requires rapid surgical intervention
        - c) Rapid extrication procedure is used in these instances
    - 2. Selection of appropriate lift and carry technique is an essential aspect of emergency care
    - 3. With spinal injury it is often the most important aspect of treatment
    - 4. Safety
        - a) Improper technique can be a hazard to your patient
        - b) Back injury can last a lifetime
        - c) Proper techniques for lifting can minimize the potential for injury
- D. Decision to transport **(Slide 16-4)**
    - 1. Not always possible to stabilize patient on scene
    - 2. Fire or other hazards
    - 3. Need for surgical care outweighs benefits of splinting
    - 4. Rapid methods which minimize chances of aggravating injuries are used
    - 5. Risk benefit ratio
        - a) Bleeding patient may exsanguinate if rapid surgical intervention is not applied
        - b) Complete airway obstruction which cannot be relieved by BLS would require rapid transport
- E. Body mechanics **(Slide 16-5)**
    - 1. Scientific methods of efficiently lifting large weights so not to injure oneself
    - 2. Body is a system of levers and support structures
        - a) Used correctly can support a great deal of weight
        - b) Used incorrectly, the result can be severe and permanent injury
    - 3. Know your physical capabilities and limitations
    - 4. Seek help when needed
    - 5. Correct technique **(Slide 16-6)**
        - a) Long bones are the strongest
        - b) Largest is the femur which is surrounded by largest and strongest muscle group
        - c) These are support units you should use when lifting heavy objects
        - d) Never lift with your back
        - e) Back muscles are relatively small and weak

Content

f) Technique **(Slide 16-7)**
(1) Squat and place one foot in front of the other
(2) Get as close as possible to the person you are lifting
(3) Keep your arms close to your body as you lift
(4) Center of gravity closer to the patient, more leverage
(5) Makes patient lighter
(6) Helps maintain your balance
g) See-saw illustrates the value of this closeness
(1) When sitting toward the center
(2) Easier for your partner to raise you
(3) Toward the very edge
(4) Much more difficult
h) Lifting a stretcher **(Slide 16-8)**
(1) Keep your back straight
(2) Tighten muscles of abdomen and buttocks
(3) Maintain a firm grip on the device or patient
(4) Lift and move slowly, smoothly in unison
(5) Maintain firm footing
(6) Try not to keep your muscles contracted for too long a period of time

II. Emergency evacuation techniques
A. One rescuer techniques
1. Clothes drag **(Slide 16-9)**
a) Simplest technique for quickly moving a patient. Grasp the shirt, sweater or jacket
b) Drag patient along the long axis of his body
c) Support head in forearms
2. Foot drag **(Slide 16-10)**
a) Grasp ankles
b) Pull patient along
c) Do not use this when traversing steps or rough terrain
3. Blanket drag **(Slide 16-11)**
a) Permits long axis pull without dragging skin on the ground
b) Log roll patient on blanket
c) Pull blanket while maintaining low profile
4. Firefighter's drag **(Slide 16-12)**
a) Allows long axis drag while maintaining a low profile
b) Used in a smoke-filled room
c) Tie victim's hands together
d) Loop arms around your neck
e) Straddle the victim
f) Crawl along the floor
5. Firefighter's carry **(Slide 16-13)**
a) Permits fastest potential exit from fire
b) More likely to aggravate injuries
c) Requires increased baseline strength
d) Stand toe to toe at the victim's feet **(Slide 16-14)**
e) Hold patient's wrists **(Slide 16-15)**
f) Pull patient up in one smooth move **(Slide 16-16)**

Content

g) Maintain low profile
h) Catch victim across your shoulder **(Slide 16-17)**
i) Hold patient's arms and legs
j) Stand to an upright position
k) Hold patient's wrists with one arm around the thigh
l) Permits free hand to hold railings as you exit

B. Two rescuer techniques

1. Extremity carry **(Slide 16-18)**
a) Practical way to remove a victim quickly
b) EMT #1 positions self at victim's head supporting victim under the armpits
c) EMT #2 grasps wrists and pulls victim up while EMT #1 lifts **(Slide 16-19)**
d) Should always be done in unison
e) EMT #1 grasps patient's wrists while EMT #2 supports victim with one hand around each knee
f) Both EMTs rise smoothly to an upright position **(Slide 16-20)**
g) EMT #2 turns 180 degrees to facilitate forward movement **(Slide 16-21)**

2. Assisting ambulatory patient
a) One or two rescuer **(Slide 16-22)**
b) EMTs provide support by placing hands behind patient with wrist over their shoulder **(Slide 16-23)**

III. General principles **(Slide 16-24)**

A. Select device best suited to provide a safe and comfortable ride for patient

B. Medical patients most often require a wheeled cot stretcher
1. Allows rolling along terrain
2. Can be adjusted for sitting, supine or lateral recumbent position
3. Comfort due to mattress
4. Allows administration of resuscitation procedures with special board

C. Trauma patient may require several different devices
1. Designed to assure immobilization of spine
2. Prevent spinal cord injury
3. Extremities are protected by splinting
4. If time does not permit, the patient may be splinted to the long spine board

IV. Wheeled cot stretcher **(Slide 16-25)**

A. Overview
1. Preferred method for transporting patients along smooth terrain
2. Permits movement without undue fatigue to EMTs
3. Unstable in upright position
4. Least effective moving over rough terrain or down stairs due to its weight and bulkiness
5. In these circumstances, folding stretcher, scoop stretcher or stokes basket are preferred

B. Types **(Slide 16-26)**

1. Multi-level cot
a) Permits adjustment of height
b) Good for CPR, ventilation and transfer in E.D.

Content

2. Two-level cots
    a) Permit easy transfer of the patient from a bed to the stretcher
    b) Less versatile than multi-level
    c) Some allow one person loading procedure
    d) Tend to be less stable
3. Single-level cots
    a) Much lighter
    b) More mobile
    c) Less versatile
4. Other features **(Slide 16-27)**
    a) Permit adjustment of head from supine to 90 degrees
    b) Allows for elevation of legs, knees or Trendelenburg position
    c) Adjunctive equipment may be attached, i.e., IV poles, oxygen and monitor-defibrillators

C. Placing a patient on a wheeled cot stretcher
1. Direct carry **(Slide 16-28)**
    a) Position cot with head at the foot of the bed, at a 90 degree angle to the bed
    b) Unfold straps, lower siderails and open sheets and blankets
    c) EMTs stand together at side of patient
    d) EMT at patient's head supports patient's shoulder and neck and lumbar region
    e) EMT at the patient's thigh supports upper portion of buttocks and just below knees
    f) Patient is lifted up toward EMTs chest
    g) EMTs rotate 90 degrees
    h) Gently place the patient on the stretcher
    i) Secure with straps and siderails prior to movement
2. Draw sheet method **(Slide 16-29)**
    a) Sheet is placed under the patient
    b) EMT stands on each side of the patient
    c) EMT #1 log rolls patient on side and close to edge of bed
    d) EMT #2 places a folded draw sheet under the patient
    e) EMT #1 lowers the patient onto the draw sheet
    f) EMT #2 log rolls patient toward self
    g) EMT #1 unfolds draw sheet
    h) Patient can be released to a supine position
    i) Cot is placed directly alongside the bed
    j) Slightly lower than the bed to facilitate movement
    k) EMTs grasp top and bottom corners of sheet
    l) Gently slide patient to stretcher
3. Direct carry at floor level **(Slide 16-30)**
    a) Stretcher placed at 90 degrees to patient
    b) Both EMTs drop to one knee on the same side
    c) Kneeling on the same knee
    d) Fold victim's arms across chest
    e) EMT #1 places arm under neck and shoulder and lower back
    f) EMT #2 places one arm under buttocks and below the patient's knees

Content

g) EMTs smoothly lift patient onto elevated thighs
h) In unison, EMT's stand to the upright position
i) Rotate until adjacent to stretcher
j) Lower patient gently to stretcher

D. Moving the wheeled cot stretcher **(Slide 16-31)**
1. Foot end should always go first, except when loading patient into ambulance
2. Particularly important when going down stairs
3. Roll stretcher along the ground with one EMT at each end of the stretcher
4. EMTs should maintain a firm grip, since the top heavy stretcher may tilt and fall
5. Movement is safer with stretcher in low position
6. On rough terrain, end to end carry may be necessary

E. Loading patient in ambulance **(Slide 16-32)**
1. Side carry method is used
2. EMTs stand on opposite sides **(Slide 16-33)**
3. Bend knees and grasp the lower bar
4. Hands positioned at each end of the lower bar
5. One hand palm-down and other hand palm-up
6. Upon command, both EMT's should rise to the upright position **(Slide 16-34)**
7. Move the front wheels onto the floor **(Slide 16-35)**
8. Stretcher is rolled forward until all wheels are on floor
9. Stretcher is guided into locking bar
10. Obstetrical patient is loaded foot-first

F. Unloading **(Slide 16-36)**
1. Unlatch lock
2. Hold bottom bar as described above
3. Remove from ambulance **(Slide 16-37)**
4. Lower to ground **(Slide 16-38)**
5. Elevate by releasing latch to facilitate transfer **(Slide 16-39)**

V. Portable stretchers **(Slide 16-40)**
A. Lightweight devices which can be folded and stored
B. Permit easier transfer down stairs and over rough terrain
C. Allow ambulance more carrying power for use in multiple injury situations
D. Can be mounted on squad bench
E. Should be carried end to end

VI. Scoop stretcher **(Slide 16-41)**
A. Specialized device which facilitates easy lifting of supine patients
B. Aluminum frame with rectangular tube and shovel-type flaps for sliding under patient
C. Splits lengthwise into two equal halves
D. Patient can be "scooped" off the ground
E. Excellent means for the initial lifting off ground
F. Not recommended for spine injury victims
G. Should be immediately transferred onto a long spine board
H. Adjust to length just longer than the patient **(Slide 16-42)**
I. Each half should then be positioned under the patient **(Slide 16-43)**

Content

J. Carefully guide the edges one side at a time
K. Head end is connected first
L. Hips must be slightly lifted to allow connection of the bottom half
M. Straps should be fastened prior to moving **(Slide 16-44)**

VII. Spine Boards
  A. Cervical collars **(Slide 16-45)**
    1. Essential adjunct to spinal immobilization
    2. Does not constitute full immobilization without spine board
    3. Come in various materials and configurations
    4. Must be rigid to provide immobilization
    5. Must be sized to the patient **(Slide 16-46)**
    6. See manufacturer's recommendations on sizing
  B. Long spine board is primary device **(Slide 16-47)**
    1. Patients who are prone supine or laterally recumbent
    2. Rapid extrication from an automobile
    3. Secondary support device for patients removed with a short spine board
  C. Long spine board using a log roll **(Slide 16-48)**
    1. Adapted from Prehospital Trauma Life Support Program
    2. Team leader assumes in-line immobilization
    3. Cervical collar is applied
    4. Three rescuers are positioned on one side of patient (shoulder, pelvis, legs) **(Slide 16-49)**
    5. Spine board is positioned on opposite side of patient
    6. On command from team leader, patient is rolled toward three rescuers **(Slide 16-50)**
    7. Board is slid under patient **(Slide 16-51)**
    8. On command from team leader, patient is rolled onto board **(Slide 16-52)**
    9. Patient is adjusted on board
    10. Body is securely attached to spine board **(Slide 16-53)**
    11. Head is securely attached to spine board **(Slide 16-54)**
  D. Rapid Extrication Procedure **(Slide 16-55)**
    1. EMT #1 maintains cervical immobilization from behind the patient
    2. EMT #2 performs primary survey and applies cervical collar **(Slide 16-56)**
    3. Car door is bent open as far as possible
    4. EMT #2 takes over in-line immobilization from outside of the car **(Slide 16-57)**
    5. EMT #1 positions a spine board in the car on a cot stretcher and slides the end under the patient's buttocks
    6. EMT #3 assumes a position on the other side of the seat from EMT #2 and supports the patients thighs **(Slide 16-58)**
    7. EMT #1 supports the patient's chest and back **(Slide 16-59)**
    8. On command from EMT #2, the patient is rotated at a 45 degree angle toward EMT #3 **(Slide 16-60)**
    9. On command, the patient is lowered down on the board **(Slide 16-61)**

Content

10. With EMT #1 supporting the axilla, EMT #2 maintaining in-line cervical immobilization and EMT #3 supporting the legs, the patient is slid up the board **(Slide 16-62)**
11. Patient's torso are secured to the board **(Slide 16-63)**
12. Patient's head and neck is secured to the board
13. Patient is secured to the stretcher **(Slide 16-64)**
14. (Adapted from the Prehospital Trauma Life Support Program)

E. Applying a short spine board **(Slide 16-65)**
1. EMT #1 maintains in-line cervical immobilization from behind the patient **(Slide 16-66)**
2. Cervical collar is applied
3. Board is positioned behind the patient **(Slide 16-67)**
4. Attach the chest and groin straps placing pads to protect the patient
5. Secure head to board **(Slide 16-68)**
6. Lift patient, not board, to long spine board
7. Release groin straps before lowering legs

F. Applying a Kendrick's Extrication Device (KED) **(Slide 16-69)**
1. EMT #1 maintains in-line cervical immobilization from behind the patient **(Slide 16-70)**
2. Cervical collar is applied
3. KED is positioned behind the patient **(Slide 16-71)**
4. KED is pulled up securely in axillary region **(Slide 16-72)**
5. Attach the chest straps **(Slide 16-73)**
6. Attach the groin straps **(Slide 16-74)**
7. Attach the head section **(Slide 16-75)**

G. Performing a Rapid Takedown
1. EMT #1 assumes immobilization from behind patient **(Slide 16-76)**
2. A cervical collar is applied **(Slide 16-77)**
3. EMT #2 slides board behind patient **(Slide 16-78)**
4. EMTs #2 and #3 stand on either side of the patient facing toward the board and slip their hands under the patient's axillary region and grasp the next highest opening on the board **(Slide 16-79)**
5. EMTs #2 and #3 support the shoulders with their other hands
6. On command from EMT #1, the board is lowered smoothly to the floor **(Slide 16-80)**
7. As the board is lowered, EMT #1 must allow the head to move slowly to the board **(Slide 16-81)**
8. The patient's torso is secured to the board **(Slide 16-82)**
9. The patient's head is secured to the board
10. (Adapted from the New York State Health Department Critical Trauma Care Program)

VIII. Stokes basket **(Slide 16-83)**

A. Extrication device that is ideal for rough terrain or high and low angle rescue
B. Where a patient must be lowered or lifted
C. Wire mesh construction with a metal frame or plastic or fiber glass
D. Must be well padded to prevent further injury

Content

IX. Stair Chair **(Slide 16-84)**
- A. Designed to remove patients who are able to assume the sitting position
- B. Primary device in urban EMS systems for medical patients
- C. Should never be used with suspected spinal injury or unconscious patients
- D. Patient should never be transported in stair chair
- E. Extremity carry is preferred method for loading a patient **(Slide 16-85)**
- F. Patient should be instructed not to grasp for the handrails
- G. When descending stairs
  - 1. EMT at head should support chair firmly at the outermost portion of the bar **(Slide 16-86)**
  - 2. EMT at the foot should elevate the lower portion
  - 3. Spotter should be utilized below the EMT at the foot
- H. Along ground level chair can be tilted back and rolled along smooth terrain **(Slide 16-87)**

X. Selecting the appropriate mode of transportation
- A. Medical patients **(Slide 16-88)**
  - 1. Most often transported on the wheeled cot stretcher
  - 2. Provides both comfort and a variety of positions
  - 3. Stair chair can used to remove conscious patient
- B. Patients with dyspnea or chest pain **(Slide 16-89)**
  - 1. Generally transported in a semi-reclining or fully upright position on a wheeled cot stretcher
  - 2. Position of comfort
  - 3. Patients with dyspnea usually prefer the full upright position
  - 4. Cardiac patients in shock may require a supine position for optimal brain perfusion
- C. Unconscious medical patient **(Slide 16-90)**
  - 1. Primary concern is airway management
  - 2. Generally placed in the left lateral recumbent position on wheeled cot stretcher **(Slide 16-91)**
  - 3. Helps to prevent aspiration
  - 4. Patients in need of resuscitation
    - a) Placed in supine position
    - b) Spine or cardiac resuscitation board.
- D. Patients complaining of abdominal pain **(Slide 16-92)**
  - 1. Usually most comfortable in the supine or lateral recumbent position with knees flexed
  - 2. Wheeled cot stretchers may permit elevation of the knees to facilitate this position
- E. Trauma patients **(Slide 16-93)**
  - 1. Extremity fractures (isolated)
    - a) Patients with upper extremity injuries
      - (1) Transported in stair chair to ambulance
      - (2) Wheeled cot during transport
    - b) Patients with lower extremity injuries
      - (1) Portable or wheeled cot stretcher
      - (2) Elevate the injured part
      - (3) Traction splints should be properly secured

Content

2. Patients with a head injury **(Slide 16-94)**
    a) Isolated head injury in absence of spinal injury in a semi-fowlers position
        (1) Reduces intracranial pressure
        (2) May decrease chances of cerebral edema
    b) Suspected spinal injury patients may be kept supine with attention to airway maintenance
3. Multiple injured patient **(Slide 16-95)**
    a) Long spine board
    b) Method of immobilization may vary
        (1) Sitting position
            (a) Removed with short spine board
            (b) Transferred to long spine board
        (2) Patients found supine or are in need of rapid extrication
            (a) Removed with long spine board
            (b) Board placed on the wheeled cot stretcher
4. Pregnant patients **(Slide 16-96)**
    a) Heavily pregnant women
        (1) Left lateral recumbent position
        (2) Reduce vena caval compression
        (3) If spinal injury is suspected, tilt spine board
    b) Patient about to deliver
        (1) Stretcher placed foot first
        (2) Facilitates delivery
    c) Threatened abortion
        (1) Hips or foot of the cot should be elevated
        (2) Prevent undue strain against the cervix

LIFTING AND MOVING PATIENTS

Examination

1. The largest bones and muscles in the body are in the:

   a. back
   b. arms
   c. thighs
   d. chest

Match the description of the carry in column B to the term in column A.

Column A	Column B
2. clothes drag	a. rescuer assumes a low profile, wraps the arms of the patient around his/her neck and slides the patient along the floor
3. blanket drag	b. one rescuer evacuation technique in which the patient is pulled from a dangerous area by his/her shirt, sweater or jacket
4. firefighters drag	c. place the victim across your shoulders, stand upright, and hold the patient's wrists with one hand across the thighs
5. firefighters carry	d. position the patient on a sheet or canvas and pull this device along the long axis of the body
6. extremity carry	e. one rescuer grasps the patient under the armpits while holding the wrists and the second rescuer supports the patient with one hand around each knee

7. When lifting a patient, you should use the muscles in your:

   a. lower back
   b. upper back
   c. legs
   d. pelvis

8. When carrying a stretcher, your back should be:

   a. flexed
   b. extended
   c. held straight
   d. slightly curved

9. Which of the following devices are best suited for moving a patient over rough terrain?

   a. wheeled cot stretcher
   b. stair chair
   c. stokes basket
   d. long spine board

10. The most commonly used and effective method for placing a wheeled cot stretcher in the ambulance is the:

    a. side carry method
    b. front and back carry method
    c. sitting position method
    d. vertical lift method

11. The obstetrical patient should be loaded into the ambulance:

    a. feet first
    b. head first

12. The two piece, aluminum frame stretcher that facilitates the easy lifting of the supine patient is the:

    a. Miller body board
    b. Kendrick extrication device
    c. vacuum stretcher
    d. scoop stretcher

13. The length of the scoop stretcher should be adjusted to a length longer than the patient:

    a. after the patient is secured to the stretcher
    b. when the loaded stretcher is on the ambulance
    c. before sliding the stretcher under the patient
    d. this is not an adjustable stretcher

14. A patient who fell 20 feet and complains of back pain is to be transported. The immobilization device of choice is the:

    a. scoop stretcher
    b. ambulance cot
    c. long spine board
    d. basket stretcher

15. When performing a log roll, the EMT positioned at the patient's __________ should supervise the movements:

    a. head
    b. shoulder
    c. hip
    d. lower legs

16. Before performing a log roll for a patient who fell 20 feet, you should always:

    a. tie the patients hands and legs together
    b. immobilize the cervical spine
    c. obtain a written consent
    d. ask the patient if they can turn their head to either side

17. A patient who fell 20 feet is to be secured to a long spine board. Which of the following should be attached **last**?

    a. the leg straps
    b. the pelvic strap
    c. the head
    d. the chest strap

18. The method of quickly removing a patient from a car who is in respiratory arrest or is extremely unstable is called:

    a. load and go
    b. scoop and run
    c. rapid extrication
    d. categorization

Match the procedure for performing rapid extrication in column B to the proper sequence of events in column A.

Column A		Column B	
19.	first step	a.	the EMT holding the chest positions both hands in opposite armpits and on command slides the patient on the board
20.	second step	b.	the EMT in the car comes out of the car and the board is placed on the wheeled cot stretcher
21.	third step	c.	first EMT positions himself behind the patient and maintains immobilization of the cervical spine
22.	fourth step	d.	the EMT who performed the primary survey takes over in-line immobilization from outside of the car
23.	fifth step	e.	the patient is rotated with the patient's back toward the board so that the legs come in contact with the front of the seat
24.	sixth step	f.	one EMT grasps the patient under the armpit with one hand and in the mid-posterior thorax with the other hand

25. The proper procedure to immobilize a patient complaining of neck pain who is walking is:

    a. place a long spine board on the stretcher and have the patient lie down
    b. there is no need to immobilize any patient who is ambulatory
    c. to utilize the standing takedown technique
    d. have the patient sit on the stretcher, no long spine board is needed

26. As the first step in the standing takedown, manual spinal immobilization should be performed ________.

    a. facing the patient
    b. on the side of the patient
    c. behind the patient
    d. on both sides of the patient

27. When performing the standing takedown the EMTs at the side support the patient:

    a. at the elbow and chest
    b. under the armpit and outer arm
    c. at the chest and back
    d. at the shoulder and hip regions

28. In general, when performing the standing takedown the EMT who is the tallest should be positioned:

    a. at the left side of the patient
    b. at the right side of the patient
    c. at either side of the patient
    d. behind the patient

29. When moving and lifting a patient who is attached to a short spine board from a car to a stretcher, you should lift the:

    a. board
    b. patient
    c. straps
    d. clothing

30. When performing the helmet removal, the head should be supported at the base of the occipital bone and at the:

    a. temporal region
    b. maxilla and orbital regions
    c. lower margin of the mandible
    d. frontal bone region

Match the problem in column B to the appropriate removal and/or transportation method in column A.

Column A		Column B	
31.	stair chair	a.	conscious chest pain in a 5 floor walkup
32.	sitting upright on a cot stretcher	b.	stable auto victim with suspected spine injury
33.	rapid extrication procedure	c.	unstable auto accident victim
34.	log roll onto long spine board	d.	patient with abdominal pain
35.	KED	e.	patient on street who was struck by a car
36.	supine on cot with legs flexed	f.	8 month pregnant patient with severe vaginal bleeding
37.	left lateral recumbent position	g.	patient complaining of dyspnea

38. A stokes basket is an excellent device for:

    a. spinal immobilization
    b. extricating a patient from a car
    c. use in conjunction with the standing takedown procedure
    d. removal of a patient from rough terrain

39. Patients complaining of dyspnea are generally more comfortable if transported in a ________ position.

    a. semi-reclining or fully upright
    b. prone
    c. supine
    d. left or right lateral recumbent

40. The left lateral recumbent position is the position of choice for:

a. patients with suspected spinal injuries
b. unconscious medical patients who do not require resuscitation
c. patients with multiple injuries and fractures
d. conscious patients with an isolated head injury

41. Patients in need of CPR must be placed:

a. supine on a spine board
b. prone on a spine board
c. supine in a stair chair
d. prone in a stair chair

42. Patients in acute abdominal distress will usually be more comfortable:

a. if they are prone
b. with their knees bent
c. if they drink milk
d. on a spine board

43. Patients with multiple fractures of the lower extremities and suspected head injury should be transported on the:

a. wheeled ambulance stretcher
b. scoop stretcher
c. long spine board
d. stair chair

44. Pregnant trauma patients showing signs of hypovolemic shock (without suspected spinal injury) should be placed:

a. supine with legs elevated
b. in the left lateral recumbent position
c. in the prone position
d. in the semi-reclining position

45. Patients complaining of chest pain are generally more comfortable transported in a _______ position.

a. semi-reclining or fully upright
b. prone
c. supine
d. left or right lateral recumbent

Match the procedure for applying the Kendrick extrication device in column B to the proper sequence of events in column A.

Column A		Column B	
46.	first step	a.	pull the KED securely into the axillary region
47.	second step	b.	secure the head using the velcro fasteners
48.	third step	c.	one EMT maintains cervical spine immobilization from behind the patient
49.	fourth step	d.	apply a rigid cervical collar and position the KED behind the patient
50.	fifth step	e.	attach the bottom two straps followed by the groin straps

Chapter 16

Skill Performance Sheet

Long Spine Board Using a Log Roll Procedure

Student's Name_________________________ Date_________

Performance Standard	**Performed**	**Failed**
Team leader maintains in-line immobilization		
Cervical collar is applied		
Three rescuers positioned on one side of patient (shoulder, pelvis, legs)		
Spine board positioned on opposite side of patient		
On command from team leader, patient is rolled toward three rescuers		
Board is slid under patient		
On command from team leader, patient is rolled onto board		
Patient is adjusted on board		
Securely attach body then head to spine board		

Comments____

____

____

____

Instructor __________________ Circle One: Pass Fail

Skill Performance Sheet

Rapid Extrication Procedure

Student's Name____________________________ Date_________

Performance Standard	**Performed**	**Failed**
EMT #1 maintains cervical immobilization from behind the patient		
EMT #2 performs primary survey		
The car door is bent open as far as possible		
EMT #2 takes over in-line from outside of the car		
EMT #1 positions a spine board in the car on a cot stretcher and slides the end under the patient's buttocks		
EMT #3 assumes a position of the side of the seat from EMT #2 and supports the patients thighs		
EMT #1 supports the patient's chest and back		
On command from EMT #2 the patient is rotated at a 45 degree angle toward EMT #3 and his back toward the board		
On command the patient is rotated down on the board		

CONTINUED ON NEXT PAGE

Chapter 16

Skill Performance Sheet

Rapid Extrication Procedure (continued)

Student's Name____________________________ Date_________

Performance Standard	**Performed**	**Failed**
With EMT #1 supporting the axilla, EMT #2 maintaining in-line cervical immobilization, and EMT #3 supporting the legs, the patient is slid up the board		
The patient's torso is secured to the board		
The patient's head and neck are secured to the board		
The patient is secured to the stretcher		

Comments____

____

____

____

Instructor _________________ Circle One: Pass Fail

Skill Performance Sheet

Applying a Kendrick's Extrication Device

Student's Name____________________________ Date_________

Performance Standard	Performed	Failed
EMT #1 maintains in-line cervical immobilization from behind the patient		
Cervical collar is applied		
KED is positioned behind the patient		
KED is pulled up securely in axillary region		
Attach the chest straps		
Attach the groin straps		
Attach the head section		

(adapted from The Prehospital Trauma Life Support Program)

Comments____

Instructor __________________ Circle One: Pass Fail

Chapter 16

Skill Performance Sheet

Applying a Short Spine Board

Student's Name____________________________ Date__________

Performance Standard	**Performed**	**Failed**
EMT #1 maintains in-line cervical immobilization from behind the patient		
Cervical collar is applied		
Board is positioned behind the patient		
Attach the chest and groin straps placing pads to protect the patient		
Secure head to board		
Lifts patient, not board, to long spine board		
Releases groin straps before lowering legs		

Comments____

____

____

____

Instructor __________________ Circle One: Pass Fail

Skill Performance Sheet

Performing a Rapid Takedown

Student's Name______________________________ Date__________

Performance Standard	**Performed**	**Failed**
EMT #1 assumes immobilization from behind patient		
A cervical collar is applied		
EMT #2 slides board behind patient		
EMTs #2 and #3 stand on both sides of the patient facing toward the board and slip their hands under the patient's axillary region and grasp the next highest opening on the board.		
EMTs #2 and #3 support the shoulders with their other hands		
On command from EMT #1, the board is lowered smoothly to the floor		
As the board is lowered, EMT #1 must allow the head to move slowly to the board		
The patient's torso is secured to the board		
The patient's head is secured to the board		

(Adapted from the New York State Health Department Critical Trauma Care Program)

Comments____

____

____

Instructor ________________ Circle One: Pass Fail

Chapter 17

DISASTERS AND TRIAGE

Materials and Equipment for Lesson

1. Slides or overhead transparencies
2. Handouts
   - Disasters
   - Helicopter protocol
   - Triage tags
   - Disaster kit
3. Slide projector, overhead projector and/or blackboard

Disasters and Triage

Objectives
(Slide 17-1)

At the conclusion of the chapter the students will be able to:

1. Define the following terms:

Disaster	**Command post**
Multiple casualty incident (MCI)	**Mutual aid**
Triage	

2. List three important initial steps that EMS personnel should take upon arrival at the disaster scene.

3. Describe the roles of the following participants in disaster:

Triage officer	**Communications officer**
Staging officer	**Police**
EMS command	**Fire**

4. Describe function of the following areas within a disaster plan:
- **Command post**
- **First stage triage area**
- **Second stage triage area**
- **Third stage triage - (field hospital)**

5. Describe the proper use of disaster tag.

6. Define convergence and discuss its importance at the disaster scene.

7. Describe the phases of a disaster.

8. Explain debriefing and its importance at the disaster scene.

Chapter 17

Instructor Preparation

Reading preparation for the lesson:

EMT Prehospital Care, Chapter 17, pages 717-733
Local disaster plan

Suggested Learning Activities
Using a lecture format with the aid of slides, overhead transparencies or charts, provide an overview of disaster operations.
Demonstrate the basic use of a triage tag.
Provide case histories or video footage of disasters.

Content

I. Scenario **(Slide 17-2)**

- A. Disaster
  1. Large school bus on its side
  2. Other vehicle on fire
  3. People are running past you
  4. Some are injured
  5. At least 25 children are in bus
  6. Not sure of severity or extent of injuries
- B. Action plan **(Slide 17-3)**
  1. What is your overall plan of action?
  2. How would you activate your disaster plan?
  3. What resources are needed?
  4. With whom do you have to communicate?
  5. What roles would you assume as the first responders on the scene?
  6. What steps can you, the EMT, take
     - a) To prevent further injury
     - b) To reduce the number of deaths
     - c) To transport the patients in an appropriate time frame
- C. Purpose of this presentation is to answer these questions

II. Definitions **(Slide 17-4)**

- A. Disaster (The American Heritage Dictionary of the English Language)
  1. Occurrence inflicting widespread destruction and distress
  2. A grave misfortune
  3. A total failure
- B. EMS definition
  1. Any instance where situation overwhelms resources available
  2. Multiple casualty incidents where the number of victims exceeds capability of transporting unit
  3. EMT routinely determines the need for additional resources
  4. Disaster requires a multi-agency response in order to limit death and destruction
- C. Closed vs open **(Slide 17-5)**
  1. Open
     - a) Situation allows easy access to victims from different directions
     - b) Could be spread over large area
     - c) Placing additional demands on rescuers to search a large territory
     - d) For example, plane crash in a field
  2. Closed
     - a) Physical or geographic boundaries preventing speedy access or evacuation of patients
     - b) Victims pinned in a bus accident
     - c) High-rise fire with victims trapped on the top floor
     - d) Building collapsed with victims beneath debris
     - e) Plane crash in woods with no usable roads

Content

f) Requires specialized resources to gain access,
(1) Helicopters
(2) Search and rescue teams
(3) Self-contained breathing apparatus
(4) Specialized extrication equipment

D. Active vs contained
1. Active
a) Forces contributed or associated with disaster are active, evolving, and ongoing
b) Poses further threat to the rescuers, public and victims
c) Active fire or flood
2. Contained
a) Forces responsible for disaster are exhausted or contained
b) Extinguished fire

E. Mutual aid
1. Predetermined response system with neighboring communities
2. Ensures a large scale response of emergency vehicles
3. Regular needs of the community must be met
4. Outside units will cover the normal response

F. EMS command
1. Disaster requires central authority or command responsible for emergency operations
2. EMS command represents one component of overall command
3. EMT may assume responsibility of overall command during initial stages of a disaster

G. Triage
1. To sort or to choose
2. Sorting of casualties of war or other disaster
3. Determine priority and proper place of treatment
4. Require change in thinking on part of EMTs
5. Cardinal rule is to save the most people possible
6. Cardiac arrest would have the lowest priority

H. Transport
1. Encompasses more than the movement of patients
2. Movement of vehicles and supplies
3. Selection of traffic routes
4. Traffic control
5. Selection of staging areas
6. Supplies and communication coordination

III. Essential components of disaster management

A. Command **(Slide 17-6)**
1. Person ultimately in charge of the disaster response
2. Fire or police chief, EMS chief, mayor or county executive
3. May vary with type of incident or political structure
a) Riot--police may be primary command
b) Fire scene--fire chief
c) Medical emergency--EMS chief

Content

4. EMS command
    a) May be primary or secondary command role
    b) Responsible for the coordination of EMS resources
    c) Transport, triage, hospital destination

B. Roles and interagency relationships **(Slide 17-7)**
1. Police
    a) Protect and serve
    b) Scene security
    c) Traffic control
    d) Investigation
    e) Identification of the dead
    f) Notification of families
2. Fire **(Slide 17-8)**
    a) Protection of life and property
    b) Rescue and extrication
    c) Fire suppression
    d) Hazard elimination
    e) Scene safety
3. Other Agencies **(Slide 17-9)**
    a) Red Cross
    b) Salvation army
    c) Social agencies, hospitals
    d) Military

C. Communications **(Slide 17-10)**
1. EMS communications should be separated from other disaster communications
2. Plans identify specific communication channels
3. EMS communications is a function unto itself
4. Dispatcher or someone at scene may coordinate
5. Radio silence unless information is requested
6. Communications public information
7. EMTs should maintain patient confidentiality

D. Documentation **(Slide 17-11)**
1. Maintain information about individual patients
2. Key events and progress of the incident
3. Specific records
    a) Major event log **(Slide 17-12)**
    b) Numbers of patients
    c) Conditions and triage categories
    d) Vehicles on scene
    e) Personnel on scene
    f) Hospital availability
    g) Individuals transported
    h) Hospital disposition
    i) Mode of transport

E. Safety **(Slide 17-13)**
1. EMS command oversees scene safety of EMS personnel
2. Responsibility of all rescuers

Content

3. Safety concerns are prioritized
    a) Rescuer
    b) Public
    c) Victim
4. Primary concern is not to add to the number of victims
5. Injury prevention factors
    a) Protective clothing
    b) Fire suppression
    c) Lighting
    d) Crowd and traffic

F. Resource recruitment and allocation **(Slide 17-14)**
1. EMS command notifies central communication
2. Specialized equipment and personnel

G. Traffic control
1. Traffic routes to insure rapid access and egress
2. EMTs arriving first may identify routes for responders
3. Information should be sent by first responding EMS or police units

IV. Triage **(Slide 17-15)**

A. Stages
1. First stage triage **(Slide 17-16)**
    a) No treatment rendered
    b) Victims are tagged with colored surveyor's tape
    c) Or tagged by category of injury
2. Second stage triage **(Slide 17-17)**
    a) Begins when patients are removed to a safe area
    b) Area should be central and free of debris
    c) Close proximity to transport area
    d) Protected from weather
    e) Medical supplies available
    f) Thorough assessment and medical care are given
    g) Patients may be recategorized
    h) Collection point for appropriate priority and transport
3. Third stage triage **(Slide 17-18)**
    a) Field hospital may be developed on site
    b) Extraordinary delays in securing hospital care
        (1) Isolation
        (2) Weather conditions
        (3) Earthquakes
        (4) Floods
    c) Advanced life support occurs during the second and third stages

B. Disaster triage system **(Slide 17-19)**
1. Red
    a) Critical patients with life threatening conditions
    b) Hypotension or hypoxia
    c) Survive only with early stabilization and transport
    d) Require hospital care within one hour
2. Yellow
    a) Potentially life threatening injuries
    b) Must be treated within few hours

Content

c) Do not have signs of shock
d) If not cared for, injuries can cause death
e) If unable to walk, patients may be categorized as yellow in some systems

3. Green
   a) Have no life threatening injuries
   b) Generally are ambulatory
   c) Should be directed to secondary triage for further triage
4. Black
   a) Patients without signs of life
   b) Obvious mortal injuries
5. Other triage methods exist in EMS systems

C. Sequence of triage **(Slide 17-20)**
   1. Initial triage at accident site
   2. Victims are moved in priority to secondary triage
      a) Triage tags may be filled out at this time
      b) Identifying information elicited
      c) Patients should be immobilized
         (1) May have been done at first triage
         (2) Conditions can exist where this is not possible
      d) Oxygen is administered
      e) Major fractures splinted
      f) Shock treatment begun
      g) Patients transported or transferred to third stage triage

D. Special considerations for triage **(Slide 17-21)**
   1. Children may have to be removed early
      a) Regardless of status
      b) Should be kept with parents when possible
   2. Panicky or hysterical patients and injured rescuers
      a) Reduces confusion at disaster site
      b) To avoid diverting attention from the general rescue effort
   3. Panic
      a) Occurs when three conditions exist
         (1) Victim fears death
         (2) Perceives limited escape
         (3) Has no information about what has happened
      b) EMT can reduce panic by providing information, direction and care
      c) Hysterical patients should be separated from other victims

V. Transport **(Slide 17-22)**

A. Transport officer activities
   1. Coordinates ambulance staging and dispatch
   2. Responsible for personnel and vehicles
   3. Ensures smooth traffic flow
   4. Supplies and manpower are stockpiled by the transport officer
   5. Drivers should remain with vehicles
   6. Notifies receiving hospital

Content

B. Helicopters **(Slide 17-23)**
1. Represent a rapid method of evacuation
2. Landing zone should be established
3. Protocols should be strictly adhered to avoid accidents
4. EMTs should stay clear until advised by pilot or crew member

C. Hospital selection **(Slide 17-24)**
1. Performed according to local protocol
2. Patients should be distributed to minimize overloading of hospitals
3. Transfer of patients to other facilities may be necessary

D. Convergence
1. Obstruction of response or egress due to onlookers, rescuers and press
2. Must be anticipated to ensure traffic routes remain clear
3. Rescue personnel may be asked to wait for instructions from the command post
4. Staging areas for vehicles are essential to prevent convergence

VI. Steps of disaster management **(Slide 17-25)**

A. Planning
1. Essential for coordination of resources and manpower
2. Without planning, success of management is limited

B. Warning and evacuation
1. May or may not occur
2. Depends on the type of disaster
3. Smoke alarms, hurricane warning systems and the emergency broadcast system
4. No warning is possible in many situations

C. Event
1. Actual disaster occurs
2. Most events are out of control of the rescuer
3. EMT must anticipate that these conditions will exist

D. Response
1. Organized dispatched response of emergency personnel
2. May last from hours to days

E. Recovery
1. Process of demobilizing response
2. Returning the community to normal

F. Restoration
1. Rebuilding of the community in a physical and emotional sense
2. Includes critical incident stress debriefing, reconstruction and restoration of services

VII. Role and responsibilities of EMT **(Slide 17-26)**

A. Scene assessment
1. Perform a windshield survey
2. Obtain basic information for type of equipment and resources needed

B. Type of incident **(Slide 17-27)**
1. Establish the type of incident
2. Determine if further injuries may occur
   a) Fire

Content

b) Hazardous materials
c) Vehicle positioned safely
d) Open or closed
e) Active or contained
3. Determine specific location
4. Identify the best access routes
5. One EMT should walk the scene **(Slide 17-28)**
a) Estimate patient numbers and injury types
b) Identify if incident is open or closed, active or contained.
6. Second EMT stays with ambulance
a) Identifies staging areas and traffic routes
b) May be necessary move the ambulance to expedite traffic control
c) Contact communications center with preliminary information
7. Provide communications with following information **(Slide 17-29)**
a) Number of victims
b) Specific location of incident
c) Open or closed
d) Active (continuing) or contained
e) Need for special resources
(1) Lights
(2) Cranes
(3) Boats
(4) Helicopters
f) Number of additional ambulances required
g) Any other relevant information.

C. Communications and command **(Slide 17-30)**
1. One EMT will initiate first triage
a) Do not stop and treat
b) Tag patient with colored tape or tag
c) Assign EMTs as they arrive
2. Second EMT will remain with ambulance **(Slide 17-31)**
a) Assume command and transport functions
b) Major event log should be initiated
c) Transportation log should be established
d) Resource list that specifies
(1) Personnel available on the scene
(2) Requested resources yet to arrive
(3) Hospital availability
e) Contact supervising police officer and fire chief
f) Establish a centralized command post **(Slide 17-32)**
g) Hospitals notified about incoming patients
h) Traffic pattern is established
i) Ambulance staging area selected
j) Scene safety plan to minimize injuries to rescuers
(1) Placement of lights
(2) Fire suppression
(3) Placement of ladders
(4) Safe extrication and rescue

Content

        k) Continue coordination until relieved
    3. As other units arrive on the scene
        a) Directed to staging area
        b) Driver is identified as transport officer

VIII. Psychological aspects **(Slide 17-33)**
  A. Extreme stress for victims, families, rescuers and community
  B. EMT must treat stress and control emotions
  C. Victims will look at the EMT for signs (spoken and unspoken) of reassurance
  D. EMT should offer positive and encouraging feedback
  E. Debriefing exercises
    1. Venting of emotions
    2. Sharing common human reactions
    3. Professional counselors may be available
    4. Rescuers should avail themselves of services
    5. Failure to acknowledge stress can result in being unable to perform
    6. Opportunity to learn from the disaster experience
    7. Used in future disaster planning and shared with other systems
    8. Important to maintain patient confidentiality

IX. Disaster drills **(Slide 17-34)**
  A. Method of preparing and training personnel
  B. Five types
    1. Orientation
        a) Presentation of plan
        b) Lecture only
    2. Discussion
        a) Hypothetical situation review
        b) Feedback to analyze approach
    3. Table top
        a) Problem solving
        b) Round table forum
    4. Emergency coordination simulation
        a) Utilizes communication equipment
        b) Physical movement of personnel
        c) No mock victims are used
    5. Full scale field
        a) Mock victims
        b) Actual personnel
        c) Hospitals and other agencies
        d) Participants should be notified

Chapter 17

DISASTERS AND TRIAGE

Examination

Match the description in column B to the appropriate term in column A.

	Column A		Column B
1.	open disaster scene	a.	the forces that contributed to or were associated with the disaster are still active, evolving and ongoing
2.	closed disaster scene	b.	physical or geographic boundaries that prevent speedy access to or evacuation of patients
3.	active disaster situation	c.	easy access to the victims from different directions is possible
4.	contained disaster situation	d.	the likelihood of further injury is low, since the forces responsible for the disaster are exhausted

Match the appropriate term in column B to the scenario in column A.

	Column A		Column B
5.	a plane crash on a mountain with no access road	a.	open disaster scene
		b.	closed disaster scene

6. A predetermined response system with neighboring communities that insures a large scale response of emergency vehicles during a disaster best describe:

   a. a transfer agreement
   b. a mutual aid agreement
   c. a disaster plan
   d. an MCI strategy

7. The sorting of casualties of war or other disaster to determine the priority of need and proper place of treatment best defines:

   a. categorization
   b. stacking
   c. triage
   d. designation

Match the condition in column B to the appropriate color triage tag in column A.

Column A		Column B	
8.	red	a.	an unconscious patient with a head injury
9.	yellow	b.	traumatic cardiac arrest patient
10.	green	c.	a patient with a multiple pelvic fractures
11.	black	d.	fractured humerus

12. At a scene of a disaster command signifies:

    a. the highest ranking officer present
    b. the staging area for additional personnel
    c. the person ultimately in charge
    d. the staging area for additional equipment

13. It is imperative that at the site of a disaster, drivers of emergency vehicles should:

    a. participate in early triage and treatment
    b. park as close to the accident as possible
    c. remain with their vehicles
    d. report to the triage officer

14. When relating to the disaster situation the term *convergence* means the:

    a. rapid response of onlookers, rescuers and press upon the scene of a disaster, which results in the blockage of traffic
    b. process of demobilizing response vehicles and apparatus for the purposes of returning them to normal community service
    c. rebuilding of the community in a physical and emotional sense after a disaster, a process which includes critical incident stress debriefing
    d. the feeling of the victims when they see a large group of rescuers arriving to render aid

15. When relating to the disaster situation the term *restoration* means the:

    a. rapid response of onlookers, rescuers and press upon the scene of a disaster, this results in the blockage of traffic
    b. process of demobilizing response vehicles and apparatus for the purposes of returning them to normal community service
    c. rebuilding of the community in a physical and emotional sense after a disaster, a process which includes critical incident stress debriefing
    d. the feeling of the victims when they see a large group of rescuers arriving to render aid

16. When relating to the disaster situation the term recovery means the:

    a. rapid response of onlookers, rescuers and press upon the scene of a disaster, this results in the blockage of traffic
    b. process of demobilizing response vehicles and apparatus for the purposes of returning them to normal community service
    c. rebuilding of the community in a physical and emotional sense after a disaster, a process which includes critical incident stress debriefing
    d. the feeling of the victims when they see a large group of rescuers arriving to render aid

17. The three primary functions of disaster management are:

    a. command, triage and patient care
    b. triage, patient care and transport
    c. triage, communications and patient care
    d. command, control and triage

18. At a disaster scene, the person whose function is to control traffic flow, gather supplies, stage additional vehicles and communicate ambulance availability to the command post is the:

    a. supply officer
    b. transport officer
    c. communication officer
    d. triage officer

19. The process by which participants are allowed to express their feelings about the incident and thereby relieve stress associated with the situation is called the:

    a. catharsis
    b. debriefing
    c. critique
    d. field exercise

Match the description in column B to the type of disaster drill in column A.

Column A		Column B	
20.	orientation	a.	requires the use of communications equipment and the physical movement of personnel and vehicles without role-playing victims
21.	discussion		
22.	tabletop exercise		
23.	emergency coordination simulation	b.	participants try to solve a problem in a round table forum
24.	full scale field simulation	c.	where the disaster plan is presented
		d.	role-playing victims are used for realism and are transported to the hospital
		e.	hypothetical situations are gone over in relation to the plan and feedback is encouraged to analyze the overall approach

25. The log that records the patient distribution to ambulances and hospital destination is called the:

    a. major event log
    b. logistics sheet
    c. transportation log
    d. disposition log

Chapter 18

EXTRICATION

Materials and Equipment for Lesson

1. Slides or overhead transparencies
2. Handouts
   - Extrication
   - List of local tools
   - Local extrication protocols
3. Slide projector, overhead projector and/or blackboard

Extrication

Objectives
(Slide 18-1)

At the conclusion of the chapter the students will be able to:

1. **Describe the basic uses of the following devices used in the extrication process:**

Reflectors	**Wrench - 12" Adjustable Crescent**
Hacksaw	**Screwdrivers**
Vise grip pliers	**Hammer**
Fire axe	**Wrecking Bar and Crowbar**
Bolt cutters	**Shovel**
Tin snips	**Ropes**
Blankets	**Mastic knife**
Pruning saw	**Spring loaded center punch**
Bale hooks	**Cold chisels**
Jacks	**Storage and maintenance**
Air chisel	**Hand winch or come-long**

2. **Describe the basic components of self-protection gear used at a rescue site.**

3. **Describe the basic methods for gaining access through the following routes:**

Door	**Window**
Roof	**Floor**

4. **Describe the techniques for the following extrication techniques:**
   - **Displacing a brake pedal**
   - **Removing a steering wheel**

5. **List three routes of removal from an automobile.**

Instructor Preparation

Reading preparation for the lesson:

EMT Prehospital Care, Chapter 18, pages 735-753
Local disaster plan

Suggested Learning Activities
Using a lecture format with the aid of slides, overhead transparencies or charts, provide an overview of extrication procedures.
Demonstrate the use of basic tools.
Provide case histories or video footage of extrication scenarios.

Content

I. Scenario **(Slide 18-2)**
   A. Two-vehicle accident
   B. Victim pinned by steering wheel in vehicle one
   C. Victims in vehicle two
      1. Arm of driver is trapped between seat and door, feet caught beneath brake petal
      2. Head of passenger has been thrust through windshield
   D. How do you rescue these patients?

II. Role of EMT **(Slide 18-3)**
   A. Primary role is evaluation and emergency care
   B. If rescue crews are not available
      1. EMT should be confident to perform extrication
      2. Done with minimal light equipment
      3. Provided heavy equipment is not needed
   C. EMT should be familiar with hand tools for light rescue
   D. Light rescue can be accomplished with **(Slide 18-4)**
      1. Hand tools
      2. Manual skills
         a) Moving seat by sliding back
         b) Opening locked doors
         c) Breaking windows
         d) Removing windshield
   E. Heavy rescue uses power tools
   F. If rescue personnel are available, EMT roles are **(Slide 18-5)**
      1. Ensuring proper assessment
      2. Treatment
      3. Immobilization
      4. Removal
   G. Scene safety **(Slide 18-6)**
      1. Significant hazards to both rescuers and the public in rescue situations
      2. EMTs must analyze risk prior to initiating rescue
      3. Example of failure to assess hazards:
         Several years ago in Lancaster, Pennsylvania a child became trapped in a toxic environment. An EMT entered a toxic environment without protective gear and was overcome by toxic environment. A second EMT proceeded to attempt rescue and was also overcome. Finallly, a firefighter, who knew both EMTs, entered without protective gear and succumbed to atmosphere. The child, was retrieved and resuscitated and the three rescue personnel died
      4. Protective envelope is single most important factor in reducing injury
      5. Complete protective envelope **(Slide 18-7)**
         a) Headgear
         b) Eye protection
         c) Respiratory protection (if required)

Content

(1) Gloves
(2) Boots and coat
d) Safety hazard must be dealt with prior to accessing the patient

H. Treatment **(Slide 18-8)**
1. Medical treatment becomes priority
2. Most auto accidents do not involve single patients
3. Triage is an essential part of rescue
4. French word meaning "to sort or to choose"
5. Extrication time may alter triage
   a) Patients with fractures who may experience blood loss during rescue
   b) Compensated patients may decompensate

I. Time on the Scene **(Slide 18-9)**
1. Time is an important consideration in every rescue
2. Time must be foremost in the mind of the rescuer
3. Golden hour
   a) Refers to optimal time from accident to arrival at operating room
   b) Not always achievable due to factors beyond the EMTs control
   c) EMTs should target ten minutes on scene as goal

III. Basic tools

A. Traffic delineation devices **(Slide 18-10)**
1. Essential in maintaining the safety of the scene
2. Reflectors, traffic cones and battery operated lights are recommended
3. Flares represent a fire hazard
   a) Due to gasoline spills
   b) Flares are small and may not affect the sleeping driver
   c) Are sometimes used due to their size and storage ability
4. Traffic cones
   a) Effective in alerting sleeping or distracted drivers
   b) Hitting a traffic cone makes a sound at time of impact
   c) Alerts sleeping driver and jogs him/her back to consciousness
5. Placement of traffic delineation devices
   a) Relative to posted speed limit on roadway
   b) First device should be placed one and a half times the stopping distance of the vehicle
   c) When turn precedes accident scene, devices should be placed before turn

B. Wrench - 12" adjustable crescent **(Slide 18-11)**
1. Useful in opening the nuts and bolts
2. Usually easier to disengage metal than to distort or displace
3. Screwdrivers (12" flat-head, 8" Phillips
4. Disengage car parts
5. Blade to cut through metal
6. Prying tool to open windows

C. Hacksaw
1. Cut through steering wheels, window posts, brake pedals and other metal obstacles
2. Extra blades are essential

Content

D. Vise grip pliers
   1. Removal of nuts and bolts
   2. Stripping of plastic covering from steering wheels
E. Tin snips
   1. Cut through sheet metal
   2. Ideal for roofs or door panels
F. Cold chisels
   1. Used with a sledge hammer
   2. Distort and sever with surprising accuracy
G. Hammer **(Slide 18-12)**
   1. Striking device to drive shearing instruments through metal
   2. Used to bend or distort metal
H. Fire axe
   1. Bend metal
   2. Strike through glass
I. Bolt cutters
   1. Cut through metal objects
   2. Minimal effort needed
J. Wrecking bar and crowbar **(Slide 18-13)**
   1. Prying metal
   2. Leverage in moving objects
K. Shovel **(Slide 18-14)**
   1. Move dirt or snow
   2. Create dikes to contain spills
L. Ropes **(Slide 18-15)**
   1. Creating hand-holds on steep hills
   2. Rescue from ditches
   3. Throw-lines for water rescue
   4. Care should be taken in selection of ropes
   5. Tensile strength appropriate for task
   6. Require significant maintenance and protection (bag)
M. Blankets
   1. Should be thick and fire retardant
   2. Protecting victims from glass shards
   3. Ambulance blankets sometimes do not meet this requirement
   4. Rescue blanket should be acquired and maintained
N. Mastic knife **(Slide 18-16)**
   1. Useful tool for removal of windshield and seat belts
   2. Curved blade is an asset in protection when cutting is required
O. Spring-loaded center punch **(Slide 18-17)**
   1. Device carried by individual EMT
   2. Breaks window glass (with exception of windshield)
   3. Minimizes risk of injury to the patient
   4. Initiates force at a focal point that shatters glass without forcing the glass to fall
P. Pruning saw
   1. Cutting wooden objects that present obstacles
   2. Tree limbs and fences

Content

Q. Bale hooks **(Slide 18-18)**
 1. Pulling and tearing operations
 2. Useful in removal of windshields

R. Jacks
 1. Jacks that accompany most cars are capable of assisting in many rescue operations
 2. Lift, stabilize and distort effectively

S. Storage and maintenance of tools **(Slide 18-19)**
 1. Signs of a good mechanic are clean and dirt-free tools
 2. Tool box should be dry
 3. Tools should be kept neat and clean
 4. Periodically checked
 5. Total familiarity is essential in order to be effective in those situations where minutes count
 6. Practice with junk vehicle on a regular basis

T. Additional tools that may be used in light rescue
 1. Hydraulic jack spreader **(Slide 18-20)**
  a) Spreader or Port Power should have a minimum of 2 to 4 ton capacity
  b) Provides lifting and pulling capability
 2. Hand winch or come-along **(Slide 18-21)**
  a) Should have 5 ton capacity and breakaway handle
  b) Greatly assists in pulling and distorting operations
 3. Air chisel
  a) should have a minimum generating pressure of 90 psi
  b) Should carry additional cylinders and chisels
  c) Cuts panels of metal, glass and plastic almost effortlessly

IV. Additional rescue equipment **(Slide 18-22)**

A. Power hydraulic jack spreader combination **(Slide 18-23)**

B. 2 x 4' wood cribbing sufficient to stabilize vehicles; various lengths may be required.

C. Two ropes, 150' length, 5/8"
 1. Kernmantle construction
 2. Maximum 2% stretch factor
 3. 11,000 lbs. minimum tensile strength
 4. Must be carried in a protective bag

D. Swiss seat

E. Carabiners, locking type, minimum rod stock 10 mm (minimum of 10)

F. Stokes basket

G. Additional come-along (minimum 5 ton)

H. Chain, 15 feet, grab hook, running hook

I. Hydraulic truck jack (minimum 4 tons)

J. Rappelling harness, one per rescuer

K. Local extrication needs
 1. Scuba gear **(Slide 18-24)**
 2. Equipment for mountain rescue equipment

Content

V. Stages of extrication
  A. Scene safety **(Slide 18-25)**
    1. Gain immediate access and provide life saving intervention
    2. Assess need for additional assistance and specialized help
    3. Protective clothing **(Slide 18-26)**
      a) Headgear
      b) Eye protection
      c) Body and foot protection
      d) Protective clothing is often bulky, hot and not conducive with providing treatment
      e) Decision to remove protective gear is an individual one
      f) Potential for injury is expanded
      g) Uniform should be flame resistant and retardant
      h) Reflective capability of clothing is important
    4. Respiratory protection **(Slide 18-27)**
      a) Self-contained breathing apparatus
      b) Frequent concern to EMTs
      c) Should be restricted to individuals with hands-on training
    5. Approach to the scene **(Slide 18-28)**
      a) Approach scene 100 feet, up hill and upwind and look and listen
        (1) What is happening?
        (2) How many cars?
        (3) How many victims?
        (4) What resources do you need?
      b) Perform risk-benefit analysis
        (1) Evaluate risk of attempting rescue
        (2) If risk is greater than benefit, take those actions to reduce risk
        (3) Example:
          (a) Car in flames
          (b) Attempt rescue or put the fire out?
          (c) If risks are minimal, gain access
      c) Upon approaching the car, windshield survey **(Slide 18-29)**
        (1) Are the victims moving?
        (2) Are they conscious?
        (3) Are they attempting to exit the vehicle? Check for downed electrical wire
          (a) If wires are down, DO NOT TOUCH ANYTHING
          (b) Retreat to a position of safety
          (c) Protect all bystanders by establishing a hazard zone
          (d) Advise occupants of car not to attempt to exit
          (e) Contact support service (local utility)
        (4) Evaluate the stability of vehicle **(Slide 18-30)**
          (a) Will the vehicle turn over?
          (b) Is it on its side or its wheels?
          (c) Is it secure?
          (d) Does the vehicle rock?

Content

(e) Could movement injure the patient?
(f) If unstable
i) Block frame with cribbing
ii) Stabilize vehicle on side

6. Stabilizing the vehicle **(Slide 18-31)**
   a) Many methods of stabilizing a vehicle
   b) Purpose of stabilization
      (1) Eliminate potential of movement
      (2) Ensure structural integrity
   c) Pitfalls
      (1) Use of manpower is unsafe and foolhardy
      (2) Men may abandon effort during lift
      (3) Vehicle may fall on rescuers and occupants
   d) Cribbing **(Slide 18-32)**
      (1) Safe method of stabilizing a vehicle
      (2) Airbags quickly stabilize a vehicle
      (3) Wood should be hardwood, i.e., oak **(Slide 18-33)**
      (4) Several different sections and sizes should be carried
      (5) Base of large pieces integrating smaller pieces towards the top
7. Support operations
   a) Lighting of a darkened scene
   b) Establishing effective police lines
   c) Safety zones
   d) Traffic control

B. Gaining access **(Slide 18-34)**
1. Most expedient method possible
2. Route to reach patient not necessarily route through which patient is removed
3. Path of least resistance
   a) Doors
   b) Windows
   c) Windshield
   d) Roof
   e) Floor
4. Take rescue blanket and cover your victim
   a) Treat for shock
   b) Provide some protection during the rescue
5. Doors **(Slide 18-35)**
   a) If door is locked and victim is conscious, ask him/her to unlock the door
   b) Check all doors including hatchbacks before breaking glass
   c) Unlocking the door
      (1) Hook wire
         (a) Piece of small wire with a hoop
         (b) Car antenna usually better than a coat hanger
         (c) Use flat head screwdriver or prying tool to open window

Content

(2) "Slim jims" **(Slide 18-36)**
(a) Used by car repossession agents
(b) Effective, leaving little or no damage to the vehicle
(c) Proper technique is required
(d) Unless used on a regular basis, potential for success will be limited
(3) Anti-theft devices **(Slide 18-37)**
(a) Very common in modern vehicles
(b) 18" length of coat hanger with washer looped at end
(c) Bent to a 45 degree angle
(d) Washer with 1/2 inch hole
(e) Slip over the door button and when pulled up will snag the lock
d) Cutting door panels **(Slide 18-38)**
(1) Several devices are quite suitable for this purpose
(2) Screwdriver and hammer **(Slide 18-39)**
(3) Tin snips, panel cutters, axes and pieces of sharpened leaf springs
(4) Suitable when additional time might be taken
(5) Concern is always compromise of structural integrity of the vehicle
(6) Techniques **(Slides 18-40 to 18-42)**
6. Windows
a) Spring-loaded punch **(Slide 18-43)**
(1) If door is locked and victim is unconscious, quickest method of gaining access
(2) Select window farthest from victim
(3) Break glass with the spring-loaded window punch
b) Other methods **(Slides 18-44 to 18-47)**
(1) Hammers, axes, Halligan tools and screwdrivers
(2) May cause glass shards to spray over patient
(3) Contact paper over glass may reduce this affect
(4) Windshield is made of laminated glass
(5) Suitable to withstand significant impact
(6) Cannot be broken with a window punch
(7) Cut along the outside with an axe and fold onto the hood
(8) Disassembly of windshield **(Slide 18-48)**
(a) Windshield mountings have changed in the last 15 years
i) Prior to 1965
i) Windshields are mounted in a rubber channel
ii) Removal significantly easier
iii) Less likely to protect in a crash

Content

ii) 1965 to 1969
i) Soft adhesives replaced many channel systems
ii) Sometimes leaked and dried out
iii) 1969
i) Mastic compounds used
ii) Greatly increased the integrity of windshields
iii) Removal more difficult
iv) Reseals itself
v) Once separated must keep away from surface
vi) Small wooden wedges or screwdrivers are helpful

7. Cutting the roof
a) Impacts on structural integrity of the vehicle
b) Size of flap will be determined by the desired operation and impact on structural integrity
c) Upright car
(1) Remove windshield **(Slide 18-49)**
(2) Cut structural points surrounding the windshield
(3) Cut close to base **(Slide 18-50)**
(4) Start at the lowest corner and cut in an upward direction
(5) Make two cuts in side of roof **(Slide 18-51)**
(6) Crease roof with axe **(Slide 18-52)**
(7) Fold roof back
(8) Four-door car may require additional cuts

8. Going through floor **(Slide 18-53)**
a) Used when no other method of entrance is possible
b) Locate a section of the floor with support
c) Locate rubber drain plug in rear foot well
d) Assess victim location by direct visualization or poking out the plug and feeling
e) Using the three-side fold technique, cut an 18" square hole

C. Essential emergency care **(Slide 18-54)**
1. Assume in-line cervical immobilization
2. Conduct primary survey
3. Mechanism of injury should guide in your assessment
4. If life-threatening conditions are identified, rapidly extricate
5. If removal is not possible, attempt to stabilize victim
6. Principles remain the same
a) Airway
b) Breathing
c) Circulation
d) Disability
e) Expose
7. Lowering back of the front seat may be needed to facilitate management

Content

D. Disentanglement **(Slide 18-55)**
   1. Removing wreckage from patient; not patient from wreckage
   2. Methods
      a) Disassembly
      b) Distortion
      c) Displacement
      d) Severance
   3. Doors **(Slide 18-56)**
      a) Excellent for the rapid removal **(Slide 18-57)**
      b) Widen door opening by pushing and pulling with several rescuers
      c) Disassemble if clear removal cannot be accomplished
   4. Steering wheel entrapment **(Slide 18-58)**
      a) Seat movement
         (1) Move seat back without unduly moving the driver is the simplest method
         (2) Manually or electrically, it should be done slowly
         (3) Disconnecting or cutting of battery cables may hamper this operation
         (4) Frequently an unnecessary operation
      b) Cutting steering wheel **(Slide 18-59)**
         (1) Strip plastic from steering wheel with vise grip
         (2) Cut metal core with a hacksaw or bolt cutter **(Slides 18-60 to 18-61)**
         (3) Two locations of parallel sides
         (4) Remove loose portion of the wheel
   5. Foot pedal entrapment
      a) Pedals present small but annoying obstacles
      b) Structural integrity of the pedal from side to side is not great
      c) Easier to move a brake pedal sideways than up and down
      d) Secure chain to pedal and pull sideways
      e) If door is still intact, attach the other end of the chain to the door **(Slide 18-62)**
   6. Hydraulic jacks **(Slides 18-63 and 18-64)**
      a) Useful in operations where human strength will not meet demand
      b) Lifting and pulling of steering columns
      c) Stabilizing vehicles
      d) Raising dashboards
      e) Pulling seats back

E. Immobilization and packaging **(Slide 18-65)**
   1. While disentanglement progresses
      a) Patient can be prepared for removal
      b) Secondary survey can be conducted
      c) Serious injuries are stabilized
      d) Minor injuries can be treated at the end of the survey
      e) Application of traction splints and long board splints is sometimes not possible in automobile

Content

2. Patient should be attached to short spine board
3. Removed from the vehicle on long spine board

F. Removal **(Slide 18-66)**

1. Once immobilized, patient can be removed
2. Follow path of least resistance
3. Condition and location of wreckage dictates options
4. Manpower should be based on experience in handling patients and individual physical strength
5. Strong rescuers should be assigned positions which require the greatest effort
6. Senior EMT should hold cervical immobilization
7. Should proceed carefully without abrupt or jerky movements
8. Path and steps should be reviewed prior to execution
9. Each step should be initiated with a verbal cue from the team leader
10. Patient should be protected during removal
11. Rescuers should support the patient as one unit
12. Lift patient -- not a device
13. Rolling cot stretcher can be positioned adjacent to the exit route

Chapter 18

EXTRICATION

Examination

1. The EMTs primary role at the automobile accident is:

   a. gaining access
   b. extrication
   c. disentanglement
   d. emergency care

2. The term used to describe an extrication that can be accomplished through the use of power tools is called:

   a. disentanglement
   b. light rescue
   c. strategic access
   d. heavy rescue

3. The greatest and most common hazard encountered by EMTs is:

   a. hazardous material spills
   b. the release of toxic gases
   c. traffic surrounding auto accidents
   d. hypoxia due to rescues in closed spaces

4. Traffic devices such as flares or cones should be placed so that the first device is _____ times the distance in feet of the posted speed limit:

   a. 2
   b. 3
   c. 4
   d. 5

5. Because of the possibility of spilled gasoline at an automobile accident site, the **least** appropriate method of securing the scene is through the use of:

   a. reflectors
   b. flares
   c. road cones
   d. battery-operated lights

6. The device which can effectively break window glass (with the exception of the windshield) while minimizing the risk of injury to the patient is the:

   a. crowbar
   b. bale hook
   c. spring-loaded center punch
   d. tire iron

7. The device that is used to pull steering wheels, displace seats, and stabilize vehicles is the:

   a. bale hook
   b. cribbing
   c. mastic knife
   d. come-along

8. Blocks of wood used to stabilize vehicles is commonly called:

   a. stacking blocks
   b. cribbing
   c. stabilizers
   d. construction blocks

9. In order to bend away the roof of an automobile, you must first:

   a. cut completely through the rear posts
   b. cut completely through the front posts
   c. place a support structure inside the car
   d. remove the rear windshield

10. You are dispatched to the scene of a train derailment with a possible toxic gas release. You should approach the scene:

    a. from the upwind direction
    b. from the downwind direction
    c. it does not matter as long as no cloud of toxic gas is visible
    d. it does not matter as long as you do not get within 100 feet of the train

11. When gaining access to an automobile involved in an accident your last approach for entry would be the:

    a. door
    b. floor
    c. roof
    d. window

12. If the door is locked and the victim is unconscious, the quickest way to gain access is to:

    a. cut through the door panel
    b. remove the roof
    c. remove the front windshield
    d. break a side window in the car

13. If you have to break a side window and time permits, you can reduce the amount of glass entering the vehicle by:

    a. using only a screwdriver and a hammer to break the glass
    b. use a bale hook and pull the side window out
    c. apply contact paper to the window prior to breaking the glass
    d. place a blanket over the outside of the glass prior to breaking the glass

14. Which of the following is a useful device to create a flap necessary to gain access to a door lock?

    a. tire iron
    b. crescent wrench
    c. hacksaw
    d. spring-loaded punch

15. When creating a flap in a door to necessary to gain access to a door lock, The flap should be:

    a. circular
    b. oval
    c. "U" shaped
    d. square

16. Upon gaining access to the interior of the car you notice that the steering wheel is bent. You patient is short of breath, pale, hypotensive and has a respiratory rate of 40. Your immediate reaction is to:

    a. apply oxygen and a KED
    b. rapidly extricate the patient
    c. apply the PASG prior to extrication
    d. begin positive pressure ventilation

17. The simplest and best method for creating room between the driver and the steering wheel is to:

    a. cut the steering wheel away
    b. slide the seat back
    c. distort the steering wheel
    d. cut the steering wheel post off

18. The EMTs primary focus during the disentanglement stage is to:

    a. gain access to the patient
    b. remove the patient from the wreckage
    c. remove the wreckage from the patient
    d. minimize further damage to the vehicle

19. The extrication process can be divided into five distinct phases. Three of these five phases include:

    a. disentanglement, removal, scene safety
    b. rapid extrication, notification of police agencies, removal
    c. protective envelope, immobilization, disentanglement
    d. respiratory phase, perfusion phase, oxygenation phase

20. If rescue personnel decide that the battery should be disconnected, the procedure is to:

    a. disconnect the negative cable
    b. disconnect the positive cable
    c. cut the negative cable
    d. cut the positive cable

21. The optimal time from injury to arrival at the operating room is sometimes referred to as the:

    a. prime time
    b. critical minutes
    c. magic minutes
    d. golden hour

22. Upon approaching the scene you look to see if the patients are moving, are conscious and are attempting to exit the vehicle. These are all part of the:

    a. primary survey
    b. secondary survey
    d. MAST survey
    d. windshield survey

23. If electrical wires are down at a scene, you should do all of the following:

    a. retreat to a position of safety, establish a hazard zone, remove the wires with a pole
    b. retreat to a position of safety, establish a hazard zone, advise the occupants not to exit
    c. advise the occupants not to exit, rescue occupants with a rope, establish a hazard zone
    d. test the wires with a meter to determine if the wires are live

24. Your headgear, eye protection, gloves, boots and coat are all components of your:

    a. SCUBA system
    b. protective envelope
    c. heavy rescue equipment
    d. traffic delineation devices

25. If you are forced to move a break pedal in order to extricate a patient, you should remember that it is easier to move the pedal:

    a. up only
    b. down only
    c. sideways
    d. up or down

Chapter 19

AMBULANCE OPERATIONS

Materials and Equipment for Lesson

1. Slides or overhead transparencies
2. Handouts
   - Operating and emergency vehicle
   - Record keeping
   - Local ambulance call report
   - Communications
   - Local radio codes
   - Vehicle and equipment maintenance
3. Slide projector, overhead projector and/or blackboard

Ambulance Operations

Objectives
(Slide 19-1)

At the conclusion of the chapter the students will be able to:

1. **Quote laws relating to the operation of the ambulance and privileges in any of the following categories:**

Speed	**Siren use**	**Warning Lights**
Right of way	**Right of way**	**Turning**

2. **Describe the proper use of the siren.**

3. **Describe the considerations that should be given to:**
   Escorts — **Intersections**

4. **Describe the effect of the following "natural laws" upon driving an emergency vehicle:**
   Gravity — **Centrifugal force**
   Friction

5. **Describe the basic approach to maintaining the proper distances while driving an emergency vehicle.**

6. **Describe the basic safety procedures for the following situations:**
   Backing Up — **Approaching intersections**

7. **List four purposes of a call report.**

8. Write a paragraph discussing each of the following principles of record keeping :
   - Accuracy
   - Clarity
   - Chronology
   - Completeness

9. List four areas of patient data.

10. Give one example of an authorization form and describe its importance.

11. Discuss the importance of confidentiality with record keeping.

12. Describe the roles of the following communications components in an EMS System:
    - Receiving operators
    - Communications center
    - Dispatcher
    - Repeater systems
    - Telemetry radios

13. Describe the differences between simplex, duplex and multiplex radio systems.

14. Describe the differences between Type I, Type II and Type III ambulances.

15. Give three examples of vehicle and equipment inspection for the following areas:
    - Engine
    - Outside of vehicle
    - Cab inspection
    - Patient compartment

Instructor Preparation

Reading preparation for the lesson:

EMT Prehospital Care, Chapter 19, pages 756-793
Local vehicle operation laws
Local ambulance call report

Suggested Learning Activities

Using a lecture format with the aid of slides, overhead transparencies or charts, provide an overview of ambulances operations.

Review local emergency vehicle operation laws.

Have students complete local ambulance call report with mock case history.

Review local ambulance inspection sheet.

Content

I. Scenario **(Slide 19-2)**
  A. In 1976, fire department responded to a cardiac arrest call
  B. Two Emergency Medical Technicians aboard
  C. Resuscitation efforts continued en-route to the hospital
  D. Traveling at speeds in excess of 70 m.p.h. on local streets
  E. The ambulance mounted the curb and struck a tree during a turn
  F. Killing two firefighters, two EMT's and the patient
  G. This prompted the establishment of Emergency Vehicle Operation Course sponsored by DOT
  H. Effective emergency care is useless if EMT never arrives at scene or fails to deliver patient to hospital

II. Arch of Driver Safety **(Slide 19-3)**
  A. Mental fitness
    1. Driving is often considered a physical task
    2. Driving is dependent upon cerebral involvement
    3. Mental fitness is an integral component of the arch
    4. Good judgment is essential
    5. Dominance of good habits over bad is essential
  B. Knowledge of vehicle and laws
    1. Handling characteristics of ambulance
    2. Familiarity with traffic laws and exemptions.
  C. Attitude
    1. Operator who assumes peremptory right-of-way negates all other attributes
    2. Safe operation must be primary concern
    3. EMT should assess attitude before assuming responsibility

III. Control tasks and seatbelts **(Slide 19-4)**
  A. Directional Control
    1. Dependent upon many factors
      a) Mechanical condition of the vehicle
      b) Road condition
      c) Physical condition of the driver
      d) Hand position
    2. Hand position
      a) Two hands on the wheel whenever possible
      b) Secondary tasks should be delegated to the second EMT
      c) Position
        (1) 10:00 and 2:00 position **(Slide 19-5)**
        (2) Optimum position for evasive maneuvers
        (3) Hand-over-hand turning technique **(Slide 19-6)**
        (4) Shuffling is alternate turning technique
  B. Driving habits **(Slide 19-7)**
    1. EMTs should not vary driving habits when they enter their own personal cars
    2. Effective driving skills will be reinforced by consistency
    3. One exception is size of vehicle
      a) Ambulance is larger and heavier
      b) Cannot stop as quickly

Content

C. Speed Control **(Slide 19-8)**
  1. Depends on same factors as directional control
  2. Modern ambulances weigh up to four times the standard passenger car
    a) Average weight 10,450 pounds
    b) Ambulances are often overloaded
  3. Ambulances have different handling characteristics than cars
  4. Longer stopping distances are required **(Slide 19-9)**
  5. Weight and improper braking technique can cause skid and loss of speed control

D. Seatbelts **(Slide 19-10)**
  1. Simplest device for maintaining control of vehicle
  2. Keeps operator inside car in event of collision
  3. Keeps operator in position behind the controls
  4. Accidents have two collisions
    a) Initial impact
    b) Second crash
      (1) Driver be unable to control vehicle following impact
      (2) Frequently second impact is more severe
      (3) Contact is made with a fixed object
  5. Being "thrown clear" is a very low probability
  6. Ejected passengers sustain serious injuries
  7. Statistically, 1 out of 200 people will be injured by seatbelts
  8. Injuries will be much less severe than unrestrained occupants
  9. Should be worn by patients and those escorting patients
  10. Proper position **(Slide 19-11)**
    a) Snugly across the pelvic girdle
    b) Not lower abdomen, which is susceptible to blunt trauma
    c) Small children in approved child seats

IV. Motor vehicle laws **(Slide 19-12)**
  A. Wording differ slightly from state to state
  B. Content is generally consistent
  C. Operator should be familiar with local regulations
  D. Paraphrased examples from New York State Vehicle and Traffic Law
    1. Emergency Operation (definition)
      a) The operation or parking of an emergency vehicle, when engaged in transporting a sick or injured person
      b) Or responding to, or working at the scene of an accident, disaster, police call, alarm of fire, or other emergency
      c) Emergency operations shall not include returning from such service
    2. Specific Exemptions
      a) Driver of authorized emergency vehicle, when involved in an emergency operation, may exercise the following privileges:
      b) The operator may
        (1) Proceed past a steady red signal, a flashing red signal or a stop sign
        (2) But only after slowing down as may be necessary for safe operation.

Content

(3) Exceed the maximum speed limits so long as he does not endanger life or property
(4) Disregard regulations governing direction of movement or turning in specified directions

c) Exemptions shall apply only when the authorized emergency vehicle utilizes an audible warning device
d) And displays appropriate red warning lamps.
e) The foregoing provisions shall not relieve the driver of an authorized emergency vehicle from

(1) The duty to drive with due regard for the safety of all persons
(2) Nor shall these provisions protect the driver from the consequences of his reckless disregard for safety of others

f) This last paragraph states specifically that while there are certain privileges granted to an emergency vehicle, the operator is responsible for the outcome should an accident occur while exercising any one of them

E. Consistent response **(Slide 19-13)**

1. Operators should respond to all calls in the same manner
2. Typical "seizure" call may be the result of a serious head trauma
3. The "sick" call may very well be a cardiac arrest
4. Response back to the hospital can be adjusted according to the known condition of the patient
5. Small percentage of acute cases will warrant a rapid transport back to the hospital
6. Rapid transportation of serious multi-trauma and cardiac patients is frequently contraindicated

F. Emergency lights **(Slide 19-14)**

1. Most laws mandate use of lights and siren when exercising "privileges"
2. Lights and siren do not automatically grant right-of-way
3. Use does not relieve operator of liability in event of accident
4. Most lights ineffective during periods of low light, such as dawn and dusk
5. Complete spectrum of lamps would be required to deal with all light and weather conditions
6. Each state mandates different colors for various types of emergency vehicles
7. Red and white warning lamps are the most common
8. Rear facing red lamps blend with tail and brake lights reducing their effectiveness
9. Amber and blue rear-facing warning lamps are preferred
10. Headlights are most effective warning lamps because they are mounted at the eye-level of other drivers

Content

11. White light is most noticeable in all conditions
12. Four-way hazard lights should not be used since they negate the turn signals and the brake lights

G. Emergency Siren **(Slide 19-15)**
1. Siren is emitted in a cone ahead of the vehicle
2. Effectiveness can be reduced by number of factors
   a) Reverberation
   b) Absorption
   c) Reflection
   d) Background noise
   e) Vehicle insertion
      (1) Ambulance projects itself into siren cone the faster it goes
      (2) Limiting its advance warning
      (3) At 60 m.p.h., siren barely precedes ambulance
3. Physically affects the ambulance operator **(Slide 19-16)**
   a) Wail and yelp cause an immediate release of adrenalin in the driver's bloodstream
   b) Causing a sympathetic physiologic reaction
      (1) Pulse quickens
      (2) Vision narrows
      (3) Palms sweat
      (4) Muscles tense
      (5) Foot presses down on the accelerator
   c) Operator must make a conscious effort to overcome the effects of the adrenalin
      (1) Letting up on the accelerator
      (2) Check peripheral vision by changing focus regularly
      (3) Increase general awareness of environment
   d) Patient effects
      (1) Consider effects of adrenalin on patient with MI
      (2) Increase in myocardial oxygen demand
      (3) More heart muscle would infarct en-route.
      (4) Same if patient jogged to the hospital

H. Escorts **(Slide 19-17)**
1. Not uncommon for EMTs utilize escort vehicles
2. Generally, not a good idea
3. Driver observing emergency vehicle at intersection may proceed through intersection and collide with second vehicle
4. May be practical is when ambulance driver is not familiar with the route to the receiving hospital

V. Principles of effective operation

A. Route Planning **(Slide 19-18)**
1. First order of business after dispatch
2. Shortest route is not necessarily the quickest
3. Factors influencing route planning
   a) Traffic congestion during peak "rush hours"
   b) Construction delays

Content

c) Non-sequential traffic lights
d) Weather conditions

B. "Natural Laws"

1. Gravity **(Slide 19-19)**
   a) Most evident when operating high-top van ambulance
   b) Raises "center of gravity"
   c) Sharp turns may cause flip on its side
   d) In normal operation weight of vehicle is distributed fairly evenly over all wheels
   e) During sudden braking, weight shifts forward onto the front wheels
   f) Strain on the steering and front braking systems
   g) Rear brakes are less effective
   h) Anti-lock braking systems help considerably
2. Centrifugal force **(Slide 19-20)**
   a) Demonstrated by swinging a rock attached to a string over your head
      (1) If you let go, rock will fly off in a straight line
      (2) Same force is exerted on a vehicle in a turn
   b) Tends to pull a vehicle out of a curve
   c) Force increases with following:
      (1) Weight of the vehicle
      (2) Sharpness of the curve
      (3) Speed of the vehicle
      (4) Flatness of the "bank"
   d) Modern road design compensates by banking curves in proportion to sharpness
   e) Adding "Jersey Walls" redirect vehicles back onto the road
3. Friction **(Slide 19-21)**
   a) Rolling friction
      (1) Contact with road is essential to steer
      (2) Front wheels must be rolling in order to maintain directional control
      (3) If rolling friction is lost, directional control is lost
      (4) Inertia and centrifugal force will direct the movement of the vehicle
      (5) When "peeling rubber" rolling friction is lost
   b) Stopping friction
      (1) Contact between pads and the drums (or discs) slows vehicle
      (2) At road surface, tires require friction to both stop and steer
      (3) Shortest stopping distance is achieved when brakes do not lock up
      (4) Locked brakes cause the tires to skid

Content

4. Threshold braking **(Slide 19-22)**
    a) Brakes applied to point just before they lock is optimum
    b) Technique
        (1) Depress brake pedal to point squeal (heard on dry pavement)
        (2) Let up slightly to release the lock
        (3) Pedal is "quivered" at this lock-point for maximum braking potential without loss of friction
    c) Each tire has only 20 square inches of contact with road
    d) Same as surface area of your hand
    e) Factors negatively affecting friction
        (1) Bad weather
        (2) Poor road surface
        (3) Oil, gravel and wet leaves

C. Operation **(Slide 19-23)**
1. Advantage of ambulances is that the driver is positioned high
2. View of the road above other vehicles
3. Define the safest path well ahead of the ambulance
4. Keep a safe distance from the vehicle ahead
5. Keep your eyes moving, checking rear-view and side-view mirrors regularly
6. Make sure other drivers see you
7. Acknowledge right-of-way with drivers at intersections
8. Leave yourself an "out"
9. Lave a space to one side in case room ahead suddenly disappears

VI. Causes of motor vehicle accidents

A. Distance **(Slide 19-24)**
1. Common cause of rear end collisions
2. Maintain distance behind the vehicle in front of you
3. Two-second rule
    a) Observe vehicle in front of you passing a stationary object
    b) Your vehicle passes same object in two seconds or greater, you are traveling at a safe distance
    c) Less than two seconds, reduce speed
    d) For dry road only
4. Other road conditions
    a) Rainy = four seconds
    b) Icy or snowy = six seconds

B. Speed **(Slide 19-25)**
1. Greatest contributing factor to accidents and severity
2. Less than one percent of people survive at speeds of seventy miles per hour
3. Two mile ambulance run, the difference between averaging 30 miles per hour and 60 miles per hour is only two minutes
4. Travelling at 60 miles per hour through most streets other than major interstate highways is unsafe and imprudent
5. Risks outweigh the potential benefits

Content

C. Intersections **(Slide 19-26)**
1. Most emergency vehicle accidents occur in intersections
2. Lights and siren do not negate stopping at intersections
3. Right-of-way is established on an individual basis
4. Green lights are unsafe for emergency vehicles
    a) Right-on-red laws
    b) Impatient drivers may run red lights
    c) Pedestrians often seem to be "color blind"
5. Other emergency vehicles may be responding from other directions
6. Always leave window open at least an inch to listen for sirens

D. Backing up **(Slide 19-27)**
1. Percentage of accidents involve backing-up
2. Usually into fixed objects
3. Mandatory to check behind vehicle prior to backing
4. Second EMT may assist in this maneuver.

VII. Record keeping

A. Overview **(Slide 19-28)**
1. Essential role of an EMT
2. Call report documents all aspects of a given call
3. Represents a valuable part of a patients record
4. Important part of a legal defense
5. Effective record keeping includes
    a) Systematic collection of data
    b) Dispatch phase through the transfer of the patient over to the emergency department
    c) Times, location, assessment and treatment information
    d) Other information

VIII. Purpose of a call report **(Slide 19-29)**

A. Medical record
1. First and foremost, it is a medical record of prehospital care
2. Provides physician with history of events surrounding call for help.
3. Examples of data
    a) Mechanism of illness or accident
    b) Vital signs
    c) Chronology of signs and symptoms
    d) Drugs or poisons found on the scene

B. Legal protection
1. Critical ingredient for protection from litigation
2. Lawsuits often don't emerge until weeks or months following an incident
3. Record may provide only means of recall
4. Serve as evidence of care given

C. Quality assurance
1. Review of call reports is often used to evaluate effectiveness of prehospital care
2. Audits rely upon validity and reliability of data
3. Many changes in EMS Systems were based upon these type of reviews

Content

D. Continuing education
1. Call review is a primary means of continuing education for EMTS
2. EMTS present cases to a group of peers and physician medical director
3. Success of sessions depends on quality of documentation

E. Administrative uses of the call report
1. Planning optimal distribution of ambulances
2. Compiling annual reports
3. Billing

IX. Principles **(Slide 19-30)**

A. Accuracy
1. Should be accurate and honest about recorded data
2. Bogus or inaccurate values are jeopardizing patient care.
3. Times, diagnostic signs, treatments and other entries should be as accurate as possible
4. May be impossible to be exact about certain data
5. Times must often be approximated due to activities on scene
   a) Review of times should be done from dispatch through arrival at the hospital
   b) Develop the best possible approximation of data
6. Accuracy is important when documenting unusual behavior or events
7. For example
   a) Statement," The patient was found drunk on the floor of the apartment", is too judgmental
   b) Concludes alcohol intoxication without definitive evidence
   c) Could be recorded " The patient was found disoriented on the apartment floor with alcohol-like smell on breath"
   d) More accurately reflects the actual observations rather than conclusions of the EMT

B. Clarity **(Slide 19-31)**
1. Call report should be written for the reader
2. Developed clearly and legibly
3. Abbreviations or characters should be accurate
4. Spell words properly
   a) Words change meaning when spelled incorrectly
   b) Ileum refers to a portion of the small intestine
   c) Ilium is a section of the pelvic bone
5. Areas of pain or location of wounds should be as exact as possible
   a) "Body diagrams" are often used
   b) Can be drawn on diagrams to identify locations
   c) Some systems provide diagrams on call report

C. Chronology **(Slide 19-32)**
1. Time relationships are critical areas of documentation
2. Provide a history of events in the order in which they occurred
3. For example
   a) Patient exhibits signs of hypoxia
   b) Which are abolished following oxygen therapy

Content

c) Relationship of therapy to improvement should be noted
d) Conversely, if patient's condition deteriorates changes should be noted

D. Completeness **(Slide 19-33)**
1. Factors included in the report is most difficult task
2. All assessment, treatments and reassessment procedures should be recorded in their chronological order
3. Events that affected treatment or transport should also be noted
a) Prolonged extrication to account for delay on the scene
b) Other EMS providers or first responders
c) Physicians name and address should be recorded
d) Belligerent or aggressive actions on the part of the patient or their relatives or friends
4. Avoid being judgmental or attempting to editorialize
5. Record the behavior and its implications regarding treatment
6. If a family member rides in the ambulance it should also be noted
7. Police or family may take valuables, indicate
a) Person
b) Shield number (in the case of police)
c) Property removed

X. Components of a call report

A. Dispatch data **(Slide 19-34)**
1. Call location
2. Date and time of the call
3. Crew names or numbers
4. Type of call
5. Sequential times of response
a) Arrival at the scene
b) Removal of patient from scene
c) Arrival at hospital
d) Available
6. Most systems utilize military time
7. Call identification number
8. You should confirm information with dispatcher if it is unclear
9. Many systems the EMT may receive calls directly
a) Panic and chaos on the scene may make this difficult
b) Assure call location, nature of the problem, and callback number
10. Some systems provide phone directions in self-help procedures
a) Airway control
b) Control bleeding
c) CPR
d) Excessive conversations should be avoided if person receiving the call is also the responding EMT

Content

B. Patient data **(Slide 19-35)**
   1. Name, sex, age, date of birth and address of the patient
   2. May also include
      a) Religion
      b) Next of kin
      c) Health insurance and assistance at the scene
   3. Reasonable attempts at securing this information should be made
   4. Most systems discourage a search of personal property in the absence of police or inhospital personnel
   5. May not be time to gather this information at the scene or en route to the hospital if the patient is critically ill
   6. Prehospital record often becomes primary source of basic patient data
      a) Patient who becomes unconscious
      b) Child
      c) Incompetent patient

C. Assessment data **(Slide 19-36)**
   1. Attempt to record critical signs and symptoms
   2. Information may be forgotten if not documented early
      a) Vital signs
      b) Glasgow Coma Scores
      c) Trauma Scores
      d) Recordings should be made during transport or at the first opportunity
   3. Some systems carry recording devices (EMT-defibrillation programs) which record voice and ECG's
   4. Continuous reassessment should be recorded
   5. Some systems utilize a "check box" for recording assessment and treatment
   6. A "comments" section is often provided for additional documentation

D. Treatment data **(Slide 19-37)**
   1. Treatment should be recorded clearly
   2. Time relationship should be established
   3. Treatments done prior to your arrival should be noted
   4. If factors prevented timely treatment they should be noted
   5. Treatment data includes the transportation method, time of transport and notification of hospital

E. Patient disposition **(Slide 19-38)**
   1. Receiving hospital
   2. Special transport modes (such as helicopters)
   3. Rationale for facility selection
   4. EMTs signature
   5. Signature of receiving nurse or physician

F. Authorization forms **(Slide 19-39)**
   1. Refusal of medical aid
   2. Refusal of care such as oxygen therapy
   3. Signature of this refusal should be obtained

Content

4. Should be accompanied by the signature of a witness
   a) Relative
   b) Friend
   c) Police officer
5. Make every effort to convince the patient to accept treatment and/or transport
6. Refusal signature is of no value if the patient has not been clearly informed of potential consequences
7. If standard forms are not provided
   a) May be appropriate to write one
   b) Check local policies

G. Special situations **(Slide 19-40)**
1. Documentation of death
   a) Some systems permit EMTs to withhold resuscitative methods if evidence of irreversible brain damage exists
   b) Death must be recorded clearly
   c) Not sufficient to record "Dead on Arrival", "DOA" or other general statements
   d) Factors which demonstrate irreversible or biological death must be noted
      (1) Rigor mortis(muscle rigidity following death)
      (2) Extreme dependent lividity(mottling of the dependent areas of the body)
      (3) Time factors may also be recorded
2. Example of documentation
   a) Patient was found prone and was pulseless and not breathing
   b) With extreme dependent lividity and rigor mortis
   c) Fixed and dilated pupils
   d) According to family members patient was last seen two days ago

H. Emotionally disturbed, minors or unconscious patients **(Slide 19-41)**
1. Whenever possible, minors or unconscious patients should be accompanied by an adult relative or a police officer
2. Minimize the chance for later complaints regarding missing property or improper behavior by EMT
3. With emotionally disturbed patient, a police officer is preferable
4. Most systems have policies which define these issues clearly

I. Dying statements
1. You may find yourself sole witness to dying patient's last words
2. Comments may have a legal significance or a personal significance to family members
3. Should be properly recorded
4. Particularly important in instances of suicide or criminal acts

J. Homicide, rape and suicide
1. Must carefully document any significant findings
2. Position of the body

Content

3. Mechanisms of injury(such as the presence of an empty bottle of sleeping pills)
4. Other essential facts
5. Care should be taken not to unnecessarily disturb the scene of the crime or move the body

K. Confidentiality
1. All information recorded on call report is confidential
2. Requests by bystanders or reporters should be directed to the police, physician or administrative staff at hospital
3. Certain conditions such as communicable diseases or dog bites may warrant additional action, such as reporting

XI. Communications **(Slide 19-42)**

A. Prehospital care requires many resources to effect survival of acutely ill or injured patients
1. Police
2. Rescue personnel
3. Firefighters
4. Utility companies
5. Other specialized manpower

B. Communications systems - essential role
1. Initial notification
2. Dispatch
3. Medical control

C. "Central nervous system" of EMS

XII. Aspects of a communication systems **(Slide 19-43)**

A. Communications center
1. Responsible for receiving calls, triage, dispatch and coordination of an EMS System
2. Ambulance base may serve as communication center in small systems
3. Separate center usually exists in larger systems
4. 911 system has been established in many communities over last 20 years
a) Was developed to efficiently utilize resources
b) Provides an easily remembered number

B. Receiving operators **(Slide 19-44)**
1. Individual who receives the call for help
2. In small systems this role may be assumed by on-duty EMT or the dispatcher
3. Responsibility of collecting location and essential patient data
4. May be responsible categorizing status for priority dispatch
a) Very serious responsibility
b) Determines which patient receives ambulance first
5. Modern systems have provisions for phone-directed instructions for self-help

C. Dispatcher **(Slide 19-45)**
1. Individual who coordinates emergency response
2. May have the responsibility for prioritizing calls

Content

3. Dispatchers and receiving operators should
   a) Good communication skills
   b) Knowledgeable in emergency care
   c) Familiar with geographical nature of area
4. National training program prepares dispatch personnel

D. Hospital notification and selection **(Slide 19-46)**
1. Important function of dispatch personnel is to relay information from the field to receiving hospital
2. Information must be concise but contain all essential elements
   a) Basic description of patient status, such as "cardiac arrest"
   b) Pertinent vital signs
   c) Expected time of arrival
   d) Allows the mobilization of appropriate manpower and resources
3. Dispatchers keep track of beds available at receiving hospitals

E. Radio systems **(Slide 19-47)**
1. EMS systems transmit on UHF or VHF frequencies
2. Designated for this purpose by the federal government
3. Field communication equipment
   a) Telephone
   b) Cellular telephone
   c) Radio in the vehicle
   d) Portable radios
   e) Vehicle radio has greater range due to the availability of on board electrical power
4. Repeater systems
   a) Strategically based receivers and transmitters
   b) Accept signal from the portable unit or mobile radio
   c) Relay it with a more powerful transmitter
   d) Often located on high ground or in tall buildings
   e) May also be situated in the emergency vehicle

F. Medical control **(Slide 19-48)**
1. Many systems provide on-line medical control via radio and telephone systems
2. May utilize base stations located at hospitals
3. Telemetry
   a) Method by which biological data is transferred from one location to another via radio
   b) Utilized to transmit a EKG to a base hospital for interpretation by a physician
   c) EKG information is coded into radio waves and decoded at the base hospital

XIII. Principles of communication **(Slide 19-49)**

A. Requires special skills to assure clear and accurate transfer of information
B. Radio communications are more concise than conversations over the telephone
C. Never interrupt another radio transmission unless an emergency exists
D. Most systems use unit codes to identify each caller
E. Identify yourself by announcing your code to the dispatcher

Content

F. Speak in a normal voice
G. Microphone a few inches away from your mouth
H. Only one person may speak at a time
I. While you are speaking, you are pushing a button and cannot be interrupted
J. At the end of each exchange you will give a code to let dispatcher that you are finished speaking
  1. May be the word "over" or "kay"
  2. Wait until he the dispatcher gives you this code before you press the button to speak
  3. Standardized way to end the call i.e. 10-4 or over and out
K. Codes **(Slide 19-50)**
  1. Method used to condense radio conversations
  2. Codes to convert common messages or phrases into short, prearranged numerical sequences
  3. Most common code system is "10 Codes"
  4. Number 10 followed by a series of other numbers
  5. Review local codes

XIV. Vehicle and equipment maintenance
A. Overview **(Slide 19-51)**
  1. EMS Systems use a wide range of equipment
  2. Specific to a given patient's needs
  3. Requires careful consideration by the prehospital provider
  4. Assure familiarity with local equipment prior to the first call
B. The vehicle **(Slide 19-52)**
  1. Type I ambulance **(Slide 19-53)**
    a) Consists of a box shaped passenger compartment mounted onto a truck style chassis
    b) Tends to be more spacious and more powerful
    c) Allows for some degree of cost efficiency
    d) Can be transferred onto a new chassis as the need arises
    e) Generally has a rougher ride
    f) Cab is separated from the passenger compartment
  2. Type II ambulance **(Slide 19-54)**
    a) Van style vehicle with a raised roof
    b) Extended rear compartment
    c) Cab and patient compartments are joined
    d) Allow easy access by driver should need arise
    e) Tend to have a smoother ride
    f) Space in patient compartment is smaller
    g) Generally less storage capacity
    h) Turning radius is better than modular
    i) Value in urban areas congested traffic and narrow streets.
  3. Type III ambulance **(Slide 19-55)**
    a) Modular box mounted on a van chassis
    b) Usually access to patient compartment from cab
    c) Combination of added storage space, better gas mileage than the truck style makes this popular alternative in many systems

Content

C. Patient care equipment **(Slide 19-56)**
   1. May vary according to regional requirements and resources
   2. Certain equipment is recommended as standard by regulatory agencies
      a) State Department of Health
      b) Local EMS administrations
      c) National agencies i.e. American College of Surgeons

D. Care and maintenance **(Slide 19-57)**
   1. Care of equipment extends from beginning of your working tour, after each individual call and ends with your tour of duty
   2. Life may be lost if equipment is absent or fails
   3. Check equipment and vehicle at regularly specified intervals
   4. Vehicle **(Slide 19-58)**
      a) Should be checked at beginning and end of each tour
      b) Engine
         (1) Check fuel and oil levels
         (2) Battery is checked for fluid level, connections, and signs of corrosion
         (3) Coolant system checked for fluid levels and hoses for leaks
         (4) Wiper, brake, power steering and transmission fluid levels
      c) Outside inspection **(Slide 19-59)**
         (1) Body inspection to establish the condition prior to the first ambulance run
         (2) Tire thread wear, defects and air pressure
         (3) All light systems
         (4) Doors, windows and outside compartments
         (5) Outside should be washed and waxed at regular intervals
      d) Cab inspection **(Slide 19-60)**
         (1) Brakes can be tested by noting level brake pedal can be depressed
         (2) Turning and stopping signals should be inspected
         (3) Emergency lights, sirens and the horn
         (4) Start ambulance and check all gauges, indicator or warning lights
         (5) Windshield wipers, ventilation, cooling and heating systems
         (6) Adjust mirrors and seat
         (7) Steering wheel should move freely and soundlessly
         (8) Communication equipment should be checked by contacting dispatch
   5. Equipment maintenance **(Slide 19-61)**
      a) Check patient compartment for missing, dirty or damaged equipment
      b) Ensure that the compartment itself is clean
      c) Floor and surfaces should be cleaned at beginning of each tour and after each call when needed

Content

d) Stretcher should be wiped with disinfectant solution after each patient and clean linen applied
e) Dispose of all waste materials in appropriate receptacles
f) Body fluids, dirty bandages and needles or syringes require special attention

6. Ventilation, airway and oxygen equipment **(Slide 19-62)**
   a) Bag-valve-masks, oxygen powered resuscitators and suction equipment
      (1) Should be tested for operation
      (2) Should be disinfected or disposed after each use according to local protocols
      (3) Stored appropriately
   b) In-board and portable oxygen tanks should be checked to assure a sufficient supply
   c) Airway devices should be checked and replaced as needed
7. Bandages and sterile supplies **(Slide 19-63)**
   a) Sterile supplies should be checked to ensure sterility and quantity
   b) Should be stored in a dust-free, dry location
   c) If they become wet, they should be replaced
   d) Expiration dates must be periodically checked and outdated items pulled and discarded
   e) Newly acquired supplies should be placed under old ones to minimize waste
8. Stretchers and immobilization equipment **(Slide 19-64)**
   a) Long spine boards, short spine boards and stretchers should be stored neatly and operational
   b) Straps should be examined to insure that they are in sufficient quantity for each device
   c) Traction, rigid and other types of splinting devices should be checked
   d) Soiled immobilization equipment should be cleaned after each use

E. Safety and extrication equipment **(Slide 19-65)**
   1. Traffic cones, flares and other safety devices should be checked
   2. Protective clothing and self-contained breathing apparatus should be carefully inspected to assure that they are serviceable
   3. Extrication equipment should be tested at regular intervals

F. Other equipment
   1. Stethoscopes, sphygmomanometers they are present and working
   2. PASG should be checked for leaks on a regular interval

Chapter 19

AMBULANCE OPERATIONS

Examination

1. One of the simplest devices that can help maintain control of any vehicle is the:

   a. palming steering technique
   b. seat belt
   c. properly inflated tires
   d. properly designed suspension

2. The driver of an authorized emergency vehicle, when involved in an emergency operation, may exercise all of the following privileges <u>except</u>:

   a. exceed the maximum speed limits
   b. disregard regulations governing the direction of movement of the ambulance
   c. proceed through a red light at full speed as long as the siren is on
   d. proceed through a red light only after slowing down as necessary for safe operation

3. Ambulance personnel should respond to all calls as if they were true emergencies because:

   a. even if the call is minor the vehicle will be in service faster after the call
   b. insurance is only in effect if the siren and lights are on
   c. a fast arrival is expected by the community
   d. the lay public is unaware of the fine points of emergency medicine and any call may be serious

4. People respond to a warning sound, such as a siren, in a four step process. Indicate the proper sequence of response:

   a. attention, interpret, reaction, detect
   b. detect, attention, interpret, reaction
   c. reaction, attention, detect, interpret
   d. interpret, reaction, attention, detect

5. Generally the use of an escort vehicle to lead the ambulance to the hospital is a:

   a. good idea as it speeds the trip
   b. good idea because it is safer than driving without an escort
   c. bad idea as other motorists are more apt to see the escort first and not notice the second vehicle
   d. bad idea as it ties up two emergency vehicles at the same time

6. The natural laws that affect speed control and directional control are:

   a. gravity, centrifugal force, friction
   b. centrifugal force, friction, blind spots
   c. blind spots, gravity, friction
   d. friction, centrifugal force, warning signals

7. The most important concept in accident avoidance is to:

   a. plan your route carefully
   b. have a second set of eyes up front at all times
   c. beware of road hazards such as construction
   d. leave yourself an out

8. Although driving is considered a physical task, it is ___% cerebral in nature.

   a. 50
   b. 60
   c. 70
   d. 90

9. The superior braking technique when driving an ambulance is

   a. left foot braking
   b. right foot braking
   c. dominant foot braking
   d. alternate foot braking

10. The majority of emergency vehicle accidents occur:

    a. at night
    b. due to poor weather
    c. at intersections
    d. due to collisions with other emergency vehicles

11. Palming the wheel in a turn represents a:

    a. poor driving habit
    b. method of stable turning
    c. method for "feeling" the turn
    d. accident avoidance technique

12. The basic hand position when driving an emergency vehicle is:

    a. 11:00 and 1:00 O'clock
    b. 10:00 and 2:00 O'clock
    c. 9:00 and 3:00 O'clock
    d. 8:00 and 4:00 O'clock

13. The correct position of a lap belt is across the:

    a. umbilicus
    b. crease of the thigh
    c. iliac crests
    d. upper thigh

14. Being "thrown clear" of the accident:

    a. has a very low probability
    b. is a common event
    c. is a less serious mechanism of injury
    d. is a planned response to an accident

15. The most effective colors for rear-facing warning lamps are:

    a. amber and blue
    b. red and white
    c. red and yellow
    d. yellow and white

16. Four-way hazard lights:

    a. should not be used in a moving vehicle
    b. should be turned off when the vehicle is parked
    c. are necessary in a moving ambulance
    d. are most effective in low-light situations

17. The most effective warning lights are mounted:

    a. just above the rear bumper
    b. on the roof top
    c. at eye level to other drivers
    d. in the outermost corners of the vehicle

18. The sweaty palms, rapid pulse and tense muscles felt by the operator of an emergency vehicle when the siren is switched on can cause the operator to immediately begin speeding. This response is the result of:

    a. endorphin release
    b. adrenalin release
    c. physical demands of driving
    d. vagal stimulation

19. When suddenly braking an ambulance, the rear brakes:

    a. are considerably less effective than the front
    b. do most of the braking
    c. brake equally with the front brakes
    d. allow for better directional control

20. The physical force responsible for most rollover accidents during turns is:

    a. inertia
    b. centrifugal
    c. momentum
    d. resistance

21. The technique where the brake pedal is depressed to the point that the brakes lock, then the pedal is let up slightly to release the lock and then "quivered" at this lock-point for maximum braking potential without loss of friction:

    a. is called threshold braking
    b. is only useful with anti-lock brakes
    c. causes loss of steering control
    d. increases centrifugal force

22. A good way to judge the correct traveling distance between your ambulance and the vehicle in front of you **in dry weather** is to observe the vehicle in front of you as it passes a fixed object (such as a telephone pole) and then be able to count _______ seconds before you reach the same object.

    a. 2
    b. 5
    c. 10
    d. 15

23. On icy roads, the above rule is increased to:

    a. 6 seconds
    b. 15 seconds
    c. 20 seconds
    d. 30 seconds

24. Reviewing call reports to evaluate effectiveness of prehospital care is called:

    a. continuing education
    b. quality assurance
    c. legal protection
    d. peer review

25. The effectiveness of a call report depends upon the following four major factors:

    a. legibility, honesty, accuracy, completeness
    b. legibility, clarity, judgment, accuracy
    c. clarity, accuracy, completeness, judgment
    d. accuracy, clarity, chronology, completeness

26. The information ascertained during the treatment of the patient such as the vital signs is part of the:

    a. dispatch data
    b. patient data
    c. assessment data
    d. treatment data

27. If you are treating a minor or unconscious patient it is best to:

    a. withhold transport until a relative can be located
    b. transport the patient with an adult relative or police officer
    c. have the police place the patient into protective custody and then transport
    d. have a bystander accompany the patient to the hospital

28. Information you receive concerning the patient's condition can:

    a. be told to the general public
    b. be told only to a friend
    c. be told to reporters as requested
    d. be documented and told to the emergency department staff

29. Which of the following represents the best "non-judgmental" documentation of a suspected case of alcohol intoxication on an ambulance call report?

    a. the patient appeared intoxicated with an alcohol-like compound
    b. there was an alcohol-like smell on the patient's breath
    c. the patient was speaking as if he was intoxicated
    d. the patient was extremely intoxicated

30. Body diagrams on an ambulance call report are a useful way to document:

    a. wounds and areas of pain
    b. the patient's sex
    c. the height of the patient
    d. the position that the patient was found in

31. Which of these statements is <u>least</u> effective when documenting biological death?

    a. the patient was dead for 30 minutes prior to our arrival
    b. the patient has extreme dependent lividity on the back and posterior legs
    c. the patient has evidence of rigor mortis in all extremities
    d. the patient has suffered severe destruction of the skull and brain from the fall

32. Five o'clock P.M. is expressed in military time as:

    a. 0300 hours
    b. 1300 hours
    c. 1500 hours
    d. 1700 hours

33. Noon is expressed in military time as:

    a. 0000 hours
    b. 1200 hours
    c. 2400 hours
    d. 0100 hours

34. Directing a bystander over the phone on how to perform CPR is:

    a. a dangerous technique
    b. used in many systems
    c. against heart association standards
    d. too time consuming

35. Which of the following people is **most** effective as a witness to refusal of care?

    a. the patient's family member
    b. a bystander
    c. your partner
    d. a police officer

36. The refusal signature is of no value unless you:

    a. inform the patient of the potential consequences of refusal
    b. have at least two copies of the refusal
    c. have a police officer as a witness to the refusal
    d. have rendered at least some first aid care

37. Ecchymosis in the most dependent areas of the body which occurs long after death is called:

    a. rigor mortis
    b. dependent lividity
    c. ecchymortis
    d. death discoloration

38. The individual who communicates with field personnel and other agencies to coordinate the emergency medical response is the:

    a. field service technician
    b. receiving operator
    c. mobile data officer
    d. dispatcher

39. The initials VHF stand for:

    a. verify hailing frequency
    b. valid handling frequency
    c. very high frequency
    d. volume hailing frequency

40. The device or system used to relay the signals from portable or ambulance radios to the dispatch center is referred to as a:

    a. bi-directional antenna
    b. repeater
    c. mobile data terminal
    d. telemetry unit

41. The major disadvantage of hand-held portable radios versus the ambulance radio is:

    a. the need to carry extra equipment
    b. it has a shorter range
    c. it is more difficult to operate
    d. it only comes in simplex

42. The device that can transmit both an electrocardiogram and send voice signals to a base hospital is a __________ unit:

    a. bioscopy
    b. biogram
    c. biometrics
    d. biotelemetry

Match the descriptions of the radio system in column B to the terms in column A.

Column A	Column B
43. simplex	a. simultaneous ECG data and voice
44. duplex	b. push to talk system
45. multiplex	c. two way voice communication similar to a telephone

46. A good rule to follow when speaking into a radio microphone is to:

    a. talk louder than normal while holding the microphone right next to your mouth
    b. speak in a normal voice with the microphone a few inches away from your mouth
    c. speak more slowly than normal in a low voice
    d. speak normally with the microphone touching your lower lip

Match the descriptions in column B to the ambulance types in column A.

Column A		Column B	
47.	type I	a.	van-type ambulance
48.	type II	b.	modular patient compartment with van chassis
49.	type III	c.	modular patient compartment with truck chassis

50. The ambulance should have both a mechanical check of fluids, properly working lights and proper mechanical operations as well as a check of all medical equipment:

    a. at the beginning of each shift
    b. at least daily
    c. at least weekly
    d. only after problems are discovered

Chapter 20

APPROACH TO THE MULTIPLE TRAUMA PATIENT

Materials and Equipment for Lesson

1. Slides or overhead transparencies
2. Handouts
   - Approach to trauma patient
   - Trauma score
3. Slide projector, overhead projector and/or blackboard

Approach to The Multiple Trauma Patient

Objectives
(Slide 20-1)

At the conclusion of the chapter the students will be able to:

1. **List the steps of patient assessment and general management of a trauma patient.**

2. **List two injuries for each of the following mechanisms:**
   - **Head on collisions**
   - **Rear end collisions**
   - **Side hit collisions**
   - **Fall on feet**
   - **Fall on outstretched arm**

3. **Define the pneumonic "AVPU" and describe its components.**

4. **Define the pneumonic "AMPLE" and describe its components.**

5. **List the major components of the trauma score and explain its relevance.**

Instructor Preparation

Reading preparation for the lesson:

EMT Prehospital Care, Chapter 20, pages 795-812
Trauma score

Suggested Learning Activities

Using a lecture format with the aid of slides, overhead transparencies or charts, provide an overview of the approach to the patient with multiple trauma.

Review local trauma score.

Provide case histories and discussion.

Content

I. Overview **(Slide 20-2)**
- A. Assessment must rapid, systematic and orderly
- B. Avoids a delayed response to serious injury
- C. Extent of survey will vary with each patient
  - 1. Stable patients may require a complete primary and secondary survey
  - 2. Unstable patients may only receive the primary survey followed by resuscitation and transport
- D. Judgment comes with practice and experience
- E. Hospital destination plays an important role in the assessment and treatment process
  - 1. Many systems have trauma centers designated
  - 2. Trauma triage systems are used to decide hospital destination **(Slide 20-3)**
  - 3. Assessment criteria may include trauma scoring systems **(Slide 20-4)**

II. Dispatch review **(Slide 20-5)**
- A. Upon receipt call from dispatcher you must begin to prepare for worst possible contingencies
- B. Discuss roles of the team members
  - 1. Who will assess
  - 2. Who will secure the scene
  - 3. Who will notify the dispatcher if additional resources are needed
  - 4. Roles in resuscitation
- C. Review chronological approach in your mind so that you focus on priorities upon arrival
- D. Route selection is another priority

III. Scene survey **(Slide 20-6)**
- A. Hazards
  - 1. First priority is personal safety for yourselves and the patient and oncoming motorists
  - 2. Many well-intentioned EMTs and lay people have died on highways due to poor attention to safety
  - 3. Reflective devices should be positioned to provide warning to oncoming traffic
  - 4. Other hazards should be identified
    - a) Toxic gases
    - b) Fire
    - c) Hazardous and explosive materials
    - d) Added distance from scene is important
- B. Identify need for additional resources **(Slide 20-7)**
  - 1. Fire department
  - 2. Rescue
  - 3. Additional ambulance units
  - 4. Utility companies
  - 5. Brief description of condition is provided to dispatcher

Content

C. Triage **(Slide 20-8)**

1. Avoid random attention with multiple patients
2. Rapid review of all patients allows priority selection of those in greatest need
3. Additional units can be directed to the most seriously injured patients
4. When manpower permits the senior EMT should assume role of "triage officer"
5. Categories (American College of Surgeons)
    - a) Category 1 **(Slide 20-9)**
        - (1) Combined system injury
        - (2) Bleeding
        - (3) Open fractures
        - (4) Uncontrolled hemorrhage
        - (5) Severe maxillofacial injuries
        - (6) Severe head, neck and upper respiratory tract injuries
        - (7) Unstable chest injuries
        - (8) Pelvic fractures
        - (9) Blunt abdominal trauma with hypotension and/or penetrating abdominal wounds
        - (10) Neurological injuries producing prolonged loss of consciousness
        - (11) Abnormal posturing
        - (12) Lateralizing signs, or paralysis
    - b) Category 2 **(Slide 20-10)**
        - (1) Complicated open or closed fractures
        - (2) Soft tissue injuries with stabilized bleeding
        - (3) Multiple rib fractures without flail segments
        - (4) Blunt abdominal trauma not producing hypotension
        - (5) Transient loss of consciousness
    - c) Category 3 **(Slide 20-11)**
        - (1) Uncomplicated fractures
        - (2) No hypovolemia or hypotension
        - (3) No neurological injuries
        - (4) No abdominal injuries
        - (5) Soft tissue injuries of a moderate degree
        - (6) Chest injuries not producing respiratory distress
    - d) Review American College of Surgeons Trauma Triage Scheme
6. Mechanism of injury **(Slide 20-12)**
    - a) Allows you to anticipate injuries associated with a specific force
    - b) May suggest severity, i.e., fall from height
    - c) Forces **(Slide 20-13)**
        - (1) Velocity is critical variable
            - (a) $KE = 1/2mv^2$
            - (b) Applies to blunt and penetrating trauma
        - (2) Compression **(Slide 20-14)**
            - (a) Organs compressed and rupture
            - (b) Solid organs, i.e., spleen and liver are particularly susceptible

Content

(3) Deceleration **(Slide 20-15)**
(a) Organs continue forward during deceleration of the body
(b) Tear at sites of attachment
(c) Liver, aorta and kidneys are prone to deceleration injury
(4) Penetrating injuries **(Slide 20-16)**
(a) Depends on size, direction, location
(b) Severity of missile injury depends on velocity, location, range
d) Front end collisions **(Slide 20-17)**
(1) Head and spinal trauma
(2) Chest and abdominal
(3) Flail chest
(4) Pneumothorax
(5) Lower extremity
(6) Upper extremity protection injury
e) Side collision **(Slide 20-18)**
(1) Head and spinal trauma
(2) Lateral chest and abdominal wall injury
(3) Internal hemorrhage
(4) Upper extremity
(5) Shoulder, clavicle, humerus
(6) Hip/acetabulum
f) Rear end collision **(Slide 20-19)**
(1) Head and spinal trauma
(2) Contra coup head injury
(3) Whiplash
g) Rotational collision force **(Slide 20-20)**
(1) Varies according to direction
(2) Person closest to impact point most injured
h) Falls **(Slide 20-21)**
(1) Depend on impact point
(2) Feet first
(a) Calcaneus
(b) Lower extremity
(c) Spine
(3) Outstretched arm
(a) Wrist, elbow
(b) Humerus, shoulder

IV. Primary survey **(Slide 20-22)**
A. Airway
1. Head tilt - chin lift
a) Primary technique for non traumatic patients
b) Lift chin and tilt head
2. Jaw thrust - without head tilt
a) Patients with suspected spinal injury
b) All unconscious trauma patients
c) Mechanism of injury that may have caused spinal injury
d) Injuries above the clavicle

Content

3. Airway maintenance
   a) Oropharyngeal or nasopharyngeal airways
   b) Esophageal airway
   c) Endotracheal intubation
4. If manual maneuvers fail to open airway
   a) Suctioning can remove liquid and small particles
   b) If foreign body is suspected the airway obstruction sequence should be followed
   c) Crush injuries to the airway, rapid transport

B. Breathing **(Slide 20-23)**
1. Respiratory rate and depth
   a) Rates below 12 and above 30 usually require positive pressure
   b) Chest excursion is primary determinant of adequate depth of breathing
2. Skin color
   a) Cyanosis is indicative of poor oxygenation
   b) Provide high concentration oxygen
   c) Positive pressure if unconsciousness is present
3. Accessory muscle use
   a) Active use of neck and abdominal muscles
   b) Indicates severe respiratory distress
4. Evidence of chest trauma
   a) Open wounds
   b) Bruises
   c) Flail chest segments
   d) Signs of fractures
5. Tracheal shift and neck vein distention **(Slide 20-24)**
   a) Tension pneumothorax
   b) Flat neck veins may suggest hypovolemic shock
6. Abnormal respiratory sounds
   a) Snoring, gurgling, wheezing and stridor
   b) May suggest airway obstruction
7. Breath sounds
   a) Quickly auscultated
   b) Pneumothorax or hemothorax

C. Circulation **(Slide 20-25)**
1. Pulse
   a) Carotid pulse is checked to determine need for CPR
   b) Peripheral pulse is checked for rate, quality and regularity
2. Blood pressure
   a) Blood pressure can be estimated
      (1) Carotid = 60 mm/hg
      (2) Femoral = 70 mm/hg
      (3) Radial = 80 mm/hg
      (4) Not exact parameters
      (5) Decision-making criteria
   b) Auscultated blood pressure when time and conditions permit

Content

3. Skin color
    a) Pale, cool and sweaty skin
    b) May suggest poor perfusion
4. Capillary refill
    a) Measured by squeezing nail beds and observing refill
    b) Greater than 2 seconds or no refill is suggestive of poor perfusion
    c) Early sign of redistribution related to hypovolemic shock
    d) May be delayed normally in cold, some adult females and elderly
5. Bleeding
    a) Obvious external hemorrhage
    b) Controlled with direct pressure, elevation, pressure points and rarely a tourniquet

D. Disability - CNS function **(Slide 20-26)**
1. Evaluated by quickly evaluating the level of consciousness
2. Mental status is most sensitive indicator of CNS function
3. AVPU
    a) Alert - patient communicates clearly without any stimuli
    b) Verbal - responds to verbal stimuli
    c) Painful- does not respond to verbal stimuli but does respond to painful stimuli
    d) Unresponsive- patient is unresponsive to both verbal and painful stimuli
4. Calculate Glasgow coma scale
5. Altered mental status
    a) High index of suspicion for intracranial bleeding
    b) In the absence of other explanations, i.e., respiratory or cardiovascular problems

E. Expose **(Slide 20-27)**
1. Expose patient's body to identify specific injuries
2. Special attention should be paid to head and trunk
3. Concern for the patient's privacy should not hamper your evaluation

V. Management **(Slide 20-28)**

A. Problems identified in primary survey should be addressed immediately

B. Cervical in-line immobilization
1. Manual immobilization of the neck and head should be established
2. Cervical collar is applied
3. Cervical collar does not constitute adequate immobilization by itself
4. Patient is immobilized to short or long spine board

C. Airway
1. Manual maneuvers
2. Oropharyngeal and nasopharyngeal
3. Endotracheal intubation
4. Esophageal airway
5. Airway obstruction procedures as needed
6. Suctioning as needed

Content

D. Ventilation **(Slide 20-29)**

1. Provide positive pressure as needed
2. Ventilate slowly (less than 40 liters/minute) in order to avoid gastric distension
3. Cricoid pressure
    a) Can be maintained during mouth or mask ventilation
    b) If man power is available
4. Chest excursion to determine the adequacy of tidal volume during ventilation
5. If tidal volumes appear inadequate
    a) Airway should be evaluated or an alternate method of ventilation should be considered
    b) Particularly important when using the bag valve mask resuscitator
    c) Consider two handed technique

E. Oxygen **(Slide 20-30)**

1. High concentration oxygen should given to all patients with respiratory cardiovascular compromise
2. COPD history should be inquired about and local protocols should be followed
3. Patients with ventilatory depression or arrest
    a) Should be rapidly extricated
    b) Positive pressure ventilation should be provided

F. Control hemorrhage/manage chest injuries **(Slide 20-31)**

1. Control bleeding
2. Seal open chest wounds with an occlusive dressing
3. Stabilize impaled objects
4. Cover eviscerations

G. PASG

1. Should be applied according to local protocol
2. May call for inflation either on the scene or enroute

H. Rapid transport

1. Respiratory distress, circulatory shock, or severe central nervous system injury
2. Rapid transport should be initiated
3. Other essential treatments and continuing assessments can be performed enroute

I. Notification/Facility selection **(Slide 20-32)**

1. Hospital should be notified as soon as possible
2. Allows mobilization of manpower and resources
3. Critical information
    a) Number of patients
    b) Types of injury
    c) Vital signs including mental status
    d) Obvious severe injuries
    e) Other special information such as exposure to toxic chemicals
4. Facilities should be selected according to local protocol

Content

J. Evaluation and continued management enroute
1. Continued evaluation enroute in order to avoid undue delay at the scene
2. Trauma score should be elicited

VI. Secondary survey **(Slide 20-33)**
A. Stable patients should be carefully surveyed prior to transport
B. AMPLE history
1. Allergies
a) Avoid complications which may occur in-hospital during drug administration
b) Antibiotics and local anesthetics are specifically questioned about
2. Medications
a) Often point to preexisting disease
b) May affect care strategy
c) May blunt compensatory response
3. Past medical history
a) Significant medical conditions in the patient's past
b) Heart disease, diabetes, or COPD
c) Should be made known to the hospital personnel
d) Crucial in patient management
4. Last meal
a) Time of last oral intake
b) Vomiting and aspiration may result during management
5. Events
a) Events leading up to the injury should be ascertained
b) Accidents often precipitated by medical problems
(1) Fainting
(2) Hypoglycemia
(3) Primary cardiac arrest
c) Family members or other passengers may provide history
C. Vital signs **(Slide 20-34)**
1. Respirations
a) Rate
b) Depth
c) Rhythm
d) Breath odor
2. Pulse
a) Rate
b) Quality
c) Rhythm
3. Blood pressure
a) Blood pressure is auscultated
b) Palpated when noise or time is factor
4. Temperature
a) Evaluated by touching the skin
b) Note relative temperature, moisture and color

Content

D. Head to toe survey
  1. Head **(Slide 20-35)**
    a) Examine for contusions and open wounds
    b) Eyes and the mastoid region for presence of Battle's sign or raccoon's eyes
      (1) Suggestive of skull fractures
      (2) Relatively late findings
    c) Bones are palpated for evidence of fractures
    d) Pupils are checked for diameter, equality and reactivity
    e) Blood or fluid leaks from the ears and nose
    f) Facial bones are also examined for underlying fractures
  2. Neck **(Slide 20-36)**
    a) Observe for contusions and open wounds
    b) Accessory muscle use
    c) Distension of the neck veins
    d) Cervical spine is palpated for deformity or crepitus
  3. Chest **(Slide 20-37)**
    a) Observe for contusions and open wounds
    b) Examine for evidence of unstable segments or other signs of fractures
    c) Tenderness or paradoxical breathing
    d) Auscultate breath sounds
  4. Abdomen **(Slide 20-38)**
    a) Observe for contusions and open wounds
    b) Palpate quadrants and note tenderness and rigidity
      (1) Absence of rigidity or swelling does not rule out internal bleeding
      (2) Abdominal rigidity may take hours to develop
  5. Pelvis **(Slide 20-39)**
    a) Gently compress iliac crests medially and posteriorly
    b) Note loss of structural integrity
    c) Palpate the pubic symphysis
    d) Pelvic fractures are often associated with significant blood loss
  6. Extremities **(Slide 20-40)**
    a) Observe the upper and lower extremities for contusions and open wounds
    b) Palpate carefully and note tenderness and deformity
    c) Distal pulses are evaluated to determine if neurovascular compromise has occurred
    d) Capillary refill should be reevaluated
  7. Neurological exam **(Slide 20-41)**
    a) Mental status and Glasgow coma scale can be reevaluated
    b) Motor movement
      (1) Motor function should be evaluated in all extremities
      (2) Determine presence of lateralizing signs or paralysis
    c) Sensory
      (1) Check sensation
      (2) Key levels of the trunk and extremities

Content

VII. Management **(Slide 20-42)**
- a. Oxygen therapy
- b. Immobilization to short or long board for removal
- c. Bandage wounds
- d. Splint fractures
- e. Immobilization to long board
- f. Notification/facility selection
- g. Evaluation and continued management enroute

VIII. Case illustrations
- A. Case 1 **(Slide 20-43)**
  - 1. Overview
    - a) Head on collision at speed of approximately 40 MPH
    - b) Three injured passengers
    - c) Scene secured by police
    - d) One EMT called for an additional unit
    - e) Patient #1
      - (1) Alert and complaining localized shoulder pain
      - (2) Exhibited no evidence of serious injuries
    - f) Patient #2
      - (1) Driver was found dead
      - (2) Massive brain injury
  - 2. Patient #3 treated by EMTs **(Slide 20-44)**
    - a) Overview
      - (1) 25 year old male front seat passenger
      - (2) Alert and agitated
      - (3) Shortness of breath
      - (4) Pain in the right hip
    - b) Physical assessment revealed:
      - (1) Pulse 64 and regular
      - (2) Respirations 30 and labored
      - (3) Blood pressure 100/palpation
      - (4) Pale and profusely sweaty
      - (5) Forehead laceration
      - (6) Pupils midpositional, equal and reactive
      - (7) Paradoxical breathing, subcutaneous emphysema and absent breath sounds left chest
    - c) Treatment **(Slide 20-45)**
      - (1) In-line immobilization of the neck
      - (2) High concentration oxygen via a nonrebreather
      - (3) Rapidly extricated
      - (4) Right leg was internally rotated and flexed at hip
      - (5) Flail segment was splinted
      - (6) PASG was applied
        - (a) Only one leg of the garment could be attached
        - (b) Due to position of the leg
      - (7) Condition did not change in route
      - (8) Pulse rate remained at 64

Content

d) Questions for discussion **(Slide 20-46)**
- (1) Likely associated injuries?
- (2) Indications for positive pressure ventilations with flail chest?
- (3) Possible causes of a relatively slow pulse (64) in hypovolemic shock?

e) Discussion **(Slide 20-47)**
- (1) Typical associated injuries with front-end collisions
  - (a) Head and cervical spine injury
  - (b) Injury to airway, shoulder and clavicle
  - (c) Blunt trauma to intrathoracic and intra-abdominal organs
  - (d) Tibia, knee, femur fractures
  - (e) Dislocation of hip through acetabulum
- (2) Positive pressure ventilation **(Slide 20-48)**
  - (a) Positive pressure is an important aspect of management of flail chest
  - (b) Caution should be used with intrathoracic trauma
  - (c) Injuries can be complicated by excessive or forceful positive pressure
  - (d) Tension pneumothorax can result by forcing air into pleural space
  - (e) Ventilation systems of choice
    - i) Oxygen powered resuscitator with 40 liter/minute flow rate
    - ii) Bag-valve-mask
    - iii) Pocket mask
- (3) Causes of slow pulse **(Slide 20-49)**
  - (a) Hypovolemia or other causes of hypoxia usually result in compensatory tachycardia
  - (b) Increased intracranial pressure may result in a slow pulse
    - i) Associated with an increase in blood pressure
    - ii) Patient did not exhibit an increase in blood pressure
    - iii) No other signs of intracerebral bleeding
  - (c) Severe end stage shock may cause a slow pulse
    - i) Due to significant ischemia to the myocardium
    - ii) Unlikely since patient has relatively stable blood pressure and mental state
  - (d) Drugs that block sympathetic tone may prevent an increase in pulse
    - i) Reinforces the need to secure a medication history
    - ii) This patient was not on this type of medication

(e) Cardiac contusion
- i) Cause of slow heart rate in this patient
- ii) Contusion resulted in damage to conduction system
- iii) Lead to poor conduction and the related slowing of the heart rate
- iv) Mechanism of injury supported this possible assessment

B. Case 2

1. Overview **(Slide 20-50)**
   - a) 24 year old woman jumped six stories
   - b) Landed on grass softened by one week's rainfall
   - c) Six inch depressions in ground made by her feet and buttocks
2. History and physical assessment
   - a) Alert and oriented
   - b) No history of loss of consciousness
   - c) Complained only of pain in lumbar region
   - d) Physical exam revealed: **(Slide 20-51)**
   - e) Pulse 100 and regular
   - f) Respirations 20 and normal
   - g) Blood pressure 100/70
   - h) Skin was normal
   - i) Pupils were midpositional, equal and reactive
   - j) Breath sounds were normal
   - k) No obvious external evidence of injury
   - l) Glasgow coma scale of 15
   - m) Normal motor and sensory function
3. Treatment **(Slide 20-52)**
   - a) In-line immobilization of cervical spine
   - b) Supplemental oxygen via a nasal cannula at 6 liters per minute
   - c) Immobilized to a long spine board
   - d) Transported to the local Trauma Center
4. Questions for discussion **(Slide 20-53)**
   - a) What injuries should be presumed given the mechanisms of injury?
   - b) What is the likelihood of cervical spine injury without also having head injury?
5. Discussion of case 2 **(Slide 20-54)**
   - a) Patient suffered bilateral fractures of the talus (ankle bone)
   - b) Compression fractures of the lumbar spine
   - c) Non-displaced fracture of the odontoid portion of cervical vertebrae 2
   - d) EMTs took appropriate cervical spine precautions
   - e) No evidence of internal bleeding
   - f) EMTs maintained a suspicion of internal bleeding and provided timely but smooth transport
   - g) Patient had no spinal cord compression
   - h) No other severe internal injuries
   - i) Went on to good recovery

Content

C. Case 3

1. Overview **(Slide 20-55)**
    a) 30 year old man was struck by a van
    b) Bystanders reported that he was thrown 15 feet on impact
    c) Suffered no loss of consciousness
    d) EMTs found the patient sitting on the curb
    e) Patient asked to sign a release against medical advice
    f) Appeared agitated and refused physical assessment
    g) EMTs convinced patient to submit to brief survey
2. History and physical assessment **(Slide 20-56)**
    a) Skin appeared pale and sweaty
    b) Pupils were midpositional, equal and reactive
    c) Glasgow coma scale was 15
    d) EMTs noted dent on van from impact
    e) Inspection revealed discharge of clear fluid and blood from nose and fluid from right ear
3. Treatment **(Slide 20-57)**
    a) Police and EMTs insisted that patient accompany them to the hospital
    b) Placed patient on stretcher with moderate resistance
    c) Notified hospital that potential neurosurgical emergency was enroute
    d) Patient refused immobilization with a cervical collar and spine board
    e) EMTs maintained in-line immobilization enroute to the trauma center
4. Questions for discussion **(Slide 20-58)**
    a) What injuries are suggested by the mechanism of injury and the physical findings?
    b) What are the medicolegal implications for treatment and transport of patient in light of refusal?
    c) What percentage of epidural hematomas have no loss of consciousness initially?
5. Discussion of case 3 **(Slide 20-59)**
    a) Patient was still agitated upon arrival in the emergency department
    b) Trauma team was present upon arrival
    c) One physician asked the EMTs why they had called case as a neurosurgical emergency
    d) They indicated that the mechanism of injury and the physical findings were basis for decision
    e) Patient subsequently lost consciousness
    f) Focal neurological deficits appeared
    g) CAT scan showed an epidural hematoma which was evacuated
    h) Some patients with epidural hematoma never lose consciousness until herniation

Content

i) EMTs should respect a patient's refusal
   (1) When the patient demonstrates an intact mental state
   (2) Can understand the consequences of his actions
   (3) Neurological status of patient should be carefully documented
j) This patient might have died if allowed to refuse
k) Other causes of alteration of mental state
   (1) Intoxication from alcohol
   (2) Other drugs
   (3) Hypoxia

D. Case 4
1. Overview **(Slide 20-60)**
   a) 60 year old woman involved in front-end collision
   b) EMTs found the patient in car with weak pulse
   c) After rapid extrication pulse was no longer detectable and CPR was begun
   d) Paramedics were dispatched and arrived five minutes after CPR had been initiated
   e) Contusions of the anterior right chest were noted
2. Treatment **(Slide 20-61)**
   a) CPR was continued
   b) Esophageal airway was inserted
   c) MAST trousers were applied
   d) IV was inserted and normal saline was infused
   e) Pulse returned at 130/min, 10 minutes after the paramedics began treatment
   f) Five minutes later pulse dropped to 40
   g) Lost pulses enroute to hospital
   h) Could not be resuscitated
3. Question for discussion **(Slide 20-62)**
   a) How could prehospital care have been altered to potentially improve outcome for this patient?
4. Discussion of case 4 **(Slide 20-63)**
   a) Resuscitation from hypovolemia requires
      (1) Restoration of blood volume
      (2) Control of further bleeding
      (3) Delivery of oxygen to tissues is dependent on blood volume and hemoglobin
   b) IV solutions and MAST trousers may address volume
   c) Serve as a temporary measure
   d) Continuous bleeding must be controlled
   e) Severe hemorrhage will ultimately require replacement with whole blood
   f) Rapid transport decision by BLS unit may have provided best hope

Content

- E. Case 5
  1. Overview **(Slide 20-64)**
     - a) 14 year old boy was balancing on railing of a bridge in Central Park
     - b) Fell 20 feet into six inches of water head first
     - c) Friends dragged him 40 feet up a hill to the roadway
     - d) EMTs found patient conscious, alert and oriented
     - e) Complaining of pain in his neck.
  2. Physical exam **(Slide 20-65)**
     - a) Pulse 60
     - b) Respirations 24 and regular
     - c) Blood pressure 80/50
     - d) Skin was warm and pink
     - e) Diaphragmatic breathing with no chest excursion
     - f) Breath sounds equal
     - g) No sensation below the clavicle
     - h) Patient could not move his arms or legs
  3. Treatment **(Slide 20-66)**
     - a) Patient was immobilized manually
     - b) Oxygen was provided via a non-rebreather mask
     - c) Patient was secured to a long spine board
     - d) Transported to a trauma center
  4. Question for discussion **(Slide 20-67)**
     - a) Does mechanism of injury dictate need for early transport decision to rule out intra-abdominal or other occult hemorrhage which may be masked by spinal shock?
  5. Discussion of Case 5 **(Slide 20-68)**
     - a) Studies have demonstrated difficulty in detecting bleeding in patients with spinal shock
     - b) Pelvis, abdomen, and thorax can contain large quantities of blood
     - c) May not be readily apparent on physical exam
     - d) Long bone fractures can also produce substantial blood loss

IX. Summary **(Slide 20-69)**

- A. Review story of Mr. Jirak in textbook
- B. Discuss feeling of students regarding human side of EMS work
- C. Have students or faculty relate personal experiences

APPROACH TO THE MULTIPLE TRAUMA PATIENT

Examination

1. In areas with a comprehensive trauma system in place, assessment criteria are used in the field to identify patients who should be taken directly to the:

   a. community hospital
   b. closest hospital
   c. municipal hospital
   d. trauma center

2. The components of assessment include:

   a. dispatch review, scene survey, comprehensive survey, and treatment stage
   b. dispatch review, treatment stage, scene survey, secondary survey
   c. dispatch review, scene survey, primary survey, secondary survey
   d. dispatch review, primary survey, secondary survey, treatment stage

Match the categories in column B with the appropriate in injuries in column A (column B items can be used more than once).

Column A		Column B	
3.	uncomplicated fracture	a.	category 1
4.	unstable chest injury	b.	category 2
5.	penetrating abdominal wound	c.	category 3
6.	multiple rib fractures without a flail chest		
7.	multiple pelvic fractures		
8.	blunt abdominal trauma without hypotension		

9. In an injury from a gunshot wound the <u>most important variable</u> in determining the extent of injury is:

   a. weight of the bullet
   b. distance traveled by the bullet
   c. velocity of the bullet
   d. the material the bullet is made of

10. The airway maneuver of choice for a suspected spinal injury patient is the:

    a. head tilt-chin lift
    b. head tilt-neck lift
    c. jaw thrust without head tilt
    d. the triple airway maneuver

Match the mechanisms in column B with the injuries in column A.

Column A		Column B	
11.	aorta tears with with resulting hemorrhage	a.	compression
		b.	deceleration
12.	puncture of the heart and left lung	c.	penetrating
13.	rupture of the diaphragm		

14. Which of the following fractures are commonly associated with a hanging?

    a. lumbar spine
    b. cervical spine
    c. bilateral feet
    d. bilateral femurs

15. Respiratory rates above _____ per minute usually require positive-pressure breathing.

    a. 12
    b. 16
    c. 30
    d. 40

16. Respiratory rates below _____ per minute usually require positive-pressure breathing.

    a. 8
    b. 12
    c. 20
    d. 25

17. All of the following are key signs of inadequate ventilation and oxygenation:

    a. respiratory rate and depth, skin color, evidence of chest trauma, tracheal shift and neck vein distention
    b. skin color, evidence of chest trauma, capillary refill, blood pressure
    c. abnormal respiratory sounds, capillary refill, blood pressure, skin color
    d. bleeding, skin color, respiratory rate and depth, evidence of chest trauma

18. All of the following are key signs used to determine cardiovascular function:

    a. bleeding, skin color, respiratory rate and depth, evidence of chest trauma
    b. blood pressure, skin color, capillary refill, bleeding
    c. skin color, capillary refill, respiratory rate and depth, pulse check
    d. pulse check, bleeding, capillary refill, respiratory rate and depth

19. A quick assessment of the level of consciousness is made by using the mnemonic:

    a. CUPS
    b. TRISS
    c. AVPU
    d. GLASGOW

20. In the primary survey the last thing that is done is:

    a. establish responsiveness
    b. check for bleeding
    c. expose the patient
    d. assess the adequacy of breathing

21. The systematic collection of data from the patient to determine the mechanism of injury or illness and to identify significant medical conditions in the patient's past is called the:

    a. medic alert tag
    b. lifeline vial
    c. history
    d. primary survey

22. Key historical facts necessary to make a decision in regard to a traumatized patient, as recommended by the American College of Surgeons, is known by the mnemonic:

    a. CUPS
    b. TRISS
    c. AVPU
    d. AMPLE

23. When a group of 4 people are in a car that is involved in a left front end accident where the car rotates around the point of impact, the most likely person to be severely injured is the:

    a. driver
    b. front seat passenger
    c. rear right passenger
    d. rear left passenger

24. A dash board injury is likely to result in which of the following injuries?

    a. femur fracture
    b. posterior hip dislocation
    c. patellar fracture
    d. all of the above

25. Tracheal shift, distended neck veins and absent breath sounds on one side are most likely caused by a:

    a. pericardial tamponade
    b. injury to the large airways
    c. tension pneumothorax
    d. cardiac contusion

APPENDICES

DOT Curriculum Reading Assignment List

DOT Lesson Number	DOT Topic	EMT Prehospital Care Chapter Number	EMT Prehospital Care Chapter Title and Pages	
1	Introduction to Emergency Care and training	1	Introduction to Prehospital Care	3-21
2	Anatomy & Physiology and Patient assessment	2	Anatomy & Physiology and Patient Assessment	2-79
3	Airway obstruction and respiratory arrest	3	Respiratory emergencies	81-100 127-154
4	Cardiac arrest	4	Cardiovascular Anatomy and Physiology	157-185
		6	CPR and EMT-D	238-287
5	Manikin practice and certification	6	Cardiovascular Anatomy and Physiology	157-185
			CPR and EMT-D	238-287
6	Practical use of airway adjuncts	3	Respiratory emergencies	100-187
7	Bleeding and shock	5	Cardiovascular emergencies	187-209
8	Test and evaluation	1-6	Review previous reading	

DOT Lesson Number	DOT Topic	EMT Prehospital Care Chapter Number	EMT Prehospital Care Chapter Title and Pages	
9	Review of shock and introduction to MAST	5	Cardiovascular emergencies	187-209
10	Soft tissue injuries	9	Soft tissue injuries	387-402
11	Musculoskeletal care and fractures of the upper extremities	10	Musculoskeletal Injuries	429-485
12	Fractures of the pelvis, hip and lower extremities	10	Musculoskeletal Injuries	429-485 Review
13	Practical lab: Fracture care of the upper and lower extremities	10	Musculoskeletal Injuries	429-485 Review
14	Injuries to the head, face, neck and spine	7	Central nervous system emergencies	289-338
		9	Soft tissue injuries	402-427
15	Practical lab: patient assessment and spine immobilization		Review previous reading	
16	Injuries to the chest, abdomen and genitalia	3 8	Respiratory emergencies Abdominal emergencies	145-154 378-385
17	Practical lab: injuries	20	Approach to the multiple	795-812

DOT Lesson Number	DOT Topic	EMT Prehospital Care Chapter Number	EMT Prehospital Care Chapter Title and Pages	
18	Test and evaluation Injuries II	20	Approach to the multiple trauma patient Review previous readings	795-812
19	Medical emergencies I	3	Respiratory emergencies	141-145
		5	Cardiovascular emergencies	209-237
		7	Central nervous system emergencies	338-348
		12	Medical emergencies	552-578
20	Medical emergencies II	7	Central nervous system emergencies	338-348
		8	Abdominal emergencies	351-378
		12	Medical emergencies	538-552 578-595
		14	Pediatric patients	643-677
21	Emergency childbirth	13	Obstetrical emergencies	596-641
22	Burns and hazardous materials	11	Environmental emergencies	499-525 528-536
23	Environmental emergencies	11	Environmental emergencies	488-499 525-528
24	Psychological aspects of emergency care	15	Psychological aspects of emergency care	679-687

DOT Lesson Number	DOT Topic	EMT Prehospital Care Chapter Number	EMT Prehospital Care Chapter Title and Pages	
25	Lifting and moving patients	16	Lifting and moving patients	688-714
26	Principles of extrication	18	Extrication	735-753
27	Practical lab: extrication	18	Extrication Review previous reading	735-753
28	Test and evaluation medical emergencies, childbirth, environmental emergencies and lifting and moving	11 12 13 16	Review previous reading	
29	Ambulance operations I	19	Ambulance operations	756-793
30	Ambulance operations II	19	Disasters and triage Ambulance operations	717-733 756-793
31	Situational review		Review previous reading	
32	Final practical skills evaluation		Review previous reading	
33	Final written test			

CHAPTER 1

1. C
2. A
3. C
4. D
5. A
6. C
7. A
8. A
9. C
10. D
11. C
12. C
13. B
14. A
15. A
16. C
17. D
18. B
19. C
20. D
21. A
22. D
23. C
24. D
25. D
26. C
27. B
28. A
29. D
30. B
31. B
32. D
33. C
34. C
35. A
36. B
37. C
38. C
39. C
40. B

CHAPTER 2

1. C
2. B
3. D
4. B
5. B
6. C
7. C
8. D
9. B
10. A
11. C
12. B
13. C
14. D
15. B
16. C
17. D
18. D
19. A
20. C
21. A
22. C
23. A
24. B
25. C
26. C
27. A
28. B
29. D
30. B
31. A
32. A
33. A
34. C
35. A
36. C
37. A
38. C
39. D
40. C
41. C
42. D
43. A
44. B
45. C
46. C
47. A
48. D
49. A
50. D
51. C
52. D
53. C
54. B
55. A
56. D
57. B
58. C
59. B
60. A
61. D
62. C
63. D
64. A
65. C
66. B
67. B
68. A
69. A
70. A

CHAPTER 3

1. D
2. B
3. A
4. A
5. C
6. B
7. A
8. D
9. C
10. C
11. C
12. B
13. C
14. C
15. D
16. A
17. C
18. C
19. C
20. C
21. C
22. C
23. A
24. A
25. B
26. C
27. B
28. C
29. A
30. B
31. C
32. C
33. D
34. C
35. D
36. B
37. D
38. A
39. B
40. B
41. C
42. B
43. A
44. C
45. A
46. A
47. A
48. B
49. C
50. B
51. A
52. B
53. D

CHAPTER 4

1. B
2. C
3. B
4. B
5. A
6. B
7. D
8. C
9. A
10. A
11. C
12. B
13. B
14. B
15. A
16. C
17. B
18. B
19. C
20. A
21. C
22. C
23. B
24. D
25. D
26. A
27. B
28. A
29. A
30. B
31. A
32. D
33. A
34. D

CHAPTER 4

35. B
36. A
37. A
38. C
39. A
40. B
41. A
42. A
43. C
44. C
45. A
46. C
47. B
48. B
49. A
50. B
51. B
52. B
53. A
54. C
55. C
56. D
57. C
58. D
59. B
60. A
61. B
62. A
63. B
64. A
65. A
66. B
67. C
68. C
69. A
70. B

CHAPTER 5

1. C
2. A
3. A
4. B
5. C
6. B
7. D
8. D
9. A
10. B
11. C
12. D
13. B
14. B
15. A
16. D
17. A
18. C
19. D
20. B
21. D
22. C
23. A
24. A
25. A
26. B
27. B
28. C
29. C
30. C
31. A
32. B
33. D
34. C
35. A
36. C
37. C
38. A
39. B
40. D
41. C
42. B
43. C
44. A
45. B
46. A
47. B
48. A
49. A
50. A
51. C
52. D
53. C
54. A
55. C
56. B
57. A
58. B
59. B
60. B
61. D
62. D
63. A
64. D
65. B
66. C
67. B
68. C
69. D
70. B

CHAPTER 6

1. B
2. A
3. B
4. D
5. B
6. B
7. C
8. D
9. C
10. C
11. B
12. C
13. D
14. A
15. A
16. D
17. A
18. B
19. C
20. A
21. A
22. B
23. A
24. B
25. C
26. C
27. A
28. B
29. C
30. A
31. D
32. B
33. D
34. A
35. A
36. B
37. D
38. C
39. B
40. C
41. B
42. B
43. A
44. A
45. C
46. B
47. A
48. B
49. A
50. C
51. B
52. B
53. C
54. B
55. C
56. A
57. B
58. B
59. A
60. C
61. D
62. B
63. A
64. B
65. A
66. B
67. A
68. B
69. B
70. A
71. D
72. C
73. C
74. D
75. D
76. A
77. B
78. B
79. B
80. C
81. C
82. C
83. B
84. D

CHAPTER 7

1. A
2. D
3. B
4. B
5. D
6. A
7. B

CHAPTER 7

8. A
9. D
10. A
11. B
12. D
13. B
14. A
15. B
16. A
17. A
18. B
19. B
20. B
21. E
22. A
23. B
24. D
25. C
26. A
27. C
28. D
29. C
30. B
31. A
32. D
33. B
34. C
35. A
36. D
37. E
38. A
39. C
40. A
41. B
42. B
43. A
44. A
45. D
46. B
47. A
48. D
49. C
50. B
51. B
52. B
53. C
54. A
55. B
56. A
57. B
58. C
59. A
60. B
61. A
62. C
63. C
64. B
65. B
66. B
67. C
68. A
69. D
70. B
71. B
72. C
73. B
74. A
75. C
76. C
77. B
78. A
79. A
80. C
81. A
82. B
83. B
84. E
85. C
86. B
87. F
88. A
89. D
90. B
91. D
92. C
93. B
94. A
95. B
96. D
97. E
98. C
99. A
100. D

CHAPTER 8

1. B
2. C
3. D
4. D
5. A
6. B
7. D
8. D
9. B
10. C
11. B
12. D
13. C
14. A
15. D
16. D
17. A
18. B
19. C
20. B
21. D
22. A
23. C
24. B
25. D
26. B
27. D
28. D
29. C
30. D
31. B
32. C
33. A
34. D
35. B
36. C
37. C
38. A
39. D
40. C
41. C
42. A
43. C
44. D
45. A
46. B
47. D
48. B
49. B
50. B

CHAPTER 9

1. D
2. B
3. B
4. A
5. F
6. D
7. E
8. C
9. G
10. C
11. B
12. C
13. B
14. B
15. A
16. B
17. D
18. E
19. C
20. A
21. C
22. B
23. A
24. D
25. C
26. D
27. C
28. C
29. A
30. D
31. D
32. B
33. B
34. B
35. B
36. B
37. C
38. A
39. D
40. C
41. A
42. C
43. C
44. B
45. D
46. A
47. D
48. B
49. C
50. B

CHAPTER 10

1. D
2. C
3. A
4. B

CHAPTER 10

5. E
6. D
7. C
8. B
9. A
10. D
11. C
12. B
13. A
14. A
15. C
16. B
17. C
18. E
19. H
20. G
21. A
22. B
23. F
24. D
25. B
26. B
27. B
28. D
29. G
30. H
31. C
32. F
33. J
34. I
35. E
36. A
37. B
38. D
39. D
40. A
41. C
42. A
43. B
44. C
45. B
46. C
47. C
48. E
49. D
50. A
51. B
52. C
53. F
54. E
55. B
56. D
57. A
58. B
59. D
60. A
61. C
62. E
63. D
64. A
65. C
66. C
67. C
68. B
69. A
70. C
71. C
72. A
73. B
74. D
75. C

CHAPTER 11

1. D
2. B
3. C
4. D
5. B
6. D
7. D
8. C
9. C
10. C
11. D
12. A
13. B
14. C
15. D
16. E
17. B
18. A
19. B
20. A
21. C
22. C
23. C
24. B
25. B
26. A
27. C
28. C
29. A
30. A
31. B
32. C
33. B
34. B
35. C
36. D
37. A
38. C
39. B
40. C
41. B
42. C
43. A
44. A
45. A
46. A
47. B
48. D
49. C
50. E
51. F
52. D
53. A
54. B
55. A
56. C
57. T
58. T
59. F
60. F
61. T
62. D
63. C
64. A
65. C
66. D
67. A
68. C
69. B
70. E
71. D
72. B
73. B
74. D
75. D
76. B
77. C
78. A
79. B
80. C
81. B
82. C
83. B
84. B
85. D
86. C
87. A
88. C
89. A
90. B
91. D
92. C
93. A
94. B
95. C
96. A
97. C
98. B
99. D
100. A

CHAPTER 12

1. A
2. C
3. D
4. C
5. B
6. D
7. D
8. C
9. C
10. C
11. B
12. B
13. A
14. B
15. B
16. A
17. B
18. B
19. A
20. B
21. A
22. C
23. D
24. B
25. A
26. C
27. C
28. D

CHAPTER 12

29. A
30. B
31. B
32. C
33. C
34. C
35. C
36. A
37. D
38. B
39. B
40. B
41. D
42. C
43. C
44. A
45. C
46. B
47. C
48. C
49. D
50. A
51. A
52. B
53. A
54. B
55. B
56. B
57. D
58. C
59. A
60. F
61. E
62. D
63. A
64. B
65. C
66. B
67. C
68. D
69. D
70. D
71. A
72. C
73. B
74. C
75. C
76. B
77. C
78. C
79. A
80. D

CHAPTER 13

1. D
2. F
3. E
4. C
5. G
6. B
7. A
8. B
9. D
10. A
11. C
12. B
13. B
14. B
15. B
16. B
17. B
18. D
19. C
20. B
21. A
22. B
23. B
24. C
25. C
26. B
27. B
28. C
29. B
30. B
31. D
32. B
33. C
34. B
35. A
36. A
37. B
38. B
39. B
40. B
41. B
42. C
43. C
44. D
45. D
46. A
47. A
48. D
49. C
50. D
51. B
52. C

CHAPTER 14

1. C
2. A
3. C
4. D
5. A
6. E
7. B
8. C
9. C
10. C
11. D
12. A
13. D
14. D
15. C
16. B
17. D
18. B
19. C
20. A
21. D
22. B
23. C
24. D
25. C
26. A
27. D
28. C
29. D
30. B
31. C
32. C
33. C
34. A
35. B
36. B
37. B
38. A
39. D
40. A
41. B
42. D
43. B
44. A
45. B
46. B
47. B
48. B
49. C
50. D

CHAPTER 15

1. A
2. B
3. B
4. A
5. B
6. B
7. D
8. A
9. B
10. C
11. C
12. C
13. A
14. D
15. D
16. A
17. D
18. D
19. B
20. C
21. D
22. D
23. B
24. A
25. B

CHAPTER 16

1. C
2. A
3. D
4. A
5. C
6. E
7. C
8. C
9. C
10. A
11. A
12. D
13. C
14. C
15. A
16. B

CHAPTER 16

17. C
18. C
19. C
20. D
21. B
22. F
23. E
24. A
25. C
26. A
27. B
28. D
29. B
30. C
31. A
32. G
33. C
34. E
35. B
36. D
37. F
38. D
39. A
40. B
41. A
42. B
43. C
44. B
45. A
46. C
47. D
48. A
49. E
50. B

CHAPTER 17

1. C
2. B
3. A
4. D
5. B
6. B
7. C
8. A
9. C
10. D
11. B
12. C
13. C
14. A
15. C
16. B
17. D
18. B
19. B
20. C
21. E
22. B
23. A
24. D
25. C

CHAPTER 18

1. D
2. D
3. C
4. B
5. B
6. C
7. D
8. B
9. B
10. B
11. B
12. D
13. C
14. A
15. C
16. B
17. B
18. C
19. A
20. A
21. D
22. D
23. B
24. B
25. C

CHAPTER 19

1. B
2. C
3. D
4. B
5. C
6. A
7. D
8. D
9. B
10. C
11. A
12. B
13. C
14. A
15. A
16. A
17. C
18. B
19. A
20. B
21. A
22. A
23. A
24. B
25. D
26. C
27. B
28. A
29. B
30. A
31. A
32. D
33. B
34. B
35. A
36. A
37. B
38. D
39. C
40. B
41. B
42. D
43. B
44. C
45. A
46. B
47. C
48. A
49. B
50. A

CHAPTER 20

1. D
2. C
3. C
4. A
5. A
6. B
7. A
8. B
9. C
10. C
11. B
12. C
13. A
14. B
15. C
16. B
17. A
18. B
19. C
20. C
21. C
22. D
23. C
24. D
25. C

PHARMACOLOGY TEACHING SUPPLEMENT

This teaching supplement can be utilized when incorporating basics about pharmacology or fluid therapy into your EMT or EMT-I training program.

Objectives: At the completion of this session you should be able to:

1. Convert one unit of measure to another in the metric system.
2. Calculate the weight in kilograms given the weight in pounds.
3. Determine the correct desired dose.
4. Calculate the dose on hand of a specific drug.
5. Calculate the dose on hand of a specific drug using gram percent.
6. Calculate the dose on hand of an IV infusion.
7. Calculate and set the drip rate of an IV infusion using the universal drip rate formula.

I. Introduction

1. In order to understand and determine the correct dosages of drugs to be administered, the EMT must be thoroughly familiar with the **units** in which the drug is measured.

2. There are **three systems** of measurement applicable to drug therapy:

   a) Apothecary
   b) Avoirdupois
   c) **Metric**

A. The Apothecary System

1. Apothecary (derived from the Greek apotheke - storehouse) - a person who prepares and sells or dispenses drugs and compounds, and makes up prescriptions.

a) Apothecaries Measure - a series of **liquid** units of capacity (i.e. minim, fluid dram, fluid once, pint, and gallon).

b) Apothecaries Weight - a series of units of weight (i.e. 1 lb., 1 dram of 60 grains, and a scruple).

2. Is the older of the systems, and is seldom used.

3. **Solids** are measured in units of grains, drams, ounces, and lbs.

4. **Liquids** are measured in units of minims, fluidrams, ounces, pints, and gallons.

B. Avoirdupois

1. Avoirdupois (derived from the French - goods sold by weight).

2. Avoirdupois weight - a series of units of weight based on the lb of 16 oz. and the oz. of 16 drams

C. The Metric System

1. Is **more** frequently used in the official listings of drugs.

2. Is **logical and simply** organized (i.e. based of units of 10).

3. The primary unit of solid measurement is the **gram (gm)**.

4. The primary unit of liquid measurement is the **liter (l)**.

5. Units within one system (**solid** - gm, mg, mcgs, **liquid** - l, ml) can be converted into other units within the same system.

6. Units in the Apothecary System can be converted into the Metric System (i.e.. pounds to kilograms, and grains to milligrams). The conversions are usually only approximations.

II. Comparison of Metric to Apothecary

Metric	Apothecary
5 ml	1 teaspoon
15 ml	1 tablespoon
30 ml	1 fluid ounce
500 ml	1 pint (approximate)
1,000 ml	1 quart (approximate)
1 kg	2.2 pounds
2.54 cm	1 inch

Commonly used prefixes

Prefix	Translation	Fraction	Decimal
Deci	Tenths	1/10	0.1
Centi	Hundredths	1/100	0.01
Milli	Thousandths	1/1000	0.001
Micro	Millionths	1/1,000,000	0.000001

A common conversion that you will need to make in the field is from pounds (Apothecary) to kilograms (Metric).

a) Most patients will give their weight in lbs, but many dosages are calculated on the basis of weight or volume per kilogram of body weight.

b) To convert pounds to kilograms, you simply divide the body weight in lbs by 2.2.

$$\textbf{Weight in kilograms (kg)} = \frac{\textbf{Weight in pounds (lbs)}}{\textbf{2.2}}$$

Example - How many kilograms (kgs) does a 150 lb male weigh?

$$\textbf{Weight in kilograms (kg)} = \frac{\textbf{Weight in pounds (lbs)}}{\textbf{2.2}}$$

$$\textbf{Weight in kilograms (kg)} = \frac{220 \text{ lbs}}{2.2} = 100 \text{ kg}$$

III. A Review of Decimals

The Number Line

Hundreds	Tens	Units	.	Tenths	Hundredths	Thousandths

1. The Metric System is based on multiples or derivatives of 10; (i.e.. the decimal system).

2. The EMT must be able to work easily with the decimal system.

3. Decimals consist of:

a) a whole number (the # before the decimal point).
b) a decimal point.
c) a decimal fraction (the # after the decimal point).

Example - 4.06

4. The position of the # in relationship to the decimal point gives the # its place name.

a) one place to the right of the decimal point is called **"tenth"**.
b) two places to the right is called **"hundredths"**.
c) three places to the right is called **"thousandths"**.

Example - 0.5 = five tenths = 5/10
0.05 = five hundredths = 5/100
0.005 = five thousandths = 5/1000

5. To eliminate confusion from overlooking the decimal point and reading the **decimal fraction** as a whole #, a zero (0) should be placed to the left of the decimal point when there is no whole #.

Example - the decimal fraction 15/100 (15 hundredths) is written 0.15.

6. Adding zeros to the right of the fraction does not change its **value**.

Example - 0.5 = 0.50 = 0.500
5/10 = 50/100 = 500/1000

IV. Addition, Subtraction, Multiplication, & Division of Decimals

A. Addition & Subtraction

1. To add and subtract decimals, the decimal points should be lined up and zeroes should be added to the right of the decimal fraction.

Example - Addition

Add 1.5 + 21.65

```
        1.50
     + 21.65
ans.   23.15
```

Example - Subtraction

Subtract 23.15 - 1.5

```
       23.15
     -  1.50
ans.   21.65
```

B. Multiplication

1. Multiplication of decimals is carried out exactly the same way as multiplication of whole #'s, **except** for the placing of the decimal point in the product of the answer.

2. The # of decimal places in the #'s to be multiplied should be counted; then the # of places should be counted from the right of the product to locate the decimal point.

Example - Multiplication

```
       125      12.5      1.25      .125
     x 0.5     x 0.5     x 0.5     x 0.5
ans.  62.5      6.25      .625      .0625
```

3. When multiplying by ten (10), the decimal point should be **one** place to the right of the number being multiplied.

Example -

```
      12.5
      x 10
ans. 125.0
```

4. When multiplying a decimal by 100, move the decimal point two places to the right.

Example -

```
       12.5     1.25
      x 100    x 100
ans. 1250.0    125.0
```

Therefore, when multiplying a decimal fraction by a multiple of 10, the decimal point should be moved to the right by the # of zeroes found in the multiple of ten.

Example - -

```
          1.25
        x 1000
   ans. 1250.0
```

Division of Decimals

1. It's the same as dividing whole #'s, except that the decimal point must be considered.

Example - 24 divided by 6 = 4
24 is the dividend
6 is the divisor
4 is the quotient or answer

```
       4
6   ⌐‾‾‾‾
    |24.0
```

2. With decimals, the decimal point is kept in the quotient above the decimal point in the dividend.

Example -

```
       .6
4   ⌐‾‾‾‾
    |2.40
```

3. The divisor must always be a whole number.

Example -

```
                          6.0
.4 ⌐‾‾‾‾‾‾‾  =   4.0 ⌐‾‾‾‾‾‾‾‾
   |2.40             |24.0
```

a) The .4 must be made into a whole # by moving the decimal point one place to the right.

b) The decimal point in the divisor can not be moved without moving the decimal point in the dividend the same # of places.

c) Therefore, the 2.4 becomes 24.0.

d) The decimal point in the quotient should be kept above the new location of the decimal point in the dividend.

4. The rule for dividing decimals by multiples of 10 is the opposite of that for multiplication; the decimal point should be moved to the **left** by the # zeroes in the divisor.

Example -

0.5	0.05	0.005
10 ⟌ 5.0	100 ⟌ 5.00	1000 ⟌ 5.000

V. The Metric System

A. Metric Units For Weight

1. The units of weight, or weight measure, in the metric system are based on decimal fractions.

2. The **primary unit** of weight on the metric system is the gram (gm).

3. The **secondary unit** of weight in the metric system is the milligram (mg).

   a) milli - means thousandth.

   b) Therefore, 1 milligram is 1/1000 of a gram if there are 1,000 mgs in 1 gm.

Example -

1 gm = 1,000 mg

1 mg = 1/1000 gm

B. Conversions

1. To convert grams to milligrams, the # of grams is multiplied by 1,000.

Example -

15 gms = 15 x 1,000 mg = 15,000 mgs.

2. To convert grams to milligrams, move the decimal point three places to the right.

Example -

15 gms = 15.000 = 15,000 mgs

3. To convert milligrams to grams, the # of mg is divided by 1,000.

Example -

$$15{,}000 \text{ mgs} = \frac{15{,}000}{1{,}000} = 15 \text{ gms.}$$

4. To convert milligrams to grams, move the decimal point three places to the left.

Example -

15,000 mgs = 15,000.0 = 15 gms.

B. Metric Units For Volume

1. The units of volume, or liquid measure, in the metric system are based on decimal fractions.

2. The primary unit of volume is the liter (l).

3. The secondary unit of volume is the millimeter (ml).

4. One liter (l) is equal to one thousand milliliters (mls).

1 l = 1,000 mls.

5. A milliliter is equal to one one thousandth of a liter.

1 ml = 1/1,000 l

6. Therefore, 1,000 mls = 1 liter (l).

7. To convert liters to milliliters, the # of liters should be multiplied by 1,000; or by moving the decimal point 3 places to the right.

Example -

3 liters = 3 x 1,000 = 3,000 mls
3 liters = 3.000 = 3,000 mls

8. To convert milliliters to liters, the # of milliliters should be divided by 1,000; or by moving the decimal point 3 places to the left.

Example -

3,000 mls = 3,000/1,000 = 3 liters (l)
3,000 mls = 3,000.0 = 3.0 liters (l)

9. Another unit of volume is the cubic centimeter (cc). A cc is equivalent to a ml (One ml of water weighs 1gm and occupies 1 cc of space). Therefore, a ml and a cc both express 1/1,000 th of a liter and can be considered equivalent expressions.

VI. Desired Dose, Dose On Hand, Gram Percent, & Dilution Ratios

A. Desired Dose (DD)

1. The desired dose is the **order given** for the medication to be administered.

2. The desired dose is expressed in metric units of weight. (i.e.. grams, milligrams, micrograms).

3. The desired dose may be ordered in terms of the patients weight (i.e. 1 mg/kg of lidocaine).

4. The desired dose may be ordered over a specific time (i.e.. 5 mcg/kg/min of dopamine).

B. Dose On Hand (DOH)

1. The dose on hand is the concentration of the medication dispensed.

2. To find the dose on hand you divide the total weight of the drug by the total volume.

$$\text{DOH} = \frac{\text{Drug Weight (i.e. mg, gm, etc.)}}{\text{Total Volume of Solution}}$$

Example - Dose On Hand of a specific drug dispensed.

What is the DOH of an ampule of epinephrine, if each ampule contains 1 mg in 10 mls?

$$\text{DOH} = \frac{\text{Total Weight}}{\text{Total Volume}}$$

$$\text{DOH} = \frac{1\text{ mg}}{10\text{ mls}} = 0.1\text{ mg/ml}$$

Example - Dose On Hand of an IV infusion.

What is the DOH of a vial of dopamine diluted in a total of 250 ml of D_5W, if each vial of dopamine contains 250 mgs?

$$\text{DOH (1 ml)} = \frac{\text{Total Weight}}{\text{Total Volume}}$$

$$\text{DOH (1 ml)} = \frac{\text{250 mg}}{\text{250 mls}} = \text{1 mg/}\mathbf{1\ ml}$$

C. Gram percent

1. Gram percent is used to express the number of grams of a drug in 100mls of solution. In prehospital care one might carry 50% glucose solution. This means there are 50 grams of glucose in every 100 ml of solution.

You are asked to give 50 ml of a 50% glucose solution. How many grams of glucose will you give the patient?

If there are 50 grams of glucose in 100 ml of a 50% solution then the dose on hand is:
<u>50 gms</u> or _0.5 gms/ml

Then in 50 mls there are 0.5 gms/ml x 50 mls = 25 grams.

D. Solution Ratios of Epinephrine (for example)

1. Common solution concentration of epinephrine are 1 gm in 1,000 ml and 1 gm in 10,000 ml.

2. This may be expressed in terms of the ratio of gms to ml.

1:1,000 or 1:10,000

1 gm/1,000ml or 1gm/10,000 ml

3. The number of gms or mgs of drug remain the same, but the number of mls of solution varies from 1,000 to 10,000 ml.

4. The solution concentration administered depends on the route used to administered the medication.

a) epi 1:1,000 is given subcutaneously.
b) epi 1:10,000 is given Intravenously

VII. Drug Calculation Formulas

A. Milliliters of drug to be administered.

$$\text{Desired dose in mls.} = \frac{\text{desired dose in mg.}}{\text{dose on hand}}$$

Example -

You are ordered to give 0.3 mg. of a 1:1,000 solution of epinephrine. How many mls do you administer.

1:1,000 = 1 gm/1,000 ml.
or 1000 mg/1,000 ml.

$$\text{Dose on hand} = \frac{1000\text{ mg}}{1000\text{ ml}} = 1\text{ mg./ml.}$$

$$\text{Desired dose in mls} = \frac{\text{desired dose}}{\text{dose on hand}}$$

$$\text{Desired dose in mls} = \frac{0.3\text{ mg}}{1\text{mg}/1\text{ml}}$$

Solve the equation

Desired dose in ml = 0.3ml

You would draw up 0.3 ml. of a 1:1000 solution to administer 0.3 mg of epinephrine.

B. Universal Drip Rate Formula.

$$\text{Gtts/min} = \frac{\text{Volume (ml) x Drip Rate Factor}}{\text{Time (minutes)}}$$

Drip rate factor depends on the types of administration set.

Macrodrip used for rapid administration - 10 gtts./ml.
Microdrip used for medication admin. - 60 gtts./ml

Example -

You are ordered to give 600 ml of saline solution over 1 hr through a macrodrip. What is the correct drip rate?

$$\text{Gtts/min} = \frac{600 \times 10}{60 \text{ (min.)}} = \frac{6000}{60} = 100 \text{ gtts/minute}$$

What you need to know to safely administer a drug

What is a drug?

A drug is any chemical which influences a living system.

What are the 'five rights' of drug administration?

1. The right drug.
2. The right patient.
3. The right time.
4. The right dose.
5. The right route.

What are the 'six characteristics' of a drug you need to know before you can safely administer a drug?

1. The actions of the drug.
2. The indications for the drug.
3. The contraindications for the drug.
4. The adverse affects of the drug.
5. The correct dose of the drug.
6. The correct route of the drug.

Definitions:

1. **Pharmacology** - a branch of knowledge which deals with the actions of drugs (chemicals) on a living organism.

2. **Pharmacokinetics** - the study of how drugs get into a living system including the absorption, distribution, metabolism, and excretion of the drug.

3. **Toxicology** - the study of the adverse or poisonous effects of drugs on living systems.

4. **Biophase** - the drug produces its effect at the actual site which works to cause its effect of action.

5. **Disease state** - the drug is used to treat the cause of the disease or the effect of the disease.

6. **Minimum Therapuetic Level** - refers to the concentration of a drug which will cause a response.

7. **Volume of Distribution** - refers to the distribution of the drug in the fluids and tissues of the living organism.